MW01056504

Pediatrics Review
Core Curriculum

Seventh Edition **2016–2017**

7

Book 4 of 5

Topics in this volume:

Cardiology

Respiratory Disorders

Gastroenterology & Nutrition

Robert A. Hannaman, MD
Editor in Chief

A Note on Editorial Style

MedStudy uses a standardized approach to the naming of diseases. The previous method of naming was to use the possessive form that adds "'s" to the names of diseases and disorders, such as Lou Gehrig's disease, Klinefelter's syndrome, and others. In MedStudy material, you will not see the possessive form when the proper name is followed by a common noun; e.g., "This patient would warrant workup for Crohn disease." Exceptions include Bell's palsy and Still's murmur. The possessive form will be used, however, when an entity is referred to solely by its proper name without a following common noun; e.g., "The symptoms are classic for Crohn's." The *AMA Manual of Style*, *JAMA*®, and *Scientific Style and Format* are among the publications that promote and use the non-possessive form.

Disclaimers

NOTICE: Medicine and accepted standards of care are constantly changing. We at MedStudy do our best to review and include in this publication accurate discussions of the standards of care and methods of diagnosis. However, the authors, reviewers, section editors, editors, editor in chief, publisher, and all other parties involved with the preparation and publication of this work do not guarantee that the information contained herein is in every respect accurate or complete. We recommend that you confirm the material with current sources of medical knowledge whenever considering presentations or treating patients.

ABP: For over 10 years, MedStudy has excelled in determining and teaching what a clinically competent pediatrician should know. The American Board of Pediatrics (ABP) tests this exact same pool of knowledge. MedStudy's expertise, demonstrated by the superb pass rate of those who use it in their studies, is in the actual "teaching" of this knowledge in a clear, learner-friendly manner that results in a stronger knowledge base, improved clinical skills, and better Board results. Although what we teach is in sync with what the Board tests, MedStudy has no affiliation with the ABP, and our authors, reviewers, and editors have no access to ABP exam content. Our material is developed as original work by MedStudy physician authors, with additional input from expert contributors, based on their extensive backgrounds in professional medical education. This content is designed to include subject matter typically tested in certification and recertification exams as outlined in the ABP's publicly available exam content outline but makes no use of, and divulges no details of, ABP's proprietary exam content.

MEDSTUDY®
1455 Quail Lake Loop
Colorado Springs, Colorado 80906
(800) 841-0547
www.medstudy.com

MedStudy®

Pediatrics Review
Core Curriculum

Seventh Edition 2016–2017

7

CARDIOLOGY

Section Editor:

Arthur S. Pickoff, MD
Chief Medical Director
Wright State Research Institute
Wright State University
Dayton, OH

Editor:

Yasmine Subhi Ali, MD, MSCI, FACC, FACP
President, Nashville Preventive Cardiology, PLLC
Nashville, TN

Reviewers:

Mark Lewin, MD
Professor and Chief,
  Division of Pediatric Cardiology
University of Washington School of Medicine
Co-Director, Heart Center
Seattle Children's Hospital
Seattle, WA

Michael Ralston, MD, FACC, FASE, FAAP
Pediatric Cardiologist
Medical Director, Echocardiography Laboratory
Associate Professor of Pediatrics
Wright State University
  Boonshoft School of Medicine
Division of Cardiology
Dayton Children's Hospital
Dayton, OH

Table of Contents

Cardiology

PHYSICAL EXAMINATION

OVERVIEW

The physical examination (and history!) can provide as many clues as any diagnostic test for the diagnosis of cardiovascular disease. Thus, for testing purposes, be on the lookout for more history and physical examination clues than echo or cardiac cath results.

SKIN

Look at the color of the skin and mucous membranes. **Cyanosis** refers to a dusky blue color that occurs due to an excessive amount of reduced hemoglobin (unoxygenated) in the circulation. Most commonly, you will see this color in the lips, mucous membranes, and nail beds. Usually, it can be seen quite readily if the arterial oxygen saturation is < 85%, but it can be difficult to see with higher oxygen saturation of 88–92%.

Peripheral cyanosis may also occur with normal oxygen saturation and is due to reduced peripheral circulation, which allows the tissues to extract more oxygen, leaving the venous end of the capillaries with more reduced hemoglobin. In this situation, the extremities can be cold and blue, while the mucous membranes and tongue are pink. In infants and children, peripheral cyanosis that occurs most often with exposure to cold, with polycythemia, and sometimes even in normal newborns and young infants, is known as **acrocyanosis**, a benign condition. **Central** cyanosis is due to arterial desaturation and is best seen in the tongue, oral mucous membranes, and trunk. Note: Cyanosis of just the lower extremities and toes, and not the fingers (differential cyanosis), could indicate aortic arch obstruction or persisting pulmonary hypertension with ductal right-to-left shunting of desaturated blood. Cyanosis of the preductal structures (e.g., fingers), but not the postductal structures (e.g., toes), is termed "reverse differential cyanosis." This indicates transposition of the great vessels, with right-to-left shunting of saturated blood through the ductus.

Petechiae can indicate infective endocarditis, but this can also be indicative of other things and, thus, is rather nonspecific. **Splinter hemorrhages** of the nail beds are more indicative of endocarditis.

Other skin findings, such as **café-au-lait** (neurofibromatosis) or **ash-leaf** spots (tuberous sclerosis), may indicate disorders associated with heart defects.

ARTERIAL PULSES

Abnormalities of arterial pulses can indicate significant cardiac anomalies. Significant delay or absence of the femoral pulse, compared to the radial pulse, indicates **coarctation of the aorta**. Pulse quality can also be a helpful indicator: You see rapid rising or bounding pulses with large patent ductus arteriosus (PDA) or aortic valve insufficiency; slow-rising pulse can indicate aortic stenosis or hypertension.

VENOUS PULSES

You can observe venous pulses in the neck; the mean jugular venous pressure gives a good measure of mean right atrial pressure. Healthy pediatric patients may have minor jugular venous distention and faint pulsation. Infants commonly do not have visible neck veins. Prominent jugular veins reflect obstruction, worsened ventricular filling due to poor compliance, or abnormal backflow.

The *a* **wave** is a venous wave that occurs just before the 1st heart sound and is due to atrial contraction. A large *a* wave typically indicates elevated right ventricular, end-diastolic pressures. Think about it … if the right atrium contracts while there is higher filling pressure in the right ventricle, the blood is going to be pushed back into the neck—and you'll see it. Cannon *a* waves occur when the right atrium contracts against a closed tricuspid valve—which can occur with AV dissociation (3rd degree heart block or junctional rhythm) or ventricular tachycardia.

The *v* **wave** is due to increasing filling volume and to concomitant, increasing pressure in the right atrium. It begins late in ventricular systole and in diastole; it is large with poor ventricular compliance and in severe tricuspid regurgitation.

AUSCULTATION OF THE HEART

First Heart Sound (S$_1$)

The 1st heart sound reflects closure of the mitral valve, then the tricuspid valve. You can best hear the 1st heart sound at the apex or lower left sternal border. It is commonly single or narrowly split. 1st heart sounds are never heard better at the base than at the apex. The loudness varies, depending on the force of atrioventricular valve closure. It is loud in mitral stenosis, increased ventricular contractility, or a short PR interval—when the valves come together forcefully at the beginning of systole. By contrast, with decreased contractility, the 1st heart sound is soft, as is seen in myocarditis.

Clicks are heard near the 1st heart sound. **Ejection clicks** with pulmonary valve stenosis occur early in systole at the left base of the heart and can vary with respiration. You generally hear aortic ejection clicks at the apex. Aortic clicks do not vary with respiration. Palpation of the pulse can be helpful to differentiate between 1st heart sounds, which precede the pulse, and clicks that are usually simultaneous with the pulse. You can hear systolic ejection clicks when there is an enlarged great vessel at the base of the heart or when there is a thickened/abnormal semilunar valve. Examples of these are:

- Thickened semilunar valves (e.g., aortic stenosis, bicuspid aortic valve, pulmonic stenosis)
- Enlarged aorta (e.g., tetralogy of Fallot)
- Truncus arteriosus (multi-valved great vessel)

Nonejection clicks occur later in systole and are heard at the left lower sternal border or the apex. For example, a midsystolic click at the apex suggests mitral valve prolapse.

Second Heart Sound (S₂)

The 2ⁿᵈ heart sound reflects closure of the aortic valve, then the pulmonic valve. Normally, the 2ⁿᵈ heart sound will have "**physiologic**" splitting, which results from increased venous return with inspiration. What happens is that when you inspire deeply, you increase right ventricular volume, which, in turn, causes delayed right ventricular emptying, which causes delayed closure of the pulmonic valve. Thus, you get a widening between the aortic and pulmonic valve closure and a splitting of the 2ⁿᵈ heart sound shortly after inspiration. It is difficult (but not impossible) to discern splitting in infants because of their rapid heart and respiratory rates. Therefore, if such splitting is easily heard in an infant, suspect a large left-to-right atrial shunt (ASD) or venous shunt (anomalous pulmonary venous return).

In transposition of the great vessels, the aortic valve is anterior and directly under your stethoscope—so aortic closure is very loud and best heard at the upper left sternal border. In tetralogy of Fallot, the aorta is wide and dextroposed, and the pulmonary artery is located anterior and is smaller than usual; this results in a single, 2ⁿᵈ heart sound that is heard loudest at the lower left sternal border.

Wide splitting (persistent) is due to delayed right ventricular emptying and can indicate possible atrial septal defect (ASD), right bundle-branch block (RBBB), or severe pulmonic stenosis. **Paradoxical** splitting of S₂ (splitting during expiration rather than inspiration) is due to a delay in left ventricular emptying, with the aortic closure sound coming after the pulmonic. You hear this in severe aortic stenosis or with LBBB.

Third Heart Sound (S₃)

You can hear the 3ʳᵈ heart sound in early diastole, when there is rapid, passive filling of a "relatively stiff" ventricle. An S₃ sound can be quite normal in children and pregnant women. Pathologic conditions that cause an S₃ can include left or right ventricular dysfunction or stiffness and AV valve regurgitation.

Fourth Heart Sound (S₄)

The 4ᵗʰ heart sound occurs in late diastole, when atrial contraction fills the ventricle. S₄ is almost always abnormal. It can be heard with aortic stenosis, mitral regurgitation, hypertrophic cardiomyopathy, and hypertension with left ventricular hypertrophy.

"INNOCENT" MURMURS

Overview

These are murmurs that are due to normal slow turbulence and vibration, and they do not indicate pathology. In infancy, the most common murmur is physiologic peripheral pulmonic stenosis (PPPS) and, occasionally, a Still's murmur; but after age 2, many children have at least 1 of the murmurs described below.

Systolic Innocent Murmurs

Note

All of these murmurs are short and soft (grade III/VI or less). They get louder when the child is placed supine, because stroke volume increases with this maneuver. They also get louder with exercise, anxiety, anemia, or fever. They may get softer or disappear with a Valsalva maneuver. (If Valsalva increases the murmur, think hypertrophic cardiomyopathy or obstructive left heart lesions!)

Still's Murmur

This is a systolic ejection murmur with a musical quality or vibratory character that some describe as similar to a plucked-string instrument or the "honking" tone of a kazoo. You can hear it best in the lower precordium, not in the back. It decreases in intensity with expiration and positional changes that decrease venous return (e.g., standing). The musical quality is what makes this easily recognizable. It is very common in childhood!

Basal Ejection Systolic Murmur

You hear this murmur at the base, and it is mid-pitched and ejection in character. It does not have musical components. It can be difficult to distinguish from mild pulmonic or aortic stenosis. Stenosis is frequently harsher and longer, and there may be a systolic ejection click if there is an associated bicuspid aortic valve.

Supraclavicular Arterial Bruit

The bruit is due to turbulence in the subclavian and carotid arteries, which, in turn, is due to increased acceleration in early systole. It is very short and early, and it ends before the 1ˢᵗ third of systole. It is easy to diagnose by its shortness and supraclavicular location.

Physiologic Peripheral Pulmonic Stenosis (PPPS)

PPPS is due to the normal newborn physiologic changes in circulation through the pulmonary artery branches associated with fetal transition. For several weeks after birth, the right and left pulmonary arteries are much smaller than, and come off at a right angle to, the large main pulmonary artery. This causes turbulence and results in a soft, harsh systolic ejection murmur best heard in the axillae and both the right and left

Quick Quiz

- Differentiate peripheral from central cyanosis.
- What is acrocyanosis?
- What does significant delay or absence of the femoral pulse compared to the radial pulse indicate?
- What does a rapid rising or bounding pulse indicate?
- In what conditions might one hear a systolic ejection click?
- In what conditions do you hear wide splitting of the 2nd heart sound?
- Which is abnormal in a child: a 3rd or 4th heart sound?
- What is the most common "innocent" murmur in an infant?
- What happens to an innocent murmur when the child is placed in a supine position? With Valsalva maneuvers?
- What distinguishes Still's murmur from others?
- Where on the thorax would you usually hear peripheral pulmonic stenosis?
- What causes a venous hum murmur?

hemithoraces. By 12 months of age, the branch pulmonary arteries become larger, and the angle at which they come off opens up; thus, the murmur usually disappears during this time period.

Continuous Innocent Murmurs

Venous hum is due to blood draining down the collapsed jugular veins into the dilated intrathoracic veins. The high velocity makes the vein walls "flutter," resulting in a low-pitched murmur. It is generally absent when the patient is supine, because the neck veins are distended and there is no pressure gradient between the 2 areas. Valsalva maneuver, turning of the head, or compression of the jugular vein also makes the murmur go away. Venous hum is very common in childhood.

THE 15-LEAD ECG

Refer to Figure 12-1 as we go over the basics of ECGs.

The electrical deflection in a given ECG lead is positive if the wave of depolarization spreads toward the positive pole of that lead, and a tracing is negative if it spreads away. The tracing is isoelectric (equal forces above and below) if the wave spreads at a 90° angle to it. For instance, if II is isoelectric, look for the maximum projection to be at −30° or +150° (i.e., 90° to the left or right of II).

With the 15-lead ECG, the wave of depolarization is recorded on both the frontal and horizontal planes, giving a 3-dimensional representation of the heart. The projection of the electrical activity of the heart onto the frontal plane is recorded by the frontal leads I, II, III, aVR, aVL, and aVF. On the horizontal plane, it is recorded via electrodes placed in the V1–V6 position. In pediatrics, an additional V7 is added, as well as right chest leads to include V3R, V4R—placed the same as V3 and V4, except on the right side of the chest. These additional leads in children give you a better look at the left ventricle (V7) or a better look at the right ventricle (V3R, V4R). Depolarization moving toward the lead causes a positive deflection (P wave and R wave), as does repolarization moving away from the lead (T wave).

The frontal leads give inferior-superior, left-right information.

The horizontal leads relay anterior-posterior-lateral information. Think of V1 as looking at the right side of the heart while V6 looks at the left side. The QRS in V1 is positive when the right ventricle (RV) is depolarizing (and negative when the LV is depolarizing), whereas the QRS in V6 is positive when the LV is depolarizing (and negative when the RV is depolarizing). Because of right ventricular dominance at birth, the R in V1 is larger than the S in V1, and, with age, the R wave in V1 decreases (and increases in V6).

AXIS DEVIATIONS

At birth, the infant has a relatively thick right ventricle; the mean QRS axis points anteriorly and to the right, giving RAD (70° to 180°) and large R waves in the right precordium. The QRS axis in the frontal plane shifts to the left and, at 3 months of age, is ~ +65° (range: 0° to 125°). By older childhood, the normal mean QRS axis is −30° to +100°. In an older child, > +100° is right axis deviation (RAD), whereas < −30° is left axis deviation (LAD).

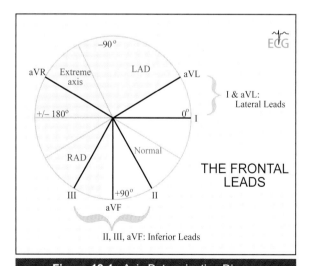

Figure 12-1: Axis Determination Diagram

For older children, a quick and fairly accurate method to determine this is to just look at I and aVF. If both are prominent, you can quickly tell in which quadrant the mean vector lies. Visualize the following:

• Both (+) = normal
• I (+) and aVF (−) = check for LAD
• I (−) and aVF (+) = check for RAD
• Both (−) = extreme axis deviation ("Northwest quadrant")

LAD in children is most often associated with tricuspid atresia, atrioventricular septal defects (AV canal), and LVH. Possible exam scenario: In a newborn with Down syndrome having an ECG with lead I (+) and lead aVF (−), think atrioventricular septal defect; this newborn needs an echo!

Causes of RAD include right ventricular hypertrophy (RVH) associated with congenital lesions; e.g., pulmonary stenosis (PS), atrial septal defect (ASD), tetralogy of Fallot (TOF), pulmonary hypertension, RBBB, or dextrocardia.

RATES AND INTERVALS

OVERVIEW

The ECG is recorded on paper with a 1-mm^2 graph, displaying a thicker line every 5 mm. Because the paper moves at 25 mm/sec, the interval between each thicker line is 1/5 of a second (or 0.2 sec—200 ms), and each mm represents 0.04 sec (40 ms). The interval covering 5 thicker lines (or 1 "big square") is 1 second.

There are a couple of quick ways to determine the heart rate. We'll discuss the RR interval, but know that any prominent wave of the standard QRS may be used to determine the interval. A quick and accurate method for determining heart rate: Calculate it as 1,500/RR interval in mm. So if the beat interval is 28 mm, the rate is 1,500/28 = 54 bpm. A less accurate but easier method is to divide 300 by the number of "big squares" in the RR interval. If the beat interval is 28 mm, this is not quite 6 big squares (since 6 x 5 mm = 30 mm). You divide 300 by 6 and get 50, but you know the heart rate is actually a little faster, because the interval is not quite 6 big squares. A derivative of this is the method in Dubin's book, *Rapid Interpretation of EKGs*, in which you memorize 2 sets of triplicates: 300–150–100 and 75–60–50. These are the corresponding heart rates for RR intervals of 1, 2, 3, 4, 5, and 6 of the "5 mm squares." (Remember: To do the math, divide 300 by the number of big squares; so, 1 corresponds to 300, 2 corresponds to 150, etc.)

Normal heart rate for newborns is 100–160 bpm. Heart rate gradually decreases with age. Mean heart rate is > 120 during the 1st year of life. By age 3, it falls to ~ 110, and by age 5, it is ~ 100. By age 12, it is, on average, 85.

Sinus tachycardia in newborns is > 160 bpm and in children > 120 bpm. Sinus bradycardia again depends on the age: < 3 years, it is < 80; > 3 years, it is generally < 60. However, it is not uncommon to see heart rates of 50–60 bpm in normal teens and preteens, especially in athletic kids.

IMPORTANT INTERVALS

The **PR interval** indicates the time between atrial and ventricular depolarization; it is a reflection of mostly AV node conduction. Normal duration is 3–5 small squares (120–200 ms, because a "small square" is defined as 40 ms). In newborns, the PR interval is, on average, shorter than in older children (i.e., 130 ms or less) and increases gradually with age. A PR interval longer than 200 ms (1 big square) in teens and adults is the definition of 1st degree AV block. Intervals shorter than 120 ms (3 small squares) at these ages may indicate Wolff-Parkinson-White (short PR interval with delta wave), junctional rhythm (with retrograde P wave—see next), or left atrial overload (widened P wave—see next).

QRS duration is usually < 100 ms (i.e., 2.5 small squares).

QRS > 120 ms may be caused by:

• Bundle-branch block (right or left)
• Ectopic ventricular beat (PVC)
• Ventricular rhythm
• Ventricular pacemaker
• Drugs that prolong conduction (such as tricyclics)
• WPW
• Electrolyte problems (hyperkalemia)

The **QT interval** varies with heart rate. The QT interval corrected for heart rate is normally 340–440 ms (450 ms in girls). The formula used to calculate the corrected QT interval is: $QT_c = QT/(RR)^{1/2}$. That is, the QT interval (in seconds) divided by the square root of the preceding beat interval in seconds. Again: The RR interval in this calculation must be in seconds. When scanning ECGs, a rule of thumb is: The QT interval normally is ~ 40% of the RR interval; do the calculation for QT_c if it appears much shorter or longer. (On exams, they will make it pretty obvious or will just tell you the patient has prolonged QT interval—you don't need to learn how to do square roots again by hand.)

With **prolonged QTc**, there is a tendency to develop recurrent syncope and/or sudden death, due to polymorphic ventricular tachycardia; i.e., *torsades de pointes*. Prolonged QTc has many causes. In a child without medications, it is most likely genetic or congenital prolonged QT syndrome. (Did the infant fail the newborn hearing screen? Long QT + sensorineural deafness = Jervell and Lange-Nielsen syndrome.)

The other etiologies for prolonged QT include:

• Tricyclic overdose (especially think about in the adolescent)
• Hypocalcemia
• Hypomagnesemia

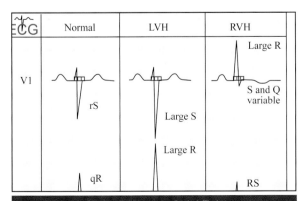

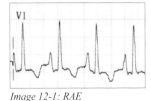
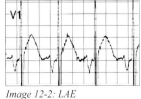

Quick Quiz

- In a 10-year-old, if the QRS is upright in lead I and down in aVF, what does this indicate about the axis?
- Know how to determine heart rates on an ECG tracing.
- What is the most common cause of prolonged QT interval in pediatrics?
- What prescribed drug may cause prolonged QT interval in a depressed adolescent?
- What P wave changes indicate right atrial enlargement? Left atrial enlargement?

- Hypokalemia
- Type Ia and III antiarrhythmics (Ia = quinidine, procainamide; III = amiodarone, sotalol)
- Starvation with electrolyte abnormalities
- CNS insult
- Non-sedating antihistamines (removed from the U.S. market)

More recently discovered causes of prolonged QT are:

- Azithromycin
- Liquid protein diet

Treatment of long QT syndrome (LQTS) may include beta blockade, pacing, an implantable defibrillator, or, rarely, surgical sympathectomy.

The Brugada syndrome is a sodium channelopathy resulting in an RV conduction delay and ST elevation in V1–V3. Like LQTS type 3, these patients have a sodium channel abnormality and are at risk for ventricular arrhythmia and sudden death. The only treatment is an implantable defibrillator.

Short QTc may be caused by hypercalcemia and digitalis; it also may just be congenitally short—but can also cause ventricular arrhythmias!

Figure 12-2: P Wave in Atrial Enlargement

WAVEFORMS AND SEGMENTS

P WAVE

The P wave results from the depolarization of the atrium. The normal P wave is < 2 mm in height and < 120 ms (3 small squares) in duration, and the normal P wave axis is 0° to +90°. (Where else have you seen 120 ms? The normal PR interval is 120–200 ms, Figure 12-2.)

Most P wave information can be derived from II, aVR, and V1. As the wave of depolarization spreads from the SA node high in the right atrium, through the right, and then left atrial myocardium, the mean vector is downward and to the patient's left—so the normal P wave is positive in II and negative in aVR.

A retrograde P wave (i.e., a P wave not originating in the sinus node) is negative in II (and III and aVF) and positive in aVR—indicating an ectopic focus, originating in the inferior part of the atrium or at the AV junction, which results in a wave of depolarization traveling toward aVR—picture this! A retrograde P wave from the AV junction often results in a short PR interval.

Because atrial depolarization traverses from the patient's right to left, the normal P wave is positive in lead I, II, and aVF and is positive or biphasic in V1.

With right atrial preponderance (enlargement, hypertrophy, overload), the right atrial (initial) portion of the P wave is delayed and overlaps onto the left atrial portion of the P wave. The P wave width stays normal (< 120 ms), but look for an increased P wave amplitude in II (also true with III and aVF, but look only at II) and in V1 (the positive portion). Actually, the P wave "peaking" in II is more important than its height. So again, RA enlargement causes peaked P waves in II and V1 (Image 12-1)!

With left atrial overload, the left atrial component of the P wave is delayed, resulting in a wide P wave taking up most of the PR interval (i.e., < 120 ms). Other typical findings are a widened, notched P wave in II and an enlargement of the negative portion of the P wave in V1. The most sensitive ECG finding for left atrial enlargement is a broad negative P wave in V1, with duration of more than 40 ms (> 1 small square wide and 1 small square deep) (Image 12-2). On the other hand, the most specific ECG finding is a notched, "M"-shaped P wave (usually in II) with an interpeak distance of > 40 ms.

Decreased P wave amplitude is seen in severe hyperkalemia.

Image 12-1: RAE   *Image 12-2: LAE*

T WAVE

The mean T wave vector changes rapidly and markedly after birth. The T wave is typically positive in V1 at birth. It remains positive for up to 7 days of age, then inverts in V1. The T wave should remain inverted in V1 until 9–10 years of age, and then it may be either inverted or upright in V1 during the teen years. If the T wave remains positive after 7 days of age and up to 10 years of age, this may indicate right ventricular hypertrophy.

T waves can be negative in the left precordial leads (V4, V5, V6) immediately at birth, and then, rapidly with aging, they can become upright.

Peaked T waves can occur with:

• Hyperkalemia
• Intracerebral hemorrhage

U WAVE

The U wave occurs just after the T wave and is mainly something to look at in adults or older adolescents. It is typically small and best seen in V2–V3. If seen, it is usually a < 1-mm, rounded deflection in the same direction as the T wave. If the U wave is prominent, there is an increased tendency for *torsades de pointes*. (If the U wave is > 50% of the height of the T wave, you should include it in your QT interval measurement.) You see prominent U waves with hypokalemia, bradycardia, digitalis, and amiodarone.

ST SEGMENT

There are 3 main causes of ST-segment elevation: acute MI, Prinzmetal angina, and pericarditis—obviously, the first 2 are almost never seen in children. Therefore, pericarditis is the most common cause of cardiac chest pain in pediatrics, and it affects the whole heart; so you see ST changes in most leads (Image 12-3).

You may also see ST-segment elevation in early repolarization (normal variant), intracerebral hemorrhage, hypertrophic cardiomyopathy, LVH, LBBB, cocaine abuse, myocarditis, and hypothermia.

ST-segment depression occurs in pediatrics with:

• Subendocardial ischemia (especially if down-sloping or flat), such as with classic angina in adults
• LVH with strain (ST depression with flipped T waves in left precordial leads)
• RVH, which may cause RAD and ST-segment depression preceding a flipped T wave in V1
• Digitalis effect
• Hypokalemia

QRS COMPLEX

Depolarization of the ventricles occurs simultaneously after the depolarization of the interventricular septum. The normal mean vector of depolarization of the interventricular septum points from the patient's left to the right, across the septum. This occurs as a small, initial deflection, which is positive in V1 (R wave) and negative in V6 (Q wave). A septal Q wave in V6 generally means normal initial depolarization.

The left ventricle is normally much more massive than the right ventricle, and, therefore, the mean QRS vector (reflecting depolarization of the ventricles) is strongly to the patient's left. You see a large negative deflection in V1 and positive deflection in V6. On the frontal plane (as mentioned under Axis Deviations on page 12-3) the mean vector is –30° to +100°.

The normal duration of the QRS is < 100 ms. We discuss QRS changes with ventricular hypertrophy and conduction disturbances in the next 2 topic areas.

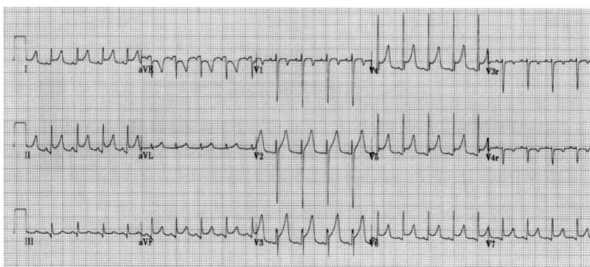

Image 12-3: Acute pericarditis

Quick Quiz

- When do you find peaked T waves?
- What is the most common cause of cardiac chest pain in pediatrics?
- What effect may hypokalemia have on the ST segment?
- How does LVH present on the ECG? RVH?
- True or false? In a term infant, what would be considered RVH in an older child or adult is a common finding and considered "normal" on a standard ECG.

VENTRICULAR HYPERTROPHY

LVH

Left ventricular hypertrophy results in the mean QRS being moved to the left and posteriorly. ECG findings are age-dependent and defined by age-group percentiles. For example, in the frontal plane, the QRS axis of the 0- to 1-month-old is usually between 30° and 90°; < 30° at this age is very uncommon and suggests LVH. The leftward shift of the QRS axis increases the R wave and decreases the S wave in V5 and V6—and the posterior shift of the QRS axis results in a decrease in the R wave and an increase in the S wave in V1.

Without an axis shift to help you, base the diagnosis of LVH mainly on voltage changes. R waves less than the 5th percentile or S waves more than the 95th percentile in V3R and V1 suggest increased posterior forces. Also

look for R waves more than the 95th percentile in V5 and V6. On an exam question, they'll have to give you a graph or the values. You won't need to memorize these for individual ages.

In older adolescents and adults, LVH causes a prolonged activation of the myocardium. LVH causes an exaggerated negative deflection in V1 and a positive deflection in V6 (Image 12-4).

Although the specificity of the various ECG criteria for LVH is pretty good (~ 95%), the sensitivity is low and varies from 25% for simple addition criteria, to 50% for a complicated point system. Note: If the prevalence of LVH in a population is 5%, there will be many more false negatives and many more false positives than true positives.

You may see a left ventricular "strain" pattern with LVH. LV strain presents with ECG changes that are precordial, ST-segment depression, and flipped T waves (particularly in inferior and lateral leads) in a patient with ECG criteria for LVH. (Is there a negative T wave in lead V6 after 7 days of life? If so, think LVH!)

RVH

The term infant has a right ventricular wall that is as thick as or thicker than the left ventricle and has physiologic "normal" right ventricular hypertrophy. For pathologic excessive RVH, the mean QRS will move farther right and anteriorly. This results in frontal plane QRS axes > 190° for infants < 1 week of age or 135° for infants > 1 month of age. RVH will produce taller R waves, with smaller S waves in right chest leads, and smaller R waves and larger S waves in left chest leads (Image 12-5 on page 12-8).

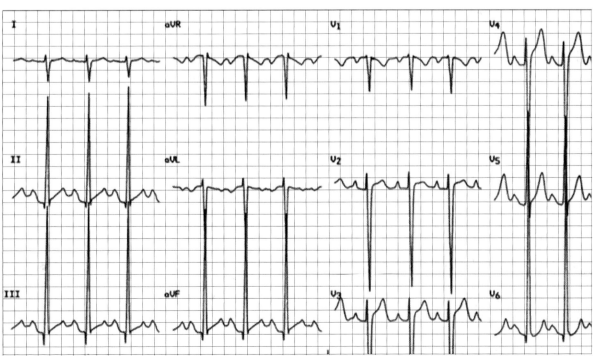

Image 12-4: LVH

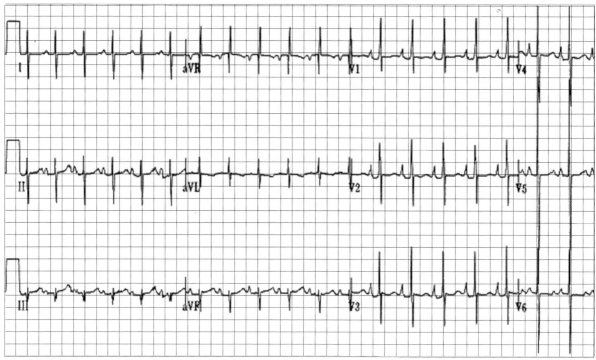

Image 12-5: RVH

Also look for a "pure" R wave, R > 25-mm voltage, or a qR pattern in the right chest leads—this suggests pathologic RVH in the newborn. It is also highly suggestive of RVH if you see an upright or even a "flat" T wave in V4R and V1 in a child between 1 week and 8 years of age.

In older adolescents and adults, ECG criteria for RVH are right axis deviation, increased R voltage in V1 or S in V6, and rsR' in V1, and again, because of repolarization changes, ST-segment depression and a flipped T wave in V1, sometimes in V2. The ST-segment depression and flipped T wave generally indicate RV stress/hypertension.

CONDUCTION DISTURBANCES

ATRIOVENTRICULAR (AV) BLOCKS

Atrioventricular blocks:

- 1° AV block prolongs the PR interval more than normal for age and by > 200 ms (1 big square) beyond 16 years (Image 12-6).
- 2° AV block results in 2 main patterns:
  - **Mobitz 1**: Wenckebach phenomenon involves progressive prolongation of the PR interval until there is a drop in QRS (ventricular beat) (Image 12-7). This effect is primarily from vagal tone on the AV node and is generally not considered malignant. Occasional follow-up is recommended. This rarely requires treatment.
  - **Mobitz 2**: Normal PR intervals, but, periodically, there is a drop in QRS. 2:1 AV block is 2 P waves for each QRS; 3:1 is 3 P waves for each QRS, etc. (Image 12-8). Mobitz 2 and higher-grade

heart block implies disease of the His-Purkinje conduction system and is an abnormal finding. This often requires a pacemaker.

- 3° AV block or complete heart block: No atrial depolarizations are conducted through the AV node. The P wave and QRS have independent regular

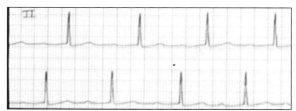

Image 12-6: 1° AV block

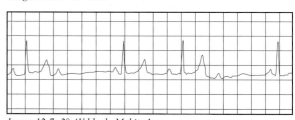

Image 12-7: 2° AV block, Mobitz 1

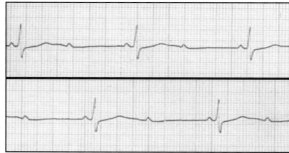

Image 12-8: 2° AV block, Mobitz 2; 2:1 AV block

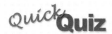

- In a term infant, what does a positive T wave in V1 indicate after 1 week of age? What does a qR pattern in V1 indicate?

- Differentiate Mobitz 1 from Mobitz 2.

- With 3° AV block, what does a narrow (normal width) QRS complex indicate? What does a wide QRS complex reflect?

rhythms at differing rates (AV dissociation). If the QRS complex has a normal width (< 100 ms), there is a junctional ectopic pacemaker. Junctional escape rate is 40–60 bpm, whereas ventricular escape rate (which also would be a wider QRS) is 20–40 bpm.

Note: The AV node has no pacemaker activity. Junctional pacing originates from the myocardial tissue at the AV junction (Image 12-9).

BUNDLE-BRANCH BLOCK

BBB Review

Just a little beyond the AV node, the bundle of His fast conduction pathway splits in two. These 2 fast conduction pathways travel down the interventricular septum, and one (the right bundle branch) then goes to the right ventricle, while the other one (the left bundle branch—functionally, if not anatomically) splits again

and proceeds to the anterior and posterior sections of the left ventricle. If conduction in 1 of these pathways is blocked, the depolarization downstream to that pathway is delayed because the myocardial tissue in that area must wait for the depolarization wave to arrive from much more slowly conducting adjacent myocardial tissue.

LBBB

Left bundle-branch block (LBBB) is rare in children and is more common in adults. The QRS is prolonged, with a duration of 120–180 ms (3–4.5 small squares). Because the left ventricle depolarization is now transmyocardial, it is depolarized over a longer period, resulting in an RR' (notched or slurred) in the lateral leads (I, aVL, and V6), and there is a corresponding SS' (also called QS) in V1. 50% of patients have a normal axis; 50% have LAD (−30° to −90°).

RBBB

Right bundle-branch block (RBBB) is more common in children, particularly after open heart surgery: The direction of septal depolarization is normal—left-to-right, but the right ventricle is depolarized over a longer period, resulting in an RR' or RSR' ("rabbit ears") in V1 and a wide S wave in V6. Visualize how the RSR' in V1 is formed: The initial R wave is due to normal, left-to-right septal depolarization, the S is depolarization of the left ventricle, and the final R' is due to the delayed depolarization of the right ventricle.

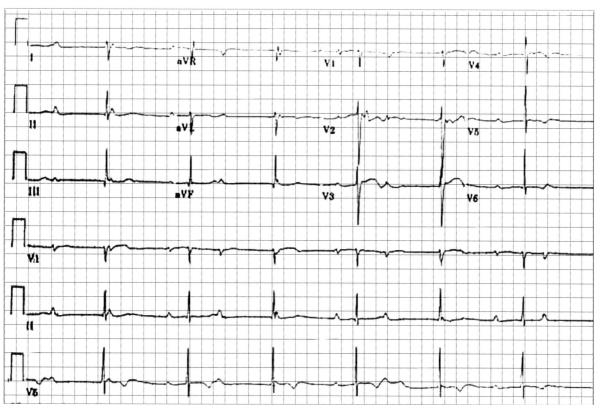

Image 12-9: 3° AV block with junctional ectopic pacemaker

In V6, the S wave is due to delayed depolarization of the right ventricle. This is often present after cardiac surgery (Image 12-10).

ARRHYTHMIAS

MECHANISMS OF ARRHYTHMIAS

The 2 usual mechanisms of abnormal cardiac rhythms are reentry and automaticity. The reentrant mechanism is the cause of most abnormal tachyarrhythmias. Reentry refers to abnormal "loops" of electricity causing arrhythmias. Atrioventricular reentry (accessory bypass tract) is the leading cause of supraventricular tachycardia (SVT) in newborns, infants, and young children; AV node reentry is the 2nd leading cause in older children. (AV node reentry is the leading cause in adolescents and adults.) Automatic rhythms are accelerated ectopic rhythms (i.e., a focus in the heart is causing the arrhythmia). Parasystole is a 3rd mechanism, which is a rare cause of PVCs. Be able to diagnose all rhythms at a glance.

SICK SINUS SYNDROME

Sick sinus syndrome (sinus node dysfunction) may manifest as 1 or more of the following: abnormal sinus bradycardia, sinus pauses, sinus blocks, sinus arrest, dominant escape rhythms, and tachy-brady syndrome. These patients usually do not need electrophysiologic testing.

Because prognosis is good, there are only 2 indications for treatment with a pacemaker in children with sick sinus syndrome:

1) The patient is symptomatic (e.g., syncope).
2) The patient has tachyarrhythmias requiring therapy, which might precipitate significant bradycardia.

Look for sick sinus syndrome in a child who has had atrial surgery—ASD repair (particularly the sinus venosus or "high" atrial septal defect with or without anomalous pulmonary venous drainage), atrial baffles in transposition of the great vessels (e.g., Mustard operation), or the Fontan procedure.

Note: If an ECG presents with sinus bradycardia in an adolescent female, don't forget that patients with anorexia nervosa will have slow heart rates. This is not true sick sinus syndrome but may look similar to it. Treat the underlying condition, and the bradycardia will improve.

HEART BLOCK

Permanent pacing is indicated for symptomatic 2nd degree (Mobitz 2) and most 3rd degree heart blocks. Patients with congenital complete heart block can remain well and asymptomatic for years. Emergency treatment consists of transcutaneous or transvenous pacing, IV atropine, isoproterenol, or other medications.

SUPRAVENTRICULAR TACHYCARDIAS

Atrial Flutter

Atrial flutter (A-flutter) has an atrial rate of 230–420 bpm (up to 500 bpm in newborns), normally with a 2:1 or 3:1 AV block resulting in a ventricular rate (or palpable pulse) in the range of 120–200 bpm (Image 12-11). It is typically due to reentry within the right atrium and around the tricuspid annulus. Isolated presentation in a healthy fetus or newborn is occasionally seen. In older patients, it is almost always an indication of disease, most often either organic heart disease or pulmonary

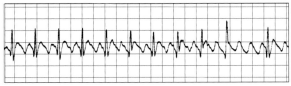

Image 12-11: Atrial flutter

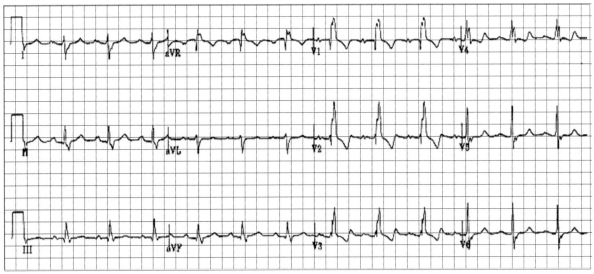

Image 12-10: RBBB

Quick Quiz

- What is the leading cause of supraventricular tachycardia (SVT) in neonates and young infants? What about older children and adolescents?
- Which children require a pacemaker for sick sinus syndrome? For heart block?
- What is the treatment for atrial flutter?
- Which antiarrhythmic drugs can you use for nonemergent conversion of atrial flutter?

disease. Atrial flutter may spontaneously convert to either atrial fibrillation or a normal sinus rhythm. Vagal maneuvers slow the rate and allow better diagnosis. Rule out pulmonary emboli (often multiple) and thyroid disease, especially if there is no identifiable heart or lung history. The normal block is 2:1. If it is ≥ 3:1, the cause is either AV node disease or drugs. For acute atrial flutter in infants < 1 year of age, do not use verapamil, because it may cause heart failure or hypotension.

The most effective treatment for atrial flutter is synchronized electrical cardioversion. (Systemic embolization may occur but is less common in atrial flutter than in atrial fibrillation.) Low energy can be used (0.5 J/kg or 10–50 Ws in older adolescents/adults). Higher energy (1–2 J/kg or 100–200 Ws in adults) is often used because it has less of a tendency than low energy to convert the rhythm to atrial fibrillation. Always shock if the patient is hemodynamically compromised. Overdrive pacing is also effective in more stable patients. Prior to cardioversion, ideally, echo imaging should be performed to assess for thrombi.

Use antiarrhythmic drugs for nonemergent cardioversion. Typically, you can control the rate by slowing AV node conduction with IV diltiazem, digoxin, or a beta-blocker; you can attempt conversion of the atrial rhythm with other agents, such as ibutilide (Corvert®), procainamide, flecainide, sotalol, or amiodarone—depending on the clinical situation. Ibutilide is a class III antiarrhythmic (intravenous only), which is particularly effective in adults for rapid cardioversion with minimal hemodynamic effects. Quinidine is a viable option but is not used much anymore. Use quinidine, flecainide, sotalol, amiodarone, and dofetilide (Tikosyn®) to prevent recurrence. Dofetilide is a class III oral agent that, due to its arrhythmogenic effects, requires special training for the prescribing physician. All class III drugs can prolong the QT interval.

Radiofrequency catheter ablation and cryoablation are treatment modalities that can cure the most common types of atrial flutter. These treatments are used for persistent or recurrent atrial flutter.

Atrial Fibrillation

Atrial fibrillation (A-fib) usually has an irregular ventricular rate of 130–200 bpm (about the same as the ventricular rate of atrial flutter with a 2:1 AV block) and is rare in children (Image 12-12). With new-onset A-fib, or in A-fib unresponsive to the usual treatment, consider hyperthyroidism, hypomagnesemia, alcoholism/cocaine abuse, and excessive caffeine and nicotine as possible causes.

Anticoagulate for 3 weeks before cardioversion if the patient is stable, and continue to anticoagulate for at least 6 months after successful cardioversion.

You can ordinarily treat the rapid ventricular response of chronic A-fib with digoxin, but also consider diltiazem,

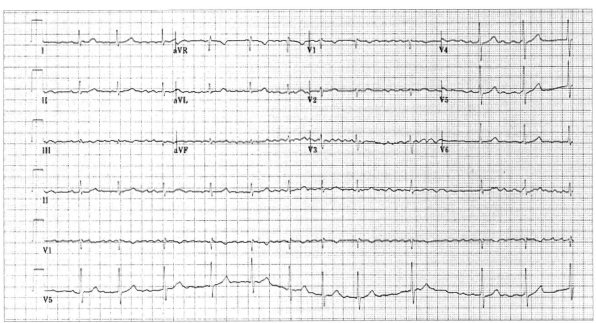

Image 12-12: Atrial fibrillation

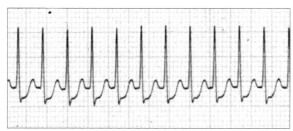

Image 12-13: PSVT

verapamil, or beta-blockers if the heart is healthy (i.e., can tolerate the negative ino-/chronotropic effects). Patients have better exercise tolerance on verapamil. These agents do not convert the abnormal rhythm; they just slow the ventricular rate!

To medically convert, after the rapid ventricular response is controlled, give dofetilide, quinidine, procainamide, flecainide, disopyramide, propafenone, sotalol, or low-dose amiodarone. IV ibutilide or amiodarone is effective in terminating acute A-fib.

Paroxysmal Supraventricular Tachycardia

Most paroxysmal SVT (PSVT) episodes are due to a reentrant rhythm (Image 12-13). This is the most common supraventricular tachycardia in children. Rate is 150–280 bpm (same as or slightly faster than A-fib or A-flutter). Usually, the P wave is not visible (buried in the QRS); but if seen, it usually is retrograde. If the monitor shows narrow complexes, treat with vagal maneuvers (diving reflex in infants—place ice bag to face for 10–20 seconds), adenosine, or verapamil. Avoid verapamil in infants < 1 year of age! Adenosine is the drug of choice because of its effectiveness and very short half-life

(~ 10 seconds). It works on the AV node, with transient AV block, which is involved in most of the SVTs .

Note: In an emergency situation with an unstable infant, treat with D/C cardioversion.

Many antiarrhythmic drugs also are effective for chronic treatment, including digoxin, beta-blockers, calcium channel blockers, class III agents, and class Ia agents. Flecainide (class Ic) is approved for SVT, but most try something else first. Radiofrequency catheter ablation or cryoablation can cure PSVT. Differential diagnosis of a wide complex tachycardia includes PSVT with aberrant conduction, PSVT with resting BBB, and V-tach (see page 12-13).

Wolff-Parkinson-White

Wolff-Parkinson-White (WPW): PR interval is < 0.12 seconds due to a delta wave (Image 12-14). Total QRS is > 0.12 seconds because of the fusion between the normal QRS and preexcited depolarization, which bypasses the AV node. This bypass tract (Kent bundle) is faster than the AV node, and therefore, a portion of the electrical current reaches the ventricle sooner (the delta wave on the ECG) and preexcites the ventricle. Another name for WPW is "preexcitation syndrome." Often, the accessory pathway is concealed, and the delta wave will not be visible when the patient is in normal sinus rhythm. An uncommon association of WPW is Ebstein anomaly of the tricuspid valve.

Treatment of WPW: Many patients have completely asymptomatic WPW and no dysrhythmias. Treat patients with WPW and a narrow complex tachycardia (rate is commonly ~ 180–240 bpm) with vagal maneuvers, cardioversion, procainamide, verapamil,

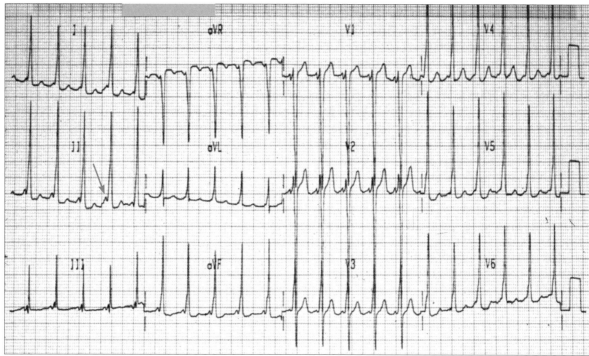

Image 12-14: WPW with delta waves (arrow)

Quick**Quiz**

- A stable infant presents with supraventricular tachycardia. What are the possible treatments? What if the infant is unstable?

- What is the drug of choice for an infant with WPW who develops atrial flutter?

- What is the treatment for simple PVCs?

- Which treatments can you use, and which can you not use for ventricular tachycardia?

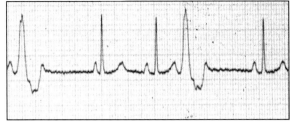

Image 12-15: PVCs

or adenosine—same as any SVT! But never ever treat acute A-fib or A-flutter (which usually has a wide QRS) in the setting of WPW with digoxin. Use extreme caution with verapamil and beta-blockers as well. Although verapamil and digoxin increase the refractory period in the AV node, they can decrease the refractory period in the bypass bundle! This can result in rapid-rate transmission to the ventricle, fibrillation, and/or sudden death.

Instead, it is better to treat acute A-fib or A-flutter in WPW with IV procainamide. [Know!] Shock if there are any signs of hemodynamic deterioration in any WPW tachyarrhythmia; especially watch those with pulse rate > 285 bpm, because they are at greatest risk of ventricular fibrillation (V-fib).

Radiofrequency ablation is now considered by many to be the treatment of choice for older children and adults with SVT and WPW and occasionally for A-fib!

Note: Most electrical cardioversion of SVTs can be terminated with low energy: 25–50 Ws. The exception is A-fib, which usually requires > 100 Ws.

VENTRICULAR ARRHYTHMIAS

PVCs

PVCs often have a compensatory pause; that is, they do not reset the sinoatrial node (i.e., the time between the sinus beats that are on either side of the PVC = 2 basic RR intervals). You do not need to treat asymptomatic, simple PVCs (even if the patient has thousands each day). Simple PVCs occur beyond the T wave, are uniform, and have constant coupling (reentrant) (Image 12-15). Also, do not treat complex PVCs (pairs, triplets) if the patient is asymptomatic and has no underlying heart disease!

(Did they give you a clue that the patient may have tuberous sclerosis? Cardiac tumors can cause multiple types of PVCs, and cardiac rhabdomyomas are associated with tuberous sclerosis.)

Ventricular Tachycardia

Ventricular tachycardia (V-tach) is defined as 3 or more sequential PVCs occurring at a regular rate of ≥ 120 bpm. Most occur at a rate of 150–200 bpm.

Differential diagnosis includes SVT with aberrant conduction, WPW, SVT with RBBB or LBBB, and severe hyperkalemia causing very large, peaked T waves (Image 12-16 on page 12-14).

A benign form of ventricular tachycardia is accelerated ventricular rhythm. This may present in infants or older children as a slow V-tach at the same or slightly faster rate as the underlying sinus rhythm. The patients are asymptomatic, and this tachycardia normally does not respond to drugs and needs no treatment. It may resolve over time.

In pediatrics, V-tach is most commonly due to:

- Electrolyte disturbances
- Myocardial disease, particularly myocarditis or hypertrophic cardiomyopathy
- Ion channel disorders (long QT syndrome)
- Postoperative states
- Ingestions
- Hypoxia or ischemia
- Idiopathic

If the V-tach lasts longer than 30 seconds or is unstable, it is usually due to organic heart disease. These patients have a high risk of sudden death; therefore, because of this danger, immediately use electrocardioversion in any patient with a wide QRS tachycardia and hemodynamic deterioration (treat like V-fib). If the patient is stable, you can use lidocaine, procainamide, or amiodarone. (Amiodarone is preferred in ACLS and PALS protocols.) Do not ever use verapamil with any wide complex tachycardias in the emergency setting—30% of those with ventricular tachycardia rapidly deteriorate! V-tach that is consistently induced by exercise is often well controlled by beta-blockers. Other V-tachs may require electrophysiologic testing.

Torsades de pointes (Image 12-17 on page 12-14) is often associated with a prolonged QT interval and a prominent U wave. Don't forget about the prolonged QT syndrome as an etiology. Also, quinidine, procainamide, other class Ia antiarrhythmics, and tricyclics are common causes. You may also see it in association with very low K+ or Mg. Treat associated bradycardia acutely by increasing the atrial rate with isoproterenol or overdrive pacing. Mg sulfate is another treatment option. Shock for sustained *torsades de pointes* because the patient will be unstable. Do not give quinidine or procainamide—any class Ia antiarrhythmic worsens *torsades de pointes*. [Know!]

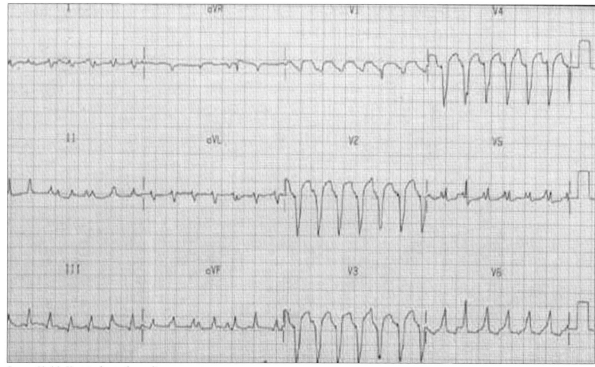

Image 12-16: Ventricular tachycardia

[Also know.] Avoid verapamil with:

- Young infants (< 1 year of age)
- Atrial fibrillation occurring in WPW
- Atrial flutter
- Wide complex tachycardias
- Beta-blockers—relative contraindication because they are both negative chronotropes and negative inotropes

Okay to use verapamil (but *never* in infants!):

- To control the ventricular response to A-fib in an otherwise healthy heart
- For PSVT (2nd choice after adenosine)

Cardiac Pacing

Temporary pacing: Single- or dual-chamber temporary pacing leads can be placed transvenously. Dual-chamber pacing is typically better but is not essential in emergency, temporary settings.

Permanent pacing is used for chronic, symptomatic sinus bradycardia and for complete heart block.

The most common dual-chamber pacemaker is called a DDD. Most clinicians use this one unless the patient is in chronic, slow atrial fibrillation. The DDD is the most physiologic and provides better exercise tolerance.

ANTIARRHYTHMIC DRUGS

With antiarrhythmic drugs (AADs), always wait 4–5 half-lives before determining whether a drug is effective. All AADs have a proarrhythmic potential.

Class I: Decreases upslope of the action potential (i.e., slows conduction primarily by blocking sodium channels).

Ia: Quinidine, procainamide, disopyramide.

Ib: Lidocaine, tocainide, mexiletine, phenytoin.

Ic: Flecainide and propafenone.

Class II: Decreases sympathetic activity—beta-blockers.

Class III: Prolongs the action-potential duration—amiodarone, sotalol, bretylium, and the newer agents, dofetilide (Tikosyn orally), and ibutilide (Corvert IV).

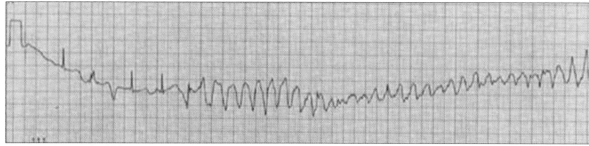

Image 12-17: Torsades de pointes

Quick **Quiz**

- For which patients should you not use verapamil to slow the heart rate?

- When is it okay to use verapamil to slow the AV nodal conduction?

- True or false? Serum digoxin concentration is usually helpful in determining toxicity.

- Know Table 12-1.

- Lithium use during pregnancy is associated with what cardiac abnormality?

Class IV: Blocks slow inward Ca^{+2} current: calcium channel blockers, especially verapamil and diltiazem.

Note: Adenosine is not in the previous grouping. It slows conduction in the SA node and AV node; it is used for conversion of SVT (AV node reentry and WPW) to normal sinus rhythm. It also induces coronary artery vasodilation and is used in cardiac perfusion imaging and stress echocardiography. Adenosine depresses LV function, but it has such a short half-life that you can use it in patients with decreased LV function.

Acute shortness of breath following adenosine can be related to bronchoconstriction; treat with a bronchodilator (e.g., terbutaline).

Major side effects of the AADs [Know]:

- **Ia**:
  ○ **Quinidine** prolongs the QRS complex and the QT interval—occasionally leading to *torsades de pointes*, diarrhea, and (rarely) autoimmune thrombocytopenic purpura. Also "cinchonism": hearing loss, tinnitus, and psychosis.
  ○ **Procainamide** prolongs QT and QRS, but also causes blood dyscrasias, such as agranulocytosis, neutropenia, and thrombocytopenia, in ~ 0.5%. It also causes drug-induced lupus and must be used with caution in heart failure patients because it has a mild, myocardial depressive effect.

- **Ib**: **Lidocaine**: seizures.

- **II**: **Beta-blockers** are commonly associated with bradycardia and can potentially aggravate asthma.

- **III**:
  ○ **Bretylium**: transient hypertension, then postural hypotension.
  ○ **Amiodarone** is the most effective drug; however, due to the extremely high iodine content (the most toxic antiarrhythmic drug in adults), do not use it chronically in children without supervision by a specialist. It has an extremely long half-life (40–55 days). Amiodarone is associated with:
    – Corneal deposits   – Sun sensitivity
    – Hyper/Hypothyroidism   – Pulmonary fibrosis
    – Hepatic toxicity   – Gray skin

Amiodarone does not cause hematologic changes. Pulmonary fibrosis can be severe and is fatal 10% of the time, but it is very rare in children.

- **Other**: **Digoxin**: arrhythmias. Digitalis toxicity is more likely in those with low K^+ or high Ca^{+2}.

Determine the toxic levels of both digoxin and quinidine by changes in the ECG, not by serum levels.

CONGENITAL HEART DISEASE

OCCURRENCE / CAUSES

Congenital heart disease occurs in ~ 7–8/1,000 live-born infants and has a much higher incidence in those who die *in utero*. VSD is the most common congenital heart lesion recognized in term newborns; pulmonic stenosis, ASD, and PDA are the next most common.

Genetic conditions are associated with specific cardiac defects. They are listed in Table 12-1.

[Know these associations!] Environmental factors can be important, too. Lithium use by the pregnant woman is associated with Ebstein anomaly of the tricuspid valve. Other drugs to be wary of during pregnancy are progesterone, retinoic acid, and alcohol (which has been associated with fetal alcohol syndrome and left-to-right shunts). Women with diabetes are at increased risk for having infants with congenital heart disease and a transient form of hypertrophic cardiomyopathy.

Table 12-1: Genetic Diseases and Their Associated Cardiac Abnormalities

I. Single Mutant Gene Syndromes (Autosomal Dominant, Recessive, or X-Linked)	
Noonan syndrome	Pulmonic stenosis Hypertrophic cardiomyopathy
Apert syndrome	VSD Coarctation of the aorta
Holt-Oram syndrome	ASD VSD
Alagille syndrome	Pulmonic stenosis, branch pulmonary artery stenosis
Ellis-van Creveld syndrome	Single atrium
II. Chromosomal Abnormalities	
Cri-du-chat syndrome	VSD
Turner syndrome (XO)	Bicuspid aortic valves Dilated aortic root Coarctation of the aorta
Trisomy 21 (Down syndrome)	Endocardial cushion defect VSD
Trisomy 13 syndrome	VSD, polyvalvular disease
Trisomy 18 syndrome	VSD

LEFT-TO-RIGHT SHUNTS

Overview

Left-to-right shunts are defined as defects where systemic circulation is shunted to the pulmonary circulation by an abnormal conduit (Table 12-2).

What determines the impact of a left-to-right shunt? Generally, 3 factors are important:

1) Size of the communication
2) Pressure differences between the 2 vessels/areas shunted
3) Total outflow (or vascular bed) resistances

If the communication is restrictive (i.e., small in size), flow will be very much reduced, and it really doesn't matter what the pressure or outflow resistances are. For atrial shunts, the pressures between left and right atria are low and almost equal, so outflow resistance and ventricular diastolic pressures will be the determining factors. Note that LV end-diastolic pressure is usually greater than RV end-diastolic pressure, so normally there is a left-to-right flow across the ASD.

At birth, systemic and pulmonary resistance and pressures are high and equal, and there is little shunting from left to right. However, as systemic vascular resistances increase, pulmonary vascular resistance decreases over 4–8 weeks; thus, a large left-to-right shunt can develop once pulmonary vascular resistance has fallen below systemic resistance/pressure—usually after a few weeks.

For VSD or PDA, where the communication is large, systolic pressures will be equal on both sides of the shunt; thus, the relative vascular bed ("outflow") resistance of each side of the shunt will determine the direction of

shunting. If left-sided vasculature resistance is higher than the right side, there will be a left-to-right shunt.

The persistence of high flow and pressures in the pulmonary arteries may lead to progressive and permanent, or fixed, elevation of pulmonary resistance, irreversible pulmonary hypertension and subsequent right-to-left shunting and cyanosis (Eisenmenger syndrome). This can be lethal.

Patent Ductus Arteriosus (PDA)

The ductus arteriosus normally closes "functionally" within 10–15 hours after birth, but complete anatomic closure may not occur for 3 weeks. Closure occurs by constriction of smooth muscle in the ductus arteriosus. Premature infants (weighing < 1,750 grams) have clinically apparent PDA ~ 40–70% of the time. Most feel that PDA is caused by the inability of the ductus arteriosus in premature infants to respond normally to both the increased oxygen tensions and to the changes in prostaglandin levels that occur at birth.

Clinically, the child presents with a continuous murmur. (Think about it—during both systole and diastole, aortic pressure will never be below pulmonary artery pressure, so blood will flow continuously from the aorta to the pulmonary artery through the ductus.) It is described as a "rumbling" or "machinery-like" murmur and commonly increases in intensity in late systole. You can hear it best below the left clavicle. If the PDA is small, the murmur is all that may occur. If it is large, the PDA increases LV output and will increase stroke volume, which causes a rise in aortic pulse pressure. Because flow continues during diastole, you get a low diastolic pressure and a "collapsing" or bounding pulse. The increased volume will result in increased left atrial and ventricular sizes; CXR may show enlargement of the cardiac silhouette, and ECG may show evidence of left ventricular hypertrophy. CXR will also show increased pulmonary markings because of the increased blood flow; eventually, irreversible pulmonary hypertension (Eisenmenger syndrome) can develop.

Echocardiogram is the best diagnostic test.

In an asymptomatic child, close a PDA either by catheter techniques or surgically. In premature infants, indomethacin therapy is used with 80% success. Even if the child is older and has no symptoms, signs, or problems from the PDA (so-called "silent PDA"), some would close the PDA to prevent endocarditis of the ductus; however, with the new endocarditis guidelines, this is controversial (since patients with a persistent ductus do not receive prophylaxis anymore for dental procedures, etc.). Latest guidelines suggest discussion between physician and patient of the risks and benefits. Transcatheter closure with a coil can be successful if the diameter of the ductus is < 5 mm, with the larger ductus needing surgery or other device closure. For further newborn management issues, see The Fetus & Newborn, Book 3.

Table 12-2: Left-to-Right Shunts Occurring in "Post-Tricuspid" Valve

Aorta to pulmonary artery shunts:
PDA
Truncus arteriosus
Aorta pulmonary window
Coronary-pulmonary fistula

Aorta to right ventricle:
Sinus of Valsalva fistula
Coronary arteriovenous fistula

Aorta to right atrium or vena cava:
Systemic arteriovenous fistula
Sinus of Valsalva fistula

Left ventricle to right ventricle:
VSD
Endocardial cushion defect

Left ventricle to right atrium:
Left ventricle to right atrium connection
Endocardial cushion defect

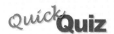

• Describe the murmur of PDA.

• What is the therapy for PDA in the premature infant? What about a 6-year-old child?

• What is the most common congenital heart defect in term newborns?

• Where do most VSDs occur in children < 1 year of age? > 1 year of age?

• How do symptomatic VSDs present? At what age would you expect symptoms to develop?

Ventricular Septal Defect (VSD)

Ventricular septal defects are the most common congenital heart defects recognized in the first few years of life and make up 25–30% of cases of congenital heart lesions in term newborns. (Bicuspid aortic valves are the most common congenital heart lesion, but often they are not recognized until teen or young adult ages.)

VSDs typically occur as isolated abnormalities but can occur with other congenital cardiac abnormalities. At birth, a majority of VSDs occur in the muscular septum, but these usually close spontaneously at ≤ 1 year of age. After 1 year, the majority of VSDs detected occur in the membranous septum. (So, to reiterate a favorite exam topic: < 1 year of age, most are in the muscular septum; > 1 year of age, most are in membranous septum—just below the aortic valve.)

Clinically, VSD is initially detected by finding a murmur, which is commonly described as "harsh" or high-pitched. (Possible scenario on an exam: An infant presents at 3–4 weeks of age with "breathing harder" and a new murmur. Think VSD. Remember: As the pulmonary resistance drops over the 1st month of life, more blood flows across the VSD leading to heart failure.) If the shunt is small, you may hear it only in early systole, but, as it increases in size, it becomes holosystolic and ends with aortic valve closure of the 2nd sound. Intensity is not related to size of the defect—loud murmurs can be heard with insignificant VSDs (known as *maladie de Roger*). Palpable thrills are common.

You can generally hear the murmur best at the lower left sternal border as it radiates through the precordium, with maximal intensity near the subxiphoid area. Variations can occur depending on where the VSD is. For example, a high subpulmonic VSD will result in a middle-to-upper left sternal border murmur, with radiation to the right side of the sternum. Additionally, if the shunt is large enough to produce a ratio of pulmonary-to-systemic flow > 2:1, a mid-diastolic murmur (the so-called "diastolic rumble" from extra blood flow across the mitral valve) will also occur at the apex, similar to a long, prominent 3rd heart sound.

If pulmonary hypertension eventually develops, the pulmonic component of the 2nd heart sound will increase in intensity; and, on CXR, there will be evidence of cardiac enlargement and increased proximal pulmonary vasculature markings (Image 12-18). The ECG can show LVH initially in large defects, and eventually RVH also will develop if the shunt is severe and persistent. If the shunt is small, CXR and ECG are frequently normal. Diagnose using echocardiogram.

Most symptoms occur in term infants 4–8 weeks of age and consist of volume overload and heart failure. The left-to-right shunt is generally greatest by about 2 months of age, when pulmonary vascular resistance has dropped to its lowest level.

You should close persistent shunts that have more than twice the normal pulmonary blood flow. Other management depends on symptoms and age.

Asymptomatic Infants

Initially, if the infant is diagnosed by murmur only and is asymptomatic with a small, quiet heart, do nothing and reevaluate periodically—as usual for "well-child" checks. At 6 months of age, if the murmur is still persistent, refer to a pediatric cardiologist, who may order an echocardiogram. If it is membranous (and thus, with a lower likelihood of closing), follow with the cardiologist and proceed to surgery in the patient with a 2:1 shunt (i.e., twice as much blood flow to the lungs as normal) and symptoms of poor weight gain or with the presence of elevated pulmonary artery pressure, in order to prevent Eisenmenger syndrome.

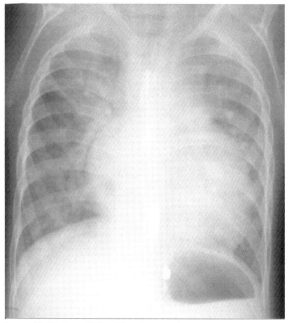

Image 12-18: Large VSD with pulmonary hypertension

Symptomatic Infants

If the infant or child has symptoms/signs of heart failure (HF) with the VSD, go straight to cardiology consultation. (If a cardiology consult is not available, order an echocardiogram.) If the echo shows an isolated VSD, management depends on the size and type: surgery for larger membranous defects with elevated right heart pressures by 6–12 months; for muscular VSDs (or smaller membranous defects), medical therapy is given a chance because these are more likely to decrease in size or even close spontaneously.

Medical therapy may include diuretics, afterload reducers, and/or digoxin.

For the medically treated: If they do not respond adequately (e.g., recurrent HF, FTT) or there is persistent pulmonary hypertension, especially with trisomy 21, proceed to surgery. Over time, for those on medical therapy and with "compensated" congestive heart failure (i.e., able to feed comfortably, grow well, and avoid frequent respiratory illnesses), evaluate and look for problems with the family in its ability to cope (e.g., can't make appointments, can't keep up with feeds). If these occur in the 1st year, consider surgery; if not, continue to monitor. At 1 year of age, repeat the echo. If the VSD has become smaller, monitor; if it is not smaller, consider surgery sometime between 1 and 2 years of age, especially if a 2:1 shunt persists.

Atrial Septal Defect (ASD)

Ostium Secundum Defect

Ostium secundum defects are the most common form of ASD and are located in the mid-septum. These are normally isolated lesions that can be very small to large in size. How much left-to-right shunting occurs depends on the size, inflow resistances (ventricular compliances) of the left and right ventricles, and the outflow resistance (vascular bed resistances) of the 2 ventricles. A large shunt results in large increases in flow through the right atrium, right ventricle, and pulmonary artery, compared to normal flow. Cardiac failure is very unusual in infancy. ASDs are twice as common in females as in males.

Older children with ASDs are usually asymptomatic. On physical examination, S_1 is normal, and S_2 is widely split without respiratory variation ("fixed splitting"). The fixed splitting of S_2 occurs because of an increase of blood flow into the right side of the heart during all phases of respiration, not just with inspiration as occurs normally. This increase of blood volume into the RV results in delayed closure of P_2 and the "fixed splitting" of P_2.

The ASD itself does not typically produce a very loud murmur—the murmur is from increased flow across the right ventricular outflow tract and pulmonic valve. It is a systolic ejection murmur that is crescendo-decrescendo and heard best at the upper left sternal border. If the shunting is large, an early or mid-diastolic murmur can occur due to increased flow across the tricuspid valve; you can best hear this at the left lower sternal border.

What does the CXR show? Before you answer, think for a moment. What is having increased volumes? That's right! The right atrium, right ventricle, and pulmonary artery—thus, the main pulmonary artery and right heart will be enlarged on CXR, and there is increased pulmonary blood flow.

ECG will show RAD, RVH, and a typical rsR or rSR' pattern in the right precordium. The S wave in the inferior leads may be notched.

Echocardiogram is diagnostic.

Pulmonary vascular disease with pulmonary hypertension (i.e., Eisenmenger syndrome) is uncommon (~ 5%), and will usually not occur until 20–30 years of age. Arrhythmias frequently occur in adults (ordinarily atrial fibrillation/flutter); also, there may be HF, as well as embolic strokes in adults. This is the reason why surgical (or a catheter device) intervention is usually indicated to prevent these complications from occurring. Usually, perform closures within the first 5 years of age to prevent complications. Most defects can be closed with catheter devices.

Ostium secundum defects do not need endocarditis prophylaxis; neither do ostium primum defects.

Ostium Primum Defect

This defect is located in the lower portion of the atrial septum in the region of the mitral and tricuspid valve rings. This is a form of AV canal defect and is also called a partial AV canal defect. The defect is typically quite large. Usually, the anterior (or septal) mitral valve leaflet is displaced and has a cleft. The tricuspid is usually not involved, but it too can have a cleft in the septal leaflet. Again, according to the 2007 endocarditis prophylaxis guidelines, ostium primum defects no longer require antibiotic prophylaxis.

Clinically, the left-to-right atrial shunt results in right ventricular hyperactivity, with increased pulmonary blood flow. There are usually a right ventricular outflow murmur, a tricuspid valve mid-diastolic flow murmur, and a widely split S_2. You may hear mitral and tricuspid regurgitation murmurs if the clefts occur in these valves.

The ECG will show left axis deviation (LAD) and right ventricular hypertrophy (RVH), demonstrated by an rsR' pattern in the right precordium. The LAD distinguishes the ostium primum defect from the ostium secundum defect.

Perform early surgical correction in childhood.

Patent Foramen Ovale

This is a normal fetal structure and is present in essentially all newborns. Remember: At birth, pulmonary blood flow and venous return increases markedly, and left atrial pressure rises. This functionally closes

Quick Quiz

- What medical therapy is used for symptomatic muscular VSDs?
- What are the most common anatomic types of ASDs?
- What is the finding of S$_2$ in an older child with ostium secundum ASD?
- What is the treatment for ostium secundum ASD?
- Does a patient with an ASD require endocarditis prophylaxis?
- What are the usual symptoms in a child with patent foramen ovale?
- What is the "defect" in complete AV canal defect?
- What is the most common heart defect seen in trisomy 21?
- By what age will heart failure occur in most children with complete AV canal defects?
- What is L-transposition of the great arteries?

the foramen ovale. In most instances, anatomic closure occurs by a few years of age. A patent foramen ovale may persist in 10–20% of children > 5 years of age and in adults. Usually, the patent foramen ovale is small and of no clinical significance in childhood. No physical findings or symptoms result. (In adults, closure of a patent foramen ovale may be indicated in cases of TIAs or strokes, if thought to be related to paradoxical emboli due to a right-to-left shunt through the foramen ovale.) There may be an association of patent foramen ovale with migraine headaches.

Complete AV Canal Defect (AV Septal Defect, Endocardial Cushion Defect)

This involves failure of the "central" heart to develop, resulting in a large hole communicating between the atria and ventricles, as well as malformation of the tricuspid and mitral valves. The anterior and posterior segments of each leaflet join each other through the defect (normally, they are separated), resulting in a common AV valve. The AV valve abnormality can result in significant mitral/tricuspid valve regurgitation. The overall result is a large left-to-right shunt and valve regurgitation, leading to a cardiac volume overload and HF. This is all due to a defect in the development of the endocardial cushions. This is the most common heart defect in Down syndrome (trisomy 21).

The child can present with the characteristic murmur of a VSD, as well as a mid-diastolic rumble that is due to increased pulmonary venous return and increased diastolic flow across the AV valve. A mitral regurgitant murmur (apical pansystolic) may also be present if the cleft in the mitral valve is significant. The same happens if the tricuspid is involved.

These infants most often present with heart failure by 2 months of age. Symptoms can start in early infancy, especially if there is a large left-ventricle-to-right-atrial shunt, or if there is significant valvular dysfunction.

ECG will usually show a left axis deviation and prominent voltages with biventricular hypertrophy. CXR reveals nonspecific, generalized cardiomegaly with increased pulmonary blood flow.

Medical management of HF can be helpful, but early surgery is necessary, within the first 6–12 months, to prevent pulmonary vascular disease (Eisenmenger syndrome). Usually, the best outcomes occur in those with balanced defects and similar-sized ventricles. Occasionally, 1 ventricle can be small/hypoplastic. Children with Down syndrome traditionally have a good chance of having compatible anatomy for correction, but they do require surgical correction early (i.e., before 6 months of age) in order to avoid irreversible pulmonary vascular disease.

L-Transposition of the Great Arteries (Ventricular Inversion or Congenitally Corrected TGA)

L-transposition occurs when the embryonic cardiac tube loops to the left instead of the right. The anatomic left ventricle ends up on the right side and connects the right atrium to the pulmonary artery. The anatomic right ventricle is now on the left side and receives oxygenated blood from the left atrium through a tricuspid valve, while the right ventricle ejects the blood to an anteriorly placed left-sided aorta.

Confusing, right? There is transposition of the great arteries (the aorta comes off the anatomic RV and the pulmonary artery from the anatomic LV) and "inversion" of the ventricles, but this allows normal flow of venous blood to the lungs and oxygenated blood to the rest of the body. Thus, this is known as "congenitally corrected" transposition. Just about all neonates with this lesion have a VSD or pulmonic stenosis. Many have conduction defects, and complete heart block develops at a rate of about 1–2% per year.

The ECG will usually show Q waves in the right chest leads and no Q waves on the left—indicating that activation of the septum occurs from right to left. CXR will show the transposed aorta as a "straight shoulder" on the left heart border.

If patients are doing well, surgery may not be indicated because it can be technically difficult and increases the risk of conduction defects. If there is significant hemodynamic load and the patient is symptomatic, perform repair with VSD closure and relief of pulmonic stenosis (PS). In higher risk situations, palliation can be done; and the pulmonary artery may be banded in the case of a large left-to-right shunt, or an aortopulmonary shunt can alleviate hypoxia when there is more severe PS. A pacemaker may be needed eventually if AV block develops.

Sinus of Valsalva Fistula

Rupture of a sinus of Valsalva into a cardiac chamber is usually due to a structural abnormality in the sinus and is uncommon. The most common fistula involves the anterior (right coronary) aortic valve sinus, which ruptures into the right ventricle or right atrium. The other, less commonly seen, fistula occurs from the noncoronary or left coronary sinus into the left atrium or left ventricle.

An associated VSD may increase risk of rupture.

Rupture is usually associated with acute chest pain and dyspnea, with sudden onset of murmur and heart failure. Echocardiogram is the best diagnostic tool. Surgical closure is necessary.

REGURGITANT LESIONS

Aortic Regurgitation

Aortic regurgitation (AR) presents with a high-pitched, early diastolic murmur that begins with the aortic component of the 2nd heart sound. An aortic systolic ejection murmur can also be present due to increased flow across the valve or to a structural abnormality of the valve itself. The **Austin Flint murmur** is associated with rheumatic fever. Austin Flint is a low-pitched, mid-diastolic murmur at the apex and is due to the regurgitant aortic jet striking the anterior leaflet of the mitral valve, preventing it from opening fully, thus causing relative "mitral stenosis."

Most children are asymptomatic unless the AR is more severe; then they'll present with fatigue or exercise intolerance. Chronic or acute AR can present with HF.

Look for a wide pulse pressure—the systolic pressure is elevated due to increased LV stroke volume, and diastolic pressure is reduced because of "runoff" into the LV and peripheral vascular dilatation.

Some causes of AR in children:

- **Congenital aortic stenosis** (AS) typically occurs due to a bicuspid aortic valve; over time, insufficiency can develop. You usually treat AS with valvulotomy (surgical) or valvuloplasty (catheterization-based)—either of which will increase the amount of AR, but generally, the degree of AR won't be clinically significant.
- **Marfan syndrome** is associated with dilated sinuses of Valsalva and ascending aorta. AR can result and can be severe.
- **Rheumatic fever** is probably the #1 cause worldwide but is less common in the U.S.
- **Infective endocarditis**, especially that due to *S. aureus*.

You can monitor most patients for signs/symptoms with periodic ECGs, and echocardiograms for those with significant AR. Use afterload reduction (ACE inhibitors, hydralazine, calcium channel blockers) with moderate or severe AR to lessen the volume and reduce the amount of regurgitant flow. Do surgery if the patient is symptomatic, if there are signs of LV dysfunction or severe dilation, or if acute regurgitation has occurred with resultant heart failure.

Mitral Regurgitation

Mitral regurgitation (MR) presents with an apical, high-pitched blowing systolic murmur. It can radiate to the left axilla and the back. The murmur commonly starts at the 1st heart sound and is holosystolic in character. With mitral valve prolapse, the murmur will usually start later (mid-to-late systolic, following the "click").

Worldwide, the most common cause of mitral regurgitation is rheumatic fever; in the U.S., it is mitral valve prolapse, which occurs in about 1–5% of the population. MR can also occur if there is a cleft in the anterior leaflet of the mitral valve, or if papillary muscle dysfunction has occurred (cardiomyopathies or ischemic infarction).

Many patients require no therapy, but in those who are symptomatic, you can use afterload reduction to postpone surgery. For those who worsen, or in whom LV function is deteriorating, perform mitral valve repair (valvuloplasty) or valve replacement.

Mitral Valve Prolapse

In mitral valve prolapse (MVP), 1 or both leaflets of the mitral valve prolapse back into the left atrium. Most of the time, there is no explanation for why this is happening. MVP occurs more frequently in those with Marfan's (they have elongated chordae tendineae), Ehlers-Danlos, or the mucopolysaccharidoses. The extent of prolapse depends mostly on an inverse relationship with LV volume; i.e., if volume is increased (as when the patient lies down), then the prolapse will decrease.

More often than not, patients with MVP have a mid- to late-systolic crescendo murmur at the apex—almost always preceded by 1 or more clicks. If you have the patient sit or stand (decrease LV volume), the murmur will get longer and the clicks move earlier in systole (i.e., the "clicks murmur" moves earlier); and when the patient squats or lies down, the murmur becomes less noticeable, shorter, and later in systole (i.e., the "clicks murmur" moves later). Know these position changes with MVP! Most older patients with MVP are asymptomatic, but some will have chest pain and/or palpitations. Studies show these are not associated with MVP in pediatric patients. Arrhythmias can also occur.

(Note: On the other hand, if they describe an increased early systolic ejection murmur with standing that disappears with squatting, think hypertrophic cardiomyopathy!)

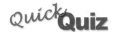

- Describe the murmur of aortic regurgitation.
- What are some causes of aortic regurgitation in children?
- Worldwide, what is the most common cause of mitral regurgitation? In the U.S. proper?
- Describe mitral valve prolapse. Which conditions carry an increased risk of having MVP?
- What is the 2nd most common congenital cardiac defect?
- An infant suddenly becomes cyanotic, with signs of cardiac collapse when the ductus arteriosus closes. What is a possible explanation? What would be the most important drug to administer to this infant?
- True or false? Most children with pulmonic stenosis are asymptomatic.
- Describe the murmur of pulmonic stenosis.

Pulmonary Regurgitation

The murmur of pulmonary regurgitation is an early, low-pitched, decrescendo diastolic murmur that starts with the pulmonary component of the 2nd heart sound. It can become high-pitched if pulmonary artery diastolic pressure is increased, such as with pulmonary hypertension. The regurgitation is usually not a clinical problem because of the lower pulmonary pressures. If the regurgitant volume is 2x normal, a soft pulmonary systolic ejection murmur may develop, and the 2nd heart sound may widen but is not fixed.

The most common cause of pulmonary regurgitation is surgery for either pulmonary stenosis or tetralogy of Fallot. Congenital pulmonary regurgitation is rare.

Manage most patients who develop pulmonary regurgitation after valvuloplasty or valvular surgery on a stenotic valve with periodic follow-up. Most do not require any special therapy. If symptoms worsen, or RV function is compromised, seriously consider valve replacement. This may be an increasingly seen problem in postoperative tetralogy of Fallot.

Tricuspid Regurgitation

The murmur of tricuspid regurgitation is a pansystolic murmur that is loudest along the lower left sternal border, with radiation to the right. You may also hear a low-pitched, mid-diastolic murmur in the tricuspid area. The CXR may show a right lower cardiac border that is large, and the ECG may also show right atrial enlargement. If the right atrium is very enlarged, you may see distended jugular veins or an enlarged liver. Isolated trace or mild tricuspid regurgitation is common. Up to moderate tricuspid regurgitation is typically well tolerated. Pretty much anything that dilates the right ventricle and increases pressure/volume will result in some tricuspid regurgitation. Rare causes include endocarditis (suspect this in an adolescent who is injecting IV drugs), pulmonary hypertension, Ebstein anomaly, and carcinoid syndrome.

OBSTRUCTIVE LESIONS

Pulmonic Stenosis

Pulmonic stenosis (PS) is the 2nd most common of the congenital cardiac defects recognized early in life. Again, VSD is the most common. Usually, PS is due to abnormalities of the valve leaflets. RVH occurs because of the valve obstruction. The overall formation and size of the right ventricle and tricuspid valve are related to the time in gestation at which pulmonic stenosis occurs. If it is early, venous return is likely to be diverted across the foramen ovale and results in a relatively small RV and tricuspid valve, with eventual pulmonary atresia. If the stenosis occurs later in gestation, RV formation is likely to be normal.

After birth, presentation depends on the extent of the stenosis and the degree to which RV and tricuspid valve development have been affected. In critical pulmonic stenosis, the RV cannot eject the total systemic venous return; thus, pulmonary blood flow from the pulmonic valve is markedly diminished. There is right-to-left atrial shunting (typically through a patent foramen ovale or ASD) away from the thickened, noncompliant, right ventricle, and cyanosis will be present. These infants appear as though they have complete pulmonary valve atresia, and most of the pulmonary blood flow has to come from the aorta to the pulmonary artery through a patent ductus arteriosus. Clinically, infants with severe pulmonic stenosis present in early infancy with severe cyanosis with cardiac collapse as the ductus closes. The need for prostaglandin E_1 (PGE_1) therapy to maintain a patent ductus arteriosus and sufficient pulmonary blood flow defines "critical pulmonic stenosis."

In those with only mild-to-moderate pulmonic stenosis, mild cyanosis may develop if the foramen ovale remains open, but the cyanosis disappears if, and/or when, the foramen ovale closes or the RV obstruction is relieved. In general, isolated PS is not a cyanotic lesion except in the newborn with critical PS.

For the great majority of affected children with pulmonic stenosis, no symptoms occur. They are picked up only because of the heart murmur. A systolic ejection click (that varies with respiration) along the left sternal border is followed by a crescendo-decrescendo murmur. You can hear this murmur best at the left upper sternal border, and it radiates to below the left clavicle and often to the back.

ECG may show peaked P waves (lead II) indicating the RA enlargement, as well as RAD and RV hypertrophy. CXR will show RV prominence and prominent main pulmonary artery with normal pulmonary blood flow.

Over time, some children, even with moderate stenosis, will have little or no worsening or increase in RV systolic pressure—probably due to the fact that the valve opening has enlarged with growth. Other children, however, will have a marked increase in RV pressures, leading to high RV end-diastolic pressures and, rarely, right heart failure.

Children with mild stenosis require no treatment and no longer require endocarditis prophylaxis. Patients with more moderate (RV pressure over 50% of systemic) to severe (RV pressure greater than systemic) stenosis will develop problems over time and should have pulmonary balloon valvuloplasty or surgical valvotomy. Additionally, treat other children who are symptomatic with exercise and those with significant RV hypertrophy. Finally, consider treatment for any child with RV systolic pressure > 50 mmHg or 2/3 of systemic pressure.

To estimate RV pressure, cardiologists often use the tricuspid regurgitant jet velocity as assessed by Doppler echocardiography. The peak velocity (e.g., 3 m/s) can be used to calculate a gradient from the right atrium to the right ventricle using the modified Bernoulli equation (gradient = $4v^2$). If you assume a normal RA pressure of 5 mmHg, then the RV pressure = gradient + 5 mmHg; e.g., gradient = $4(3^2$ m/s) = 36 mmHg (gradient) + 5 mmHg (RA) = 41 mmHg RV pressure. They may not expect you to make the calculation, but instead may give you an echo report with a tricuspid regurgitant jet echo-Doppler gradient of X mmHg. (Normal right ventricular pressure is ~ 25 mmHg.)

Alagille syndrome (more in Genetics, Book 3) is associated with pulmonary valvular or peripheral stenosis.

Noonan syndrome is also associated with pulmonic stenosis.

Peripheral Branch Stenosis

In many infants up to 6–12 months of age, a "physiologic" branch pulmonary artery stenosis occurs and produces an innocent murmur—usually grade 1–2/6 radiating to both axilla and all lung fields. It resolves with growth. It can also occur and be severe/pathologic in infants with congenital rubella syndrome, Williams syndrome, or Alagille syndrome (arteriohepatic dysplasia).

Aortic Valve Stenosis

Almost all (> 85%) congenital stenotic aortic valves are bicuspid—1 cusp is small and 1 is large. The opening is described as "fish-mouth" in character. The remaining 15% have only 1 cusp—a monocusp—and its opening is described as being like a "teardrop." If there is severe aortic stenosis at birth and the foramen ovale closes, left atrial pressure will rise while LV output is maintained. This will result, however, in pulmonary edema as left atrial pressure continues to rise. If the foramen is open and a large left-to-right shunt occurs, cardiac output will be decreased, but the pulmonary edema will be less. Either way, whether the foramen is open or closed, LV function will eventually deteriorate and LV failure will occur. If the aortic stenosis (AS) is not that severe, most infants are able to maintain an adequate cardiac output by developing LV hypertrophy to overcome the obstruction. Unfortunately, congenital AS is often progressive. As the infant/child grows, the valve opening becomes smaller and smaller, and stenosis becomes more pronounced.

Clinically, the newborn with severe, congenital AS will present fairly quickly with a systolic murmur at the right or left upper sternal border, with an early ejection click. The newborn's perfusion and pulses will be diminished, and he/she can have the appearance of being in septic shock. CXR will usually show marked cardiomegaly with severe pulmonary edema. This newborn is described as having "critical" aortic stenosis and requires initiation of prostaglandin E_1. Echo is diagnostic.

In older children, the murmur (a crescendo-decrescendo, harsh-to-rough systolic murmur with suprasternal notch thrill) is significant, and the other clinical findings generally correlate with the degree of stenosis. You typically best hear the murmur at the right upper sternal border, and it radiates into the suprasternal notch and neck. An apical ejection click that does not vary with respiration is heard commonly. Children do not usually develop the diminished pulse volume, as seen in adults. It takes much longer for the LV volume to be ejected, so the aortic component of the 2nd heart sound is delayed, frequently resulting in narrowing or loss of the split heard with the 2nd heart sound. It is rarer in children, but, occasionally, the aortic component will occur after the pulmonic component, known as paradoxical splitting. On inspiration, the 2nd heart sound's gap will narrow, and, on expiration, the gap will widen. You will typically hear a 3rd heart sound at the apex.

Note: Physical findings, CXR, and ECG are not reliable in predicting the severity of the AS! Therefore, you must periodically assess the pressure gradient between the LV and aorta, as well as the hemodynamic status, using either Doppler echocardiogram or cardiac catheterization. You may do exercise stress testing to assess adequacy of myocardial perfusion. Usually, if Doppler indicates severe AS, or symptoms occur, consider cardiac catheterization to assess more accurately the gradient and valve competency.

If a child with known AS presents with syncope or chest pain, the next step is to treat the cause with cardiac catheterization balloon angioplasty, or surgery. Generally, a Doppler gradient of 70 mmHg correlates with > 50 mmHg peak-to-peak gradient by catheterization, indicating the need for therapy. This commonly means that valve surface area has fallen to < 0.65 cm^2/m^2 (normal is > 2 cm^2/m^2). Balloon valvoplasty is now the treatment of choice in children. Patients typically do well initially and for many years. Eventually, however, stenosis recurs, and ~ 40% require repeat treatment (including surgery) within 10 years.

Quick Quiz

- Does pulmonic stenosis warrant endocarditis prophylaxis?

- True or false? In congenital aortic stenosis, the typical valve is monocuspid.

- How will an infant present with severe aortic stenosis?

- What is the murmur of an older child with aortic stenosis?

- True or false? Clinical findings are helpful in discerning the severity of aortic stenosis.

- A child with known aortic stenosis presents with new-onset syncope. What should you do next?

- How may HCM be inherited?

- How can you differentiate between HCM and aortic stenosis?

- An athlete suddenly collapses on the basketball court. What is the most likely etiology?

- What syndrome is supravalvular aortic stenosis associated with?

When the aortic stenosis is severe, all patients will eventually require surgery, with either the Ross procedure or mechanical valve replacement. The Ross procedure consists of moving the pulmonary valve ring, with the valve intact, into the aortic annulus, and placing a homograft valve (a size-matched human pulmonary or aortic valve from a tissue donor) into the right ventricular outflow tract. Anticoagulation is not required, and there is a very low risk of restenosis of the aortic valve. Unfortunately, the new pulmonary valve (the homograft placed between the RV and PA) does not grow and often becomes stenotic and/or insufficient over time. It requires surgical replacement in 5–15 years, depending on the size of the child at the time of surgery. If possible, defer either the Ross or mechanical valve replacement until the child is fully grown to alleviate future surgeries related to the child's growth.

Hypertrophic Cardiomyopathy (HCM)

HCM is a genetic disorder of heart muscle that presents with the myofibrils arranged in an unorganized, haphazard pattern. This results in a compensatory thickening (hypertrophy) of the heart muscle in order to generate an equal amount of systolic "force." As a genetic disorder, it is transmitted as an autosomal dominant (AD) disorder with variable expression. About 50% of the mutations occur on chromosome 14. HCM has historically been called by a variety of names, such as hypertrophic obstructive cardiomyopathy (HOCM) and idiopathic hypertrophic subaortic stenosis (IHSS). Since not all patients have "obstruction" and since the etiology is no

longer "idiopathic," the current name of HCM suits the disorder best.

A systolic murmur is often present and generally correlates with the degree of obstruction present in the left ventricular outflow tract as a result of hypertrophied myocardial tissue. It is not associated with systolic clicks like AS, and there is not a suprasternal notch thrill. The murmur is delayed in onset—a grade 3–4/6 crescendo-decrescendo systolic murmur at the middle left-to-right upper sternal border. A thrill is palpable over the precordium in some patients (but again, not the suprasternal notch). Gallops (3rd and 4th heart sounds) are common. The murmur gets louder with Valsalva or rising to an erect position. Either of these reduces venous return, resulting in a decrease in LV volume and an increase in the effect of the obstruction. If you have the child squat, venous return will increase and decrease the murmur due to LV dilatation. Note: These same maneuvers in AS will produce the opposite effects. This can be your clue to make this diagnosis: Look for a child in whom the murmur gets softer with squatting. It will be HCM, not AS!

The CXR will show cardiac enlargement without an enlarged ascending aorta. The ECG is abnormal in most cases, revealing LVH, prominent septal Q waves, and abnormal repolarization or strain (look for negative T waves in V6). Echocardiogram is diagnostic. Genetic testing is now available to assist in the diagnosis of borderline cases or to assist in the screening of family members of the proband.

Children with HCM are at risk to die from arrhythmias. HCM (with or without obstruction) is the most common cardiac cause of sudden death in athletes at sporting events in the U.S.

Beta-blockers are the mainstay of therapy along with restriction from competitive athletics. Children who have symptoms of syncope, aborted sudden death, arrhythmias, or severe thickening of their interventricular septum require referral to pediatric cardiologists. They may then require placement of an implantable cardioverter-defibrillator (ICD) and/or surgical therapy (myectomy) to remove part of the thickened myocardial tissue (typically from the interventricular septum). Calcium channel blockers, and/or amiodarone can be helpful in some patients.

Supravalvular Aortic Stenosis

This condition is narrowing that occurs just above the level of the coronary arteries. The coronaries arise just proximal to the obstruction and often have thickened medial and intimal layers, with occasional fibrous tissue that compromises coronary blood flow.

You can have isolated supravalvular AS, but it is most commonly associated with Williams syndrome (which is the result of a defect in elastin). Remember that Williams syndrome involves intellectual disability, "cocktail-party personality," elf-like facies, and narrowing of the peripheral systemic and pulmonary arteries. (Also remember they can have systemic hypertension related to renal artery stenosis.)

When listening to the heart, you'll frequently hear a systolic murmur (without click) at the base and toward the neck. With supravalvular aortic stenosis, the jet directed into the innominate artery usually results in a blood pressure 15 mmHg higher in the right arm, compared to the left arm (so-called Coanda effect). Do an echo and Doppler study to quantify the severity of the supravalvular obstruction; occasionally, cardiac catheterization will be required as well. If obstruction is severe, surgery is indicated.

Aortic Hypoplasia and Interruption

Hypoplasia of the aortic arch most commonly occurs in the aortic isthmus (the part of the aorta between the origin of the left subclavian and the ductus attachment). The most severe form, obviously, is complete interruption (and most commonly occurs proximal to the left subclavian); this is almost always associated with multiple congenital and cardiac defects (VSD, aortic/subaortic stenosis, mitral abnormalities).

In cases of true interruption of the aortic arch, remember to consider a FISH test (22q11 marker) to rule out DiGeorge syndrome. If complete interruption has occurred, distal aortic blood flow is provided only by right-to-left flow through a patent ductus arteriosus. Initially, when the ductus arteriosus is dilated, there may be no difference in blood pressure between the upper and lower body, but there might be differential cyanosis between the feet and hands. Over time, however, the ductus arteriosus constricts so that flow to the lower part of the body is diminished and compromised. The LV becomes overloaded as well, and kidney and other organ function in the lower part of the body is adversely affected.

In infants, look for a clinical presentation of poor systemic output with HF, decreased lower extremity pulses, and differential cyanosis (pink above/blue below). Echocardiogram will usually show the abnormality, but cardiac catheterization may be necessary to fully elucidate the problem.

Those infants with only narrowing of the transverse arch may respond to inotropes and diuretics. With severe arch narrowing or interruption, prostaglandin E_1 (PGE$_1$) is extremely useful in dilating the ductus arteriosus and returning adequate flow to the lower body. This allows the infant to stabilize for surgery.

Coarctation of the Aorta

Coarctation of the aorta (CoA) is an obstructive lesion that can be found in otherwise asymptomatic older children and young adults during a workup of hypertension or murmur. If the obstruction is severe, it can present as HF or cardiogenic shock in newborns.

The ductus arteriosus is large during fetal development. CoA develops from a defect in the aortic media, causing a posterior infolding ("posterior shelf") of the vessel. The narrowest part is juxtaductal; therefore, coarctation is unlikely to produce significant alteration in the distribution of blood flow. After birth, the ductus constricts on the pulmonary end first, so that an aortic opening is still present—often for days. However, if the aortic end of the ductus constricts, blood flow will become obstructed.

Clinically, in infancy, severe CoA looks a lot like severe aortic stenosis, with "septic shock" appearance. If left ventricular function can be restored (usually with inotropes), you will see the classic pressure difference between the upper and lower body. Murmurs are not common, but if the ductus is patent, you may hear a continuous murmur along the left sternal border or mid back. For many infants up to 3–4 weeks of age, prostaglandin E_1 is the best stabilizing therapy because it may open up the ductus enough to relieve the acute aortic obstruction. After stabilization, surgery is required to remove the narrowed section of aorta and reconnect the normal sections of the aorta. (This is called a direct anastomosis; there are other operative choices as well.)

In those with a small aortic shelf, or slow occlusion of the aortic side of the ductus, aortic obstruction develops slowly over weeks to months. These infants are more likely to develop collaterals and have less chance for acute events. However, heart failure still may occur at 3–6 months of age because the coarctation becomes more severe. If the child has not had heart failure by 6 months of age, it is unlikely to develop before adulthood. In young children beyond 6 months of age, CoA can present with hypertension or murmur. Epistaxis, claudication-like symptoms in the lower extremities with exercise, and headaches are described but are uncommon. Stroke is rare before 7 years of age, but, if it occurs, it is likely associated with a ruptured berry aneurysm. According to the latest guidelines, antibiotic prophylaxis to prevent endocarditis is no longer recommended.

What about older children and adolescents? How do they present? Diagnose from pulses and blood pressures—not murmurs. Pulses in the upper extremity are strong with associated hypertension, while the femoral pulses are weak and delayed compared with the radial pulse. Other abnormalities can occur, including an aberrant right subclavian artery below the coarctation, which would result in the right arm's blood pressure/pulse being lower than the left arm's. A murmur may be present posteriorly at the left scapular angle, and often there are murmurs/clicks from associated aortic stenosis or bicuspid aortic valve, which are common with CoA. You may hear continuous murmurs over the collateral vessels.

CXR has some features you need to know! Look down the left upper border of the aortic arch and descending aorta. The area of dilatation below the coarctation and the dilated aortic segment just above the coarctation can

Quick Quiz

- How will infants with significant coarctation of the aorta present? Older children?

- What is the classic x-ray finding in a 7-year-old with undiagnosed coarctation of the aorta?

- What is the traditional therapy for coarctation of the aorta?

- What is the most common cyanotic heart lesion associated with congenital heart disease of infants who survive past infancy?

- Name the 4 components of tetralogy of Fallot.

- A cyanotic child who squats after exertion probably has what cardiac abnormality?

- A child with undiagnosed tetralogy of Fallot is at risk for what brain infection?

sometimes look like the "3" sign. Rib notching is classic, but may not develop for 5–6 years. It occurs at the lower margins of the ribs, at about the middle third, and is due to erosion of the bone by large intercostal arteries. It occurs in > 50% of affected older children. Do an echocardiogram 1st; MRI is also helpful in diagnosis.

Untreated CoA has several potential complications: hypertension, rupture of a berry aneurysm, HF, endocarditis, and rupture of the aorta (reported only in adults). Surgery is the traditional treatment of choice—usually excision with direct anastomosis. Balloon angioplasty has become the treatment of choice for re-coarctation and can be used at times for native coarctation.

Mitral Valve Stenosis

Congenital mitral stenosis is uncommon, normally severe, and presents early in infancy. It is most often associated with other left heart obstructions or hypoplasia (part of Shone complex, which is defined as multiple left heart obstructive lesions all present at the same time). The baby presents with pulmonary edema; HF also is possible. The pulmonic component of the 2nd heart sound is usually loud because of the associated pulmonary hypertension. Normally, you hear an apical diastolic murmur, but typically not an opening snap in infancy because the valve is so thick and immobile. Mitral insufficiency may occur with the stenosis, so you may also hear an apical systolic murmur. ECG may show broad-notched P waves, indicative of the left atrial enlargement, but RVH is seen instead of LVH due to the pulmonary hypertension.

Unfortunately, medical management of severe congenital mitral stenosis with HF in infancy is rarely successful. A prosthetic valve is sometimes indicated, but it must be replaced as growth occurs. Additionally, you must give anticoagulation to prevent thrombus formation on the valve. Infants and children may do okay with dilatation of the stenotic valve with a balloon catheter, thus deferring valve surgery or replacement until a later date.

Tricuspid Stenosis

Isolated, tricuspid stenosis is very rare and usually is associated with a more global problem, like complete underdevelopment of the right ventricle. Right atrial enlargement is common, and this frequently manifests on ECG with a large peaked P wave.

RIGHT-TO-LEFT SHUNTS

Tetralogy of Fallot

Tetralogy of Fallot (TOF) is the most common cyanotic heart lesion in children with congenital heart disease who have survived untreated beyond infancy. It makes up 7–10% of congenital defects.

4 things make up the tetralogy:

1) RV outflow tract obstruction (subpulmonary valve stenosis)
2) VSD
3) Overriding aorta
4) RVH

Why is the child cyanotic? Because he/she has a right-to-left shunt as a result of pulmonary outflow tract obstruction, which causes various amounts of systemic venous blood to be shunted across the VSD into the aorta. These children tend to develop "tet" spells or "blue" spells, which occur when there is an acute reduction in pulmonary blood flow, a drop in systemic afterload, and worsened right-to-left shunt. The attacks may last only a short while and not have any sequelae, or they can be prolonged and produce limpness, exhaustion, or collapse. In rare instances, the attacks can cause seizures or death. Fortunately, most of these children have corrective surgery by 6–12 months of age, so relatively few today have hypoxic spells.

A classic question relates to the cyanotic child who squats after exertion. Squatting causes increased arterial oxygen saturation and is probably due to increased systemic arterial resistance (and therefore increased pulmonary blood flow). Again, these children are rarely seen anymore today because of corrective surgery done more consistently at an early age. If, for some reason, the child has not had surgery, he/she is at risk for brain abscess, cerebral thrombosis with hemiplegia, and infective endocarditis.

The murmur in an untreated child is due to the right ventricular outflow obstruction. You can hear a systolic murmur best at the middle or left lower sternal border. There can be an associated aortic click in older patients due to aortic dilation. As the RV outflow obstruction becomes severe during a "tet spell," there may be very little flow across the RV outflow tract, and the murmur may disappear.

CXR classically shows the "boot-shaped" heart or "coeur en sabot" (Image 12-19). 25–30% have a right aortic arch. ECG will show RAD and RVH. Echocardiogram is diagnostic, and cardiac catheterization is often not indicated.

There is a subgroup known as "acyanotic Fallot." These children have minimal RV outflow obstruction and therefore do not have a significant right-to-left shunt.

Treatment [Know]: PGE$_1$ is helpful in the neonate with pulmonary outflow obstruction to alleviate cyanosis. Usually, you will perform corrective surgery by 6–12 months of age, but sometimes earlier. If a hyper-cyanotic "tet" episode occurs before surgery, treat by placing the infant on its abdomen in a knee-chest position or by holding the infant with its knees flexed on the abdomen. You can try oxygen, but it is typically not that helpful because the lungs are not receiving much blood to oxygenate. Sedate with morphine (0.1–0.2 mg/kg IV or subcutaneously) to relieve a protracted episode. IV beta-blockers can also be helpful.

Avoid factors that worsen agitation. You can use vasopressors, particularly phenylephrine, to raise systemic resistance and increase pulmonary blood flow. Iron deficiency anemia can set these spells off, so cyanotic infants should have hematocrits of 50–55%. The hematocrit should not exceed this value, however, because this increases risk for cerebral thrombosis. If surgery cannot be performed, give propranolol 0.5–1 mg/kg/dose orally 2–4 times daily to prevent attacks.

What happens in surgery? Close the VSD, resect the infundibular subpulmonic muscle, and, sometimes, place RV outflow and main pulmonary artery patch to enhance the flow of the outflow tract. Pulmonary valvulotomy is also sometimes done. Survival rates are ~ 95% for those with uncomplicated Fallot. About 10–15% require further surgeries for recurring pulmonary stenosis. For many in whom the pulmonary artery was spared and for virtually all in whom the valve required removal

as a part of the placement of a transannular patch, long-term significant insufficiency will develop requiring pulmonary valve replacement. Complications are rare, but the most common is post-op ventricular arrhythmias (< 1%). Remember the association of ventricular arrhythmias in post-op tetralogy of Fallot with residual PS or severe pulmonic insufficiency (PI).

Complete (d-) Transposition of the Great Arteries

Complete dextro-transposition of the great arteries (d-TGA) is the most common cardiac cause of cyanosis in the newborn during the first few days of life. It comprises 4–6% of congenital defects. Remember: Tetralogy of Fallot is the most common for all ages together. What happens with d-TGA? Because the great arteries are completely transposed, the aorta is connected to the right ventricle instead of the left ventricle, and the pulmonary artery is connected to the left atrium instead of the right atrium. The systemic venous return goes into the right atrium and the right ventricle and is then ejected out into the "transposed" aorta that is coming off of the RV. Meanwhile, the oxygen-rich pulmonary venous return is going into the LA and LV and is ejected back into the lungs via the "transposed" pulmonary artery.

So we have 2 ("parallel") different circulations—2 different circuits that must somehow connect or the infant dies quickly. (In fact, this is an easy way to remember the difference between d- and l-TGA: Think "**d**" for "**d**ies" and "**l**" for "**l**ives," because without urgent surgical correction, the infant with d-TGA will die, but the infant with l-TGA will live, since the anatomy of l-TGA is "congenitally corrected.") In ~ 50% of d-TGA cases, the connection is only through a patent foramen ovale and, more rarely, a secundum ASD. If neither allows much oxygenated blood to mix, there will be severe cyanosis at birth. VSDs may allow more mixing, so less cyanosis occurs. The ductus arteriosus is open early, but it closes very quickly after birth and doesn't help very much.

The infant with transposition but without a VSD usually presents in the first few hours after birth. The only initial presenting sign/symptom in an otherwise healthy-appearing baby may be severe cyanosis. If there is ductal right-to-left shunting, reversed differential cyanosis (blue above and pink below) can be seen. Initial CXR and ECG are frequently normal.

Physical exam will show a single, loud 2nd heart sound (because the aorta is right under the sternum). There can be a 2–3/6, nonspecific, systolic ejection murmur at the middle left sternal border. The infant who has a large associated VSD can develop HF and modest cyanosis by 3–4 weeks of age. These infants commonly have tachypnea and dyspnea.

ECG may be helpful after ~ 5 days, with a persistently positive T wave in the right precordium (lead V1). CXR can vary from normal to the classic findings—egg-shaped or oval-shaped heart with a narrow

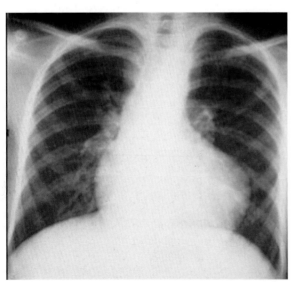

Image 12-19: Tetralogy of Fallot with "boot-shaped" heart

Quick Quiz

- What is the classic x-ray finding in tetralogy of Fallot?
- A child with tetralogy of Fallot has a prolonged, severe "tet" spell. What can you use to relieve the symptoms?
- What is the most common congenital anomaly presenting with cyanosis in the first few days of life?
- Describe the anatomy of complete transposition of the great vessels.
- What is the classic x-ray finding in complete transposition of the great vessels?
- In an infant with tricuspid atresia, when will cyanosis occur?
- How does the ECG in tricuspid atresia differ from tetralogy of Fallot and complete transposition?
- What x-ray finding is seen with Ebstein anomaly?

mediastinum and small thymus. You usually see this classic finding, though, in only ~ 33% of affected infants. Echocardiogram is diagnostic.

Balloon atrial septostomy to create an atrial septal defect offers immediate palliation and is sometimes done in conjunction with cardiac catheterization—but can be done under echo guidance right in the nursery. The use of PGE₁ infusion can be helpful. The increased pulmonary flow is across the PDA and increases venous return to the LA, enhancing atrial mixing.

Perform arterial switch surgery, the treatment of choice, once the infant is stabilized. It should be done before 2–3 weeks of age, before the LV can regress into an RV-like ventricle because of the low pressures it faces. Operative survival is 90–95%.

Double Outlet RV
(Including Taussig-Bing Anomaly)

This is a rare group of disorders in which both the aortic and pulmonary valves are positioned over the RV, and the only outflow from the LV is through a VSD. Different scenarios can occur with variable cyanosis, depending on VSD location and degree of associated PS. The RV can supply the pulmonary artery, and the aorta overrides the VSD, with subpulmonic stenosis also occurring. This results in a "tetralogy of Fallot–like" lesion. At times, the aorta can come off the RV, and the pulmonary orifice is supplied by the overriding VSD with little LV flow to the aorta (Taussig-Bing anomaly). This acts more like a transposition of the great arteries with severe cyanosis.

Coarctation is also found in ~ 25% of these patients. Surgical correction is the treatment option.

Tricuspid Atresia

Tricuspid atresia is fairly common. ~ 1% of all congenital heart disease is due to tricuspid atresia. The tricuspid opening does not exist, meaning that the only way of getting blood from the right atrium to the rest of the circulation is via a foramen ovale or ASD. Here, the systemic return and the pulmonary venous return mix.

Usually, there is a VSD. Pulmonary blood flow is across the VSD, through the hypoplastic RV, and into the PA. If there is severe PS or a small VSD, a PDA may be necessary to supply adequate flow and oxygenation. Cyanosis appears within hours to days after birth, when the ductus begins to close. Cyanosis is the key presenting sign. There is often a VSD or PS murmur.

CXR varies depending on the size of the VSD and degree of PS. Small VSD and/or severe PS will show diminished pulmonary vasculature and small heart with a round or "apple-like" shape; large VSD and/or mild PS will show increased pulmonary markings and large heart.

ECG will show left superior axis deviation (0° to –60°) and LVH with decreased RV forces for an infant. This is helpful since the other 2 common cyanotic diseases, tetralogy and complete transposition, have RAD and RVH.

Review: What are the congenital heart defects with left axis deviation? Ostium primum ASD, complete AV canal, and tricuspid atresia.

If there is significant cyanosis, initiate prostaglandin E₁ and then perform a palliative systemic-pulmonary shunt (modified Blalock-Taussig anastomosis or central anastomosis) in newborns or young infants. In older infants, replace the shunt by a cavopulmonary connection between the superior vena cava and the right pulmonary artery (called a Glenn shunt). In later years, perform the modified Fontan procedure. This diverts the inferior vena cava to the pulmonary arteries. This final procedure leads to all systemic venous return (except that from the coronary sinus) flowing into the lungs and allows the single functioning ventricle to maintain systemic output. The patient is no longer cyanotic.

Ebstein Anomaly

Ebstein anomaly (EA) is rare—except on exams! With EA, the posterior and septal leaflets of the tricuspid valve are displaced downward and attached to the RV wall. This displacement divides the RV into 2 sections—a proximal "atrial-like" segment and the distal "ventricular-like" segment. The atrial-like segment and the RA are typically huge, and tricuspid regurgitation is significant. Look for a huge RA on ECG and CXR (Image 12-20 on page 12-28).

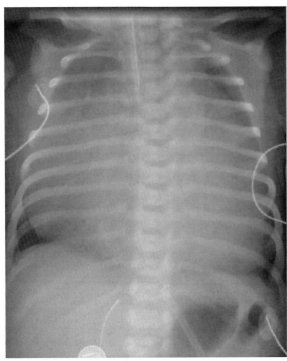

Image 12-20: Ebstein anomaly

Most EA patients are cyanotic soon after birth due to atrial right-to-left shunt, but this resolves until later childhood or young adulthood. On an exam question, look for the use of maternal lithium and development of Ebstein! Exercise tolerance gradually deteriorates during childhood. Paroxysmal supraventricular tachycardia is common. The ECG may show an RBBB or a WPW pattern.

Treat HF that is not severe with digitalis and diuretics. Surgical therapy, with tricuspid valvuloplasty or replacement, may be required at any time. Life expectancy varies widely, depending on the severity and specific conditions of each individual. Usually, however, the cause of death is HF or arrhythmia.

Pulmonary Atresia with Intact Ventricular Septum

Pulmonary atresia occurs in about 1–2% of infants with congenital heart disease during the 1st year of life. Most have a hypoplastic and thick-walled RV with a very underdeveloped tricuspid opening and valve. Systemic venous return to the lungs occurs across the atrial septum to the left heart and aorta. The pulmonary circulation is commonly maintained through a PDA.

Cyanosis is common early, but affected infants deteriorate and die unless they are given PGE_1 to keep the ductus arteriosus open. Perform an ECG because, in pulmonary atresia, you see an inferior QRS axis (0° to 90°) with LVH, while in tricuspid atresia, you see superior QRS axis with LVH.

Consider cardiac catheterization in this lesion for prognosis and therapy issues. Give PGE_1. At the time of catheterization, if the RV is of reasonable size, you can attempt pulmonary valvuloplasty. If the valvuloplasty works, keep the PGE_1 going (to keep the PDA open) for several more days, so that the RV can have time to remodel and become a useful pump to the lung. After a period of time, a 2-ventricle repair may be done. If the valvuloplasty doesn't work, perform surgery. Those defects with very poorly formed RV are treated similarly to tricuspid atresia—shunting and, later, the Fontan approach. The exact treatment depends on the severity of the lesion and is best left to the subspecialty experts.

BI-DIRECTIONAL SHUNTS (RIGHT-TO-LEFT AND LEFT-TO-RIGHT)

Total Anomalous Pulmonary Venous Return

Total anomalous pulmonary venous return makes up about 1–2% of all congenital heart lesions seen in the 1st year of life.

There is usually no direct connection between the pulmonary veins and the LA. The pulmonary veins go either to the RA or to other systemic veins that then drain into the RA.

Three main types of anatomic connections occur: supracardiac, cardiac, and infracardiac (infradiaphragmatic). 33% will have pulmonary venous return via a left vertical trunk into the left innominate vein and then into the superior vena cava. 25% will go below the diaphragm, connect with the ductus venosus, and then go into the inferior vena cava. The other 30–40% or so will connect directly to the RA or the coronary sinus.

The subdiaphragmatic form is most likely to have severe obstruction to pulmonary venous return, and the neonate presents with pulmonary edema and more severe cyanosis. The supracardiac form can also have obstructive problems, but it is much less common. Other cardiac abnormalities occur in ~ 33% of those with total anomalous pulmonary venous return.

A majority of infants present early on with tachypnea and FTT. In those without pulmonary venous return obstruction, cyanosis initially may be minimal. Murmurs are rare early. In those neonates and infants with severe obstruction to pulmonary venous return, early-onset dyspnea is prominent, with pulmonary edema developing rapidly.

In those infants with unobstructive pulmonary venous return to the innominate vein, CXR shows a classic "snowman" or "figure-8" silhouette (Image 12-21). The dilated left vertical vein, innominate vein, and the right superior vena cava sitting next to the dilated heart form the silhouette. In those with obstructive pulmonary venous return, the heart on CXR is normal in size, and the lungs show a diffuse hazy pattern resembling "ground glass," as seen with respiratory distress syndrome. Echocardiogram is diagnostic. Cardiac catheterization is rarely required.

- What drug will improve cyanosis in a child with pulmonary atresia with intact ventricular septum? Why?
- What is total anomalous pulmonary venous return?
- How do infants with total anomalous pulmonary venous return present?
- What is the CXR finding in total anomalous pulmonary venous return?
- How do most infants with hypoplastic left heart syndrome present?

Emergent surgical treatment is necessary for the severely obstructed group. You must begin symptomatic therapy early on to reverse acidemia and hypoxemia. The goal of surgical correction is to get the common pulmonary vein connected to the left atrium.

Hypoplastic Left Heart Syndrome

This name defines those disorders in which the left side of the heart is underdeveloped. The right side of the heart is dilated and hypertrophied and supports both the systemic and pulmonary circulations using a PDA. Hypoplastic left heart accounts for ~ 25% of all cardiac deaths in the 1st year of life. Frequently, associated abnormalities occur, including aortic and mitral atresia/stenoses.

Most infants are acutely ill with signs of poor perfusion (lactic acidosis, HF, and/or cardiogenic shock) within the first days or weeks of life. Infants have cyanosis with a grayish color and poor pulses, but they have hyperdynamic cardiac impulses. Pulses may become weaker and then stronger, depending on the patency of the ductus arteriosus.

CXR eventually shows cardiac enlargement and prominent pulmonary vasculature. Pulmonary edema can be present. ECG will show RA and RV hypertrophy. Echocardiogram is diagnostic.

Use PGE$_1$ to maintain the ductus arteriosus; there are 2 possible procedures:

1) Norwood procedure—1st stage: Cut the main pulmonary artery and ligate the PDA. Use the proximal pulmonary artery to reconstruct the ascending aorta and aortic arch to establish output from the RV to the aorta. A systemic-to-pulmonary shunt then reestablishes pulmonary blood flow. (Note: The Sano variant places a small RV-to-PA conduit to establish pulmonary blood flow.) If the foramen ovale is small, do an atrial septectomy. Perform a bidirectional Glenn procedure (2nd stage, SVC-to-PA shunt) 4–6 months later, followed still later with a modified Fontan procedure (3rd stage, IVC-to-PA connection).

2) Orthotopic heart transplantation has had excellent short-term results to date, but donor hearts are scarce.

Single Ventricle

Single ventricle refers to a variety of disorders in which there is 1 ventricular chamber that receives both the mitral and tricuspid openings (e.g., double inlet left ventricle), or when there is a common AV orifice. The most common of these are morphologically left ventricles without the inflow portion of the right ventricle. Typically, there is a rudimentary anterior and left-sided right ventricular outflow chamber. This connects proximally to the single ventricle through a VSD and distally with a transposed aorta. The pulmonary artery comes off the single ventricle and is posterior in position. Other cardiac anomalies are common and can include dextrocardia, common AV canal, coarctation, and either pulmonic or subaortic stenosis.

Symptoms vary, depending on the degree of PS and the other anomalies. In severe pulmonic stenosis, you will hear a loud systolic murmur and see severe cyanosis. If pulmonic stenosis is mild, there may be increased pulmonary blood flow and minimal cyanosis.

CXR may show a straightened left heart border. The ECG is nonspecific, and the echocardiogram is diagnostic. You may need to perform cardiac catheterization to fully define the abnormalities present.

Palliation is usually possible for infants with decreased pulmonary blood flow by creating either systemic pulmonary or cavopulmonary anastomoses and eventually performing the Fontan procedure. For those with increased pulmonary blood flow, effective intervention has been accomplished by banding the pulmonary artery to control pulmonary blood flow and then by proceeding to a modified Fontan procedure.

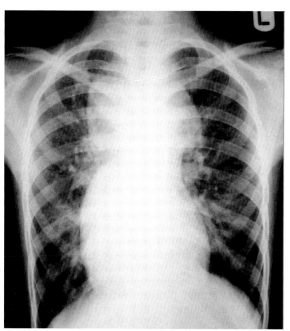

Image 12-21: Total anomalous pulmonary venous return

Truncus Arteriosus

Truncus arteriosus makes up ~ 1% of all congenital heart lesions. This abnormality occurs when a single arterial trunk comes off from the ventricular chambers. This vessel supplies the coronary, pulmonary, and systemic circulations proximal to the aortic arch. A truncal valve with 3, 4, or more leaflets is present, and this overrides a VSD. The pulmonary arteries come off as a single vessel or as 2 separate vessels from the back of the truncus. A large number of patients with truncus have an associated chromosomal abnormality—partial deletion of chromosome 22 (the "DiGeorge area" of chromosome 22). Uncommonly, they may also have an interrupted aortic arch.

Because the right and left ventricles eject blood at systemic pressure in the common arterial trunk, the coronary, pulmonary, and aortic circulations receive "mixed" venous and oxygenated blood at systemic pressures. Pulmonary blood flow is typically increased, so significant cyanosis is not common early on.

In the first weeks or months of life, the left-to-right shunt increases, and patients present with signs of congestive heart failure, dyspnea, wheezing, and FTT. Cyanosis is still not significant because pulmonary flow is often still relatively high. The heart is hyperdynamic, and the peripheral pulses are strong and bounding.

CXR in most will show cardiomegaly with increased pulmonary markings. You will see a right aortic arch in ~ 30–50%. ECG shows RV or combined ventricular hypertrophy. Echocardiogram is diagnostic.

Treatment may initially consist of medical management of HF, but surgery is necessary. Most infants will die between 3 and 12 months of age without surgery. Closing the VSD leaves the aorta coming off the left ventricle. Remove the pulmonary arteries from the truncus, and place a valved conduit from the right ventricular wall to the pulmonary arteries to form a new RV outflow tract. Generally, perform surgery at < 3 months of age. When outgrown, the valved conduit will need to be changed in childhood and again at a later age.

MALPOSITIONS

First, here's what is normal for the anatomy (when thoracic and abdominal structures are correctly placed), known as "situs solitus":

• Right lung with 3 lobes
• Left lung with 2 lobes
• Asymmetric tracheobronchial branching
• Liver with a major lobe on the right
• Left-sided stomach and spleen
• Right-sided venae cavae
• Morphologically distinct atria
• Normal, orderly arrangement of the GI tract

Now, for what's not normal …

Situs inversus: This is a "mirror-image" configuration of the asymmetric organs and includes the GI tract. Here, all of the asymmetric organs listed above are on the opposite side, so that you have a 3-lobed lung on the left side and the liver on the left. The atria are switched, but the apex may be either right or left. Interestingly, these children have no higher risk for cardiac anomalies than that of the general population. They do have a risk for dyskinetic cilia syndrome (about 25%).

Right atrial isomerism (also termed asplenia or Ivemark syndrome): This is bilateral "right-sidedness" with bilateral, 3-lobed lungs; a horizontal liver with equal-sized lobes; and bilateral morphologic right atria, each with a sinoatrial node. Usually, no spleen is present (asplenia). Bowel malrotations are common, as is complex congenital heart disease. These patients are at risk for infections like other asplenic patients.

Left atrial isomerism (polysplenia syndrome): This is bilateral "left-sidedness" involving the lungs and the atria. But there are commonly 2–30 equal-sized spleens (polysplenia) with a combined mass equal to that of a normal-sized spleen. This is not the same as "accessory" spleens, which are usually small, isolated spleens in addition to a normal spleen. These multiple spleens often function abnormally. Again, bowel malrotations are common, as is complex congenital heart disease.

Dextrocardia: If the heart is mainly in the right hemithorax, it is referred to as dextrocardia. The atrial situs can be solitus, inversus, or ambiguous (cardiosplenic). Complete "mirror-image" heart and abdomen (situs inversus totalis) makes up only 10–20% of dextrocardia.

VASCULAR RINGS AND SLINGS

Vascular rings/slings come from the abnormal persistence and/or dissolution of all, or some, of the paired embryonic aortic arches that connect the embryonic truncus arteriosus to the paired dorsal aortas. Some will produce no symptoms. Alternately, they may press on the esophagus or trachea and cause symptoms of dysphagia or breathing difficulties.

The most common aortic arch abnormality is an aberrant right subclavian artery arising from the descending aorta, but it rarely causes symptoms. The artery runs posterior to the esophagus and may indent it from the rear, but it usually does not cause any problems. (It is not even forming a real "ring" or "sling.")

Right aortic arch is very common in tetralogy of Fallot or truncus arteriosus; but, by itself, it rarely causes symptoms.

Double aortic arch (persistence of both right and left 4th embryonic arches) is the most common anomaly to cause symptoms. The anomaly results in encircling of the trachea and esophagus, resulting in tracheal compression and respiratory symptoms. The right and left arches indent the right and left sides of the trachea and

Quick **Quiz**

- What chromosomal anomalies do patients with truncus arteriosus have?
- Differentiate situs inversus from dextrocardia.
- What is the most common aortic arch abnormality? What symptoms does it usually cause?
- What is the most common aortic arch abnormality that causes significant symptoms?
- What congenital disorder is associated with aortic arch abnormalities?
- An athlete reports severe chest pain with exertion that is relieved with rest. He does not have HCM. What is the next most likely anomaly?

the esophagus. A CXR usually reveals a right aortic arch, and a barium swallow is diagnostic, revealing the esophageal compression. Look to see if the indentation or compression of the esophagus is anterior or posterior. Vascular rings will cause a posterior indentation, while a pulmonary sling will produce an anterior indentation. Open or thoracoscopic surgery can be curative, with division of the smaller, left posterior arch; this results in opening the constrictive ring.

The right aortic arch (especially if there is an aberrant left subclavian artery) can also be constricting, because of retroesophageal left-sided PDA or ligamentum arteriosum connecting to the left pulmonary artery (loose or incomplete ring). This combo makes indentations on the esophagus and trachea similar to the double arch.

Note: Look for complete or partial DiGeorge syndrome in infants with aortic arch abnormalities!

ANOMALOUS ORIGIN OF LEFT CORONARY ARTERY

With anomalous origin of the left coronary artery, the left coronary comes off the pulmonary artery, while the right continues to come off normally from the anterior aortic sinus. In the fetus, myocardial perfusion is normal. Soon after birth, however, the pulmonary artery pressure falls, and blood flows from the right coronary through collateral vessels into the left coronary, then back into the pulmonary artery. This circulation makes a small, left-to-right shunt, and the blood that should be going to the heart is diverted to the lungs. This results in ischemia of the anterolateral wall of the left ventricle.

Infants present at 2 weeks to 6 months of age with heart failure from MI or ischemia. Poor feeding, tachypnea, and respiratory symptoms are most common, although some will have episodes of restlessness/crying, as though in pain. Cardiomegaly is prominent. ECG will

show an anterolateral infarct pattern with abnormal Q waves in I, aVL, and the left anterior chest leads; additionally, ST and T wave changes are common. Echo may be diagnostic, but occasionally cardiac catheterization is required. Treatment requires reconnecting the aberrant coronary artery to the aorta.

Lastly, there is a condition that can occur wherein the left or right coronary artery arises from the opposite cusp. In either condition, the affected artery may pass between the aorta and the pulmonary artery. This results in pain, syncope, or sudden death if the artery becomes dilated and compresses the coronary artery. Consider anomalous left coronary artery from the opposite cusp as a possibility in an athlete who reports chest pain with exercise, or a sports event in which a young person "passes out" and dies. (HCM is most common, but coronary artery anomalies are the 2nd most frequent cause of sudden death among participating athletes.)

PULMONARY HYPERTENSION

Pulmonary hypertension has 2 etiologies. The most common etiology is increased pulmonary blood flow, as seen in large left-to-right shunts (e.g., VSD). (Think of a garden hose with very high flow through it.) Pulmonary hypertension can also occur as a result of an increase in pulmonary vascular resistance. (Think of the same garden hose but with a restriction or narrowing at the end of the hose.) This may be seen over time in large left-to-right shunts and is secondary to a decrease in the total cross-sectional area of the resistance vessels (either because of fewer vessels or a narrowing of normal vessels) and increased, abnormal muscle development in the small arterioles. Pulmonary hypertension from increased resistance may result from a variety of diseases—secondary to congenital heart defects with pulmonary overflow, cor pulmonale, recurrent pulmonary emboli, idiopathic/primary, or other disease states, such as SLE. Increased blood viscosity and polycythemia most often result from chronic hypoxia.

Clinically, pulmonary hypertension may present as a narrowly split or single 2nd heart sound with a loud, pulmonic component. A diastolic decrescendo murmur from pulmonary valvular regurgitation may be present. RV failure can occur. Syncope and chest pain are common only in later stages. If pulmonary hypertension is severe, sudden death can occur. CXR may show a large, proximal pulmonary artery. RA and RV hypertrophy may be apparent on the CXR and ECG.

Direct treatment toward correcting the underlying cause, if present. An example is chronic hypoxia due to persistent severe tonsillar enlargement. Once the obstruction is removed, the hypoxia resolves and the pulmonary hypertension slowly resolves. Vasodilators have a variable effect on pulmonary hypertension. Chronic IV prostacyclin (PGI$_2$) infusions may produce long-term reduction in pulmonary vascular resistance. Sildenafil citrate (Viagra®) and endothelial receptor antagonists (such as bosentan) are also used.

PERICARDIAL DISEASES

ACUTE PERICARDITIS

Acute pericarditis is an inflammation of the parietal pericardium and superficial myocardium that occurs with rapid onset. It presents with chest pain and sometimes fever. A pericardial friction rub, if present, is virtually pathognomonic. The rub is in phase with the heart sounds and usually has 3 components: atrial systole, ventricular systole, and ventricular relaxation. On an ECG, look for elevation of ST segments in most leads as the initial finding, followed by a return to normal of ST segments with T wave flattening and inversion.

Etiologies of pericarditis vary, but infections are common in children—especially viral infections (coxsackie A and B, echovirus, adenovirus). In certain areas of the U.S., histoplasmosis and coccidioidomycosis can cause pericarditis. Common childhood bacteria, such as staphylococci and pneumococci, also can be responsible. Tuberculosis is generally going to cause more of a chronic scenario. Drugs (phenytoin, hydralazine, and procainamide) have been implicated, as well as chest trauma/surgery.

Treatment includes nonsteroidal, antiinflammatory agents; occasionally, prednisone is required. If there is significant compression of the heart with tamponade, pericardiocentesis may be needed. Use antibiotics if the etiology is bacterial, and perform drainage for purulent effusions. For tuberculosis disease, some also recommend an early pericardiectomy because of the eventual high risk of constrictive pericarditis. Uremic pericarditis is treated by dialysis.

PERICARDIAL EFFUSION

Pericardial effusion (Image 12-22) can vary in character as serous, purulent, or bloody. It pushes the parietal pericardium away from the heart. Pericarditis can be associated with effusion. If the effusion is large, the

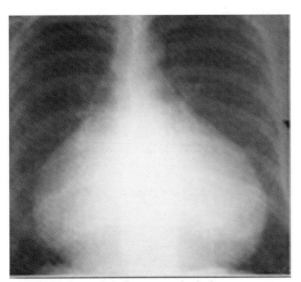

Image 12-22: Pericardial effusion; water bottle shape

heart sounds may sound muffled. Pericardial effusions have the same etiologies and treatments as mentioned above with pericarditis.

CARDIAC TAMPONADE

Cardiac tamponade is a life-threatening emergency. It can occur with just a little bit, or a large amount, of fluid present. The pericardium itself becomes "tense," causing the pressure in the pericardial cavity to increase, resulting in impaired filling and relaxation during the cardiac cycle. Ventricular end-diastolic, atrial, and venous pressures all rise on both sides of the heart by equal amounts.

Cardiac output falls with tachycardia, and hypotension occurs with a narrow pulse pressure.

Remember: Normally, with inspiration the pressure in the intrathoracic cavity drops and abdominal pressure increases, so that systemic venous return increases. With tamponade, however, the increase in venous return cannot be accommodated. This causes the jugular venous pressure to rise with inspiration, known as **Kussmaul sign**. (More commonly, it is seen in constrictive pericarditis.) Also remember: Normally with inspiration, aortic blood pressure can fall 4–10 mmHg. With tamponade, the aortic pressure will fall > 10–15 mmHg, resulting in pulsus paradoxus.

A clinical scenario may present a patient with rising jugular venous pressure (above), dropping systolic blood pressures, and quiet, muffled heart sounds. These 3 findings are known as **Beck's triad** and are associated with tamponade physiology.

Jugular venous distention with no collapse during diastole along with pulsus paradoxus is a strong clinical indicator that tamponade is occurring.

A classic question is to give you diastolic pressure readings in the heart that are all the same. This occurs in either tamponade or constrictive pericarditis. Kussmaul's is more commonly seen with constrictive pericarditis.

Treatment of tamponade is removal of the fluid via pericardiocentesis.

CONSTRICTIVE PERICARDITIS

This is uncommon in children, but if it occurs, it is most likely due to tuberculosis, previous bacterial pericarditis, or mediastinal radiation. Kussmaul sign occurs frequently, and pulsus paradoxus can also be present. End-diastolic pressures in all 4 chambers are equal. CT or MRI shows the thickened pericardium best; CXR also may show calcified pericardium. Treat by removing the restrictive fibrous tissue.

POSTPERICARDIOTOMY SYNDROME

Postpericardiotomy syndrome can follow any surgery in which the pericardium is disturbed or opened. This

Quick Quiz

- What does a pericardial friction rub almost always indicate?
- What are the classic ECG findings in acute pericarditis?
- Muffled heart sounds may be indicative of what disorder?
- What is Kussmaul sign?
- What is Beck's triad?
- During cardiac tamponade, what would you expect the end-diastolic pressures to be in the 4 chambers of the heart?
- In which pericardial diseases are you likely to see Kussmaul sign?
- Differentiate the effects of low-dose and high-dose dopamine.
- What does epinephrine do?

syndrome results from an immune-mediated inflammation occurring postoperatively. Most of the attacks occur within the first 1–4 weeks post-surgery, but they can occur as far out as 6 months. It presents as acute pericarditis, pericardial effusion, and fever. Pleural effusions also are common. ESR is increased. Patients who develop this have high titers of heat-reactive antibody, and ~ 75% have an acute rise of antibodies to adenoviruses, coxsackie B, or CMV.

Treat with aspirin 80–100 mg/kg/day. Once the acute attack is under control, gradually wean off the aspirin over 6 weeks. Recurrences occur in up to 10–15% of patients. Steroids are needed on occasion.

HEART FAILURE

TREATMENTS

Because heart failure (HF) is covered under the specific causes scattered throughout the text, we're not going to spend a lot of time discussing the specific etiologies. Realize that just about anything that disrupts myocardial function can cause HF. We will discuss the drugs in cardiac care because you may be asked about the pharmacologic effects of these agents. We'll break them down by class.

INOTROPIC AGENTS

Mechanism

Inotropic agents improve the contractility of the heart. The goal is to increase cardiac output and improve perfusion to vital organs and tissues.

Dopamine

Dopamine is used extensively to manage acute "low-output" states. It increases myocardial contractility by stimulating norepinephrine release from cardiac adrenergic receptor sites. It also dilates peripheral vascular beds where it acts on dopamine receptors. This occurs at low doses. At these lower doses, coronary and renal perfusions are enhanced. At higher doses, α-adrenoreceptor stimulation causes vasoconstriction, increased afterload, and a decrease in renal blood flow.

Dobutamine

Dobutamine is a synthetic analog of dopamine. Dobutamine has β_1-adrenergic effects that stimulate myocardial contractility. It is also a mild vasodilator. Dobutamine usually increases cardiac output without increasing heart rate or blood pressure.

Epinephrine

Epinephrine stimulates both α- and β-adrenoreceptors. It is commonly used postoperatively, when dopamine and dobutamine are ineffective. In low-output states, such as the post-op setting, it will dilate vasoconstricted beds and has potent, inotropic effects. At higher doses, it can cause systemic vasoconstriction.

Milrinone

This drug belongs to the class of nonglycoside, noncatecholamine drugs. It has both positive inotropic and vasodilator effects by inhibiting phosphodiesterase type III. It can be useful in those patients who become desensitized to dopamine and who have had repeated infusions, because these drugs act beyond the receptor site. It can also provide afterload reduction, in addition to inotropic support, in selected patients.

Digoxin (Digitalis Glycosides)

Digoxin works by inhibiting the sodium pump (Na^+-K^+ ATPase) at its receptor site; this causes intracellular sodium increases, which then causes increased intracellular calcium due to activation of the Na^+-Ca^{2+} exchange mechanism. Increases in intracellular calcium cause greater inotropic response. Another effect of digoxin is to inhibit sympathetic responses and increase parasympathetic tone, which thus decreases metabolic demands on the heart.

Monitoring of digoxin use has gotten away from looking at digoxin levels. Generally, look for clinical response and ECG changes that might indicate digoxin toxicity. Levels are more useful if you are concerned with drug interactions.

Know that digoxin levels are increased with quinidine, verapamil, amiodarone, beta-blockers, tetracycline, and erythromycin. Alternatively, digoxin levels can be decreased by rifampin, neomycin, and cholestyramine.

Acute digoxin toxicity typically presents with nausea, vomiting, and diarrhea. Be especially aware of color-vision changes, confusion, or vertigo. Palpitations and arrhythmias (AV block, SVT, or VT) are common also. If toxicity is severe, you may give digoxin antibodies (Fab fragments, Digibind®).

DIURETICS

Overview

Diuretics are the principal agents for control of pulmonary as well as systemic venous congestion. They increase sodium loss by increasing renal excretion of sodium and other ions by inhibiting tubular resorption of sodium at various sites in the nephron.

Loop Diuretics

These include furosemide and bumetanide. These inhibit the Na-K-Cl cotransporter in the ascending limb of the loop of Henle to block sodium and chloride resorption. Doing this causes sodium, potassium, hydrogen, and chloride ions to accumulate in the tubular lumen and then flush out in the urine. Side effects can include hypokalemia, hypochloremia, hyponatremia, and metabolic alkalosis. Loop diuretics also increase calcium excretion. Furosemide has been associated with nephrocalcinosis when used in the premature infant.

Agents that Affect the Cortical Diluting Segment

These diuretics are the thiazides and metolazone. They block sodium and chloride resorption in the cortical diluting segment of the renal tubule and the proximal portion of the distal convoluted tubule. Because of this action, more sodium reaches the distal tubules, where it can be exchanged with potassium. Metolazone is rarely used outside the hospital except for unusual cases, because it can cause a profound diuresis with volume depletion. Thiazides increase potassium loss and decrease calcium excretion.

Potassium-Sparing Diuretics

Spironolactone is the most commonly used potassium-sparing diuretic. It acts on the distal tubule at the site of aldosterone activity and inhibits sodium-potassium exchange. Spironolactone impairs both the resorption of sodium and the excretion of potassium and hydrogen ions, resulting in less potassium loss. It recently has been shown to be effective in reducing mortality in severe HF in adults. Monitor patients for hyperkalemia, especially if you are supplementing potassium or using an ACE inhibitor (see below). A much less common side effect (but shows up on exams!) is gynecomastia developing from the neurohormonal interactions.

Brain Natriuretic Peptide (BNP)

BNP is a hormone secreted by the heart to help regulate blood pressure. It and its prohormone (pro-BNP) are elevated in patients with HF, and the use of serum BNP or pro-BNP levels may be helpful as a screen. Elevated serum BNP levels indicate when dyspnea is due to pulmonary congestion caused by cardiac failure. They are not elevated with lung diseases.

VASODILATORS

Note

These agents are important in remodeling or manipulating ventricular load.

ACE Inhibitors

ACE inhibitors constrain the maladaptive neurohumoral forces initiated by the renin-angiotensin-aldosterone system. ACE inhibitors cause favorable ventricular remodeling and increase ventricular efficiency. They also decrease afterload. They are useful in patients with chronic, severe HF, as in dilated cardiomyopathies, in left-to-right shunts, and in other causes of HF. They are not useful in restrictive cardiomyopathies or in those with diastolic dysfunction. Side effects to look out for: hyperkalemia, elevated creatinine, and angioedema. You may see cough in adults, but this is less common in children.

Sodium Nitroprusside

This agent is used as an acute vasodilator when afterload reduction needs to occur quickly. It probably works by forming nitric oxide, which is a potent vasodilator. Cyanide toxicity is a concern if given for > 48 hours. If a patient is in the ICU with an unexplained metabolic acidosis, consider a cause to be prolonged use of sodium nitroprusside. Treatment options, after discontinuing the drug, would be sodium thiosulfate or hydroxocobalamin (vitamin B_{12}).

BETA-BLOCKERS

Beta-blockers for HF? This used to be a contraindication. Now we know that low doses of beta-blockers can be very helpful in those with dilated cardiomyopathy and chronic HF. It appears that they decrease deleterious sympathetic activity, with workload and ventricular relaxation both improving. Selective β_1-blockers, such as metoprolol succinate, have become the most commonly used in adults and are increasingly used in children. Another agent, carvedilol, has both β_1-blockade and vasodilator effects and is used commonly as well.

Quick Quiz

- How does acute digoxin toxicity present clinically?
- Which electrolytes may be depleted with loop diuretics?
- Which diuretic may actually increase serum potassium levels?
- What is the most common cause of syncope in children?
- If you suspect an arrhythmia as an etiology for syncope, what testing should you perform?
- What do you do if you suspect vasodepressor syncope?

SYNCOPE

Syncope is defined as a transient, complete loss of consciousness and postural tone. It is fairly common in childhood; ~ 20% will experience it at some point.

With syncope, the brain basically has an acute transient loss of cerebral perfusion. Lots of things can do this, and not all are cardiac in nature.

The most common cause in children is vasovagal, (a.k.a. vasodepressor, neurocardiogenic) syncope—the "simple fainting attack." It is most commonly seen in adolescents and can be triggered by injury, fear, pain, anger, disgust, or the sight of blood, among other things. The patient feels dizzy or weak but does not have true vertigo. Often, it is accompanied by a prodrome of nausea, blurred vision, and a "rushing of water–like" sound in the ears. BP falls and the patient becomes pale and clammy and has either tachycardia or, more commonly, can have profound bradycardia (cardioinhibitory) and loss of consciousness. Injury is rare because, usually, the patient can tell it is coming. Lying down alleviates the symptoms. Orthostatic hypotension is also quite common, typically occurring with prolonged standing in a warm environment or on quickly arising from a supine to standing position. It is more likely in those with volume depletion, impaired autonomic nervous systems, and with certain drugs (vasodilators, antiarrhythmics, antidepressants, cocaine, or alcohol). Postural orthostatic tachycardia syndrome (POTS) is a related disorder in which tachycardia is the dominant finding.

Cardiac etiologies are less common and include obstructive heart lesions (severe aortic or pulmonic stenosis, HCM, tetralogy of Fallot, abnormal coronary arteries) and arrhythmias (SVT, VT, sinus node dysfunction, AV block, long QT syndrome).

Vasovagal syncope can occur when a susceptible patient swallows cold food/liquid, has sudden decompression of a full bladder, or brushes their hair. These quickly result in severe bradycardia.

The nonvascular etiologies include atypical seizures, migraines, hyperventilation, cough syncope, hysterical syncope, and sudden rises in intracranial pressure. Breath-holding spells do not usually present as simple syncope.

Diagnose by using the history and physical examination to get to the underlying cause. If there are no findings of heart disease or gross autonomic dysfunction, simple vasovagal or vasodepressor syncope is most likely. If you suspect arrhythmia, order a 24-hour Holter and ECG. Echocardiography is of little benefit unless you suspect a cardiac abnormality.

In the past, to confirm vasovagal syncope, the tilt-table test was often ordered; today, it is rarely needed except in cases where the diagnosis is unclear by simple history and physical examination or the patient is not responding to medical therapy. Increasing fluid and salt intake treats vasodepressor syncope. Discourage caffeine. Beta-blockers may (or may not) be helpful. Fludrocortisone, a mineralocorticoid, and α-agonists, such as midodrine, have been used successfully.

CHEST PAIN

ACUTE vs. CHRONIC

The patient's complaint of "my chest hurts" is very common in children. Adult chest pain immediately makes one think of cardiac etiologies. With children, this frequently becomes the greatest concern to the parent (and/or child) as well. It is best to think of chest pain in 2 categories—the "acute-onset, severe" and the "chronic and recurrent." Using this as a guide, you can usually sort things out fairly quickly.

ACUTE-ONSET, SEVERE CHEST PAIN

Presentation

These kids come in looking upset and distressed. They have that "I'm going to die" look on their face. They more likely show up in emergency departments or acute care settings. Generally, they are having the chest pain when you see them. Focus on the pain and associated symptoms and determine if there are any predisposing medical conditions. Remember: Chest pain in children is most likely noncardiac!

Pericarditis

Pericarditis is described as severe, substernal chest pain that is squeezing or tightening in character. This aspect resembles angina. The pain, however, is worse with movement, and even breathing exacerbates it. Usually, the patient prefers to lean forward and does not want to lie down. Typically, there is a pericardial friction rub. Pericarditis is the most common cause of cardiac chest pain in children. For more, see the pericarditis discussion on page 12-32.

Angina / MI

This is the most feared, right? But it is very, very rare in children. Pain is severe, pressure-like, and substernal. It can radiate to the neck or arms. Usually, it is exertional in character and relieved with rest. Look for signs of ischemia on the ECG: ST-segment elevation and T wave changes in the area of affected myocardium and reciprocal ST-segment depression in the corresponding "opposite" leads. Look for cocaine/crack use in the adolescent or a history of Kawasaki disease. If coronary ischemia is suspected, use of troponin and CK isoenzymes may be helpful.

Arrhythmia

SVT is the most likely cause of acute chest pain if an arrhythmia is the etiology. Myocardial ischemia can occur with very fast rates and be similar to angina in character. Syncope or lightheadedness is common. The pain should go away as quickly as the arrhythmia resolves. Perform an ECG when the chest pain is occurring, or document very fast heart rates for diagnosis.

Aortic Dissection

The pain in aortic dissection is described as sharp and "tearing." Look for history or findings of Marfan or Ehlers-Danlos syndromes. Also look for it in any child with severe chest pain after trauma or hemopericardium. Quick surgical intervention is mandatory. Diagnose with an MRI, CT, or transesophageal echo.

Noncardiac Causes

Spontaneous pneumothorax causes severe, unilateral chest pain that is accompanied by dyspnea. Findings on physical exam are typically diagnostic, with unilateral or absent breath sounds on the affected side. A history of asthma, CF, Marfan syndrome, or trauma increases the likelihood. In adolescents with HIV risk factors, also think of *Pneumocystis* as an etiology. Viruses can also be responsible and produce mini-epidemics in community settings.

Gastroesophageal reflux (GE reflux) can produce symptoms that mimic angina. Usually, there is a strong relationship to meals and aggravation with lying supine. Esophageal spasm or foreign body can also cause chest pain.

Irritation of the diaphragm can radiate to the shoulder and lower chest. Lower lobe pneumonia can cause this. Hepatic and splenic abscesses can present with chest pain. Pancreatitis can also present this way, though more rarely.

CHRONIC AND RECURRENT CHEST PAIN

Note

Typically, these children do not have the pain when you see them in the office setting. Examination is usually normal.

Musculoskeletal Chest Wall Pain

This is the most common cause of identifiable chest pain in children. The pain is usually very localized and does not radiate. It is sometimes reproducible with chest wall palpation. The pain frequently becomes exacerbated with exercise, raising the anxiety level about cardiac pain. Athletes frequently have localized pain from working out/exercising. Treatment is reassurance for most and mild analgesics (acetaminophen or nonsteroidal antiinflammatory drug).

Costochondritis is pain and tenderness of the anterior chest at the costochondral or costosternal articulations. No swelling is noted. The pain can be mild or severe and is almost always unilateral. Most commonly, it occurs at the left 4th–6th costochondral junctions. It can follow a viral illness or exercise. It is always reproducible with palpation over the area and commonly resolves in a week or less. Treatment with NSAIDs can be helpful.

Tietze syndrome is pain and swelling of the anterior chest wall, normally involving the 2nd or 3rd costochondral junction on one side. Pain and swelling come and go and can last months to years. Look for varicella zoster in particular!

Precordial catch is the sudden onset of severe, sharp, or shooting chest pain that is localized at the cardiac apex area. Many cardiologists feel it is one of the most common etiologies for chest pain. It lasts 30 seconds to a few minutes and then resolves. It typically occurs at rest and can recur several times a day. It is worse with deep inspiration. Its etiology is unknown.

Slipping rib syndrome occurs in the 8th, 9th, or 10th ribs at the anterior tip of each. These ribs do not attach to the sternum directly, but are attached by fibrous tissue. A lower rib can move up and override the upper rib, resulting in severe pain that may last for hours or days.

Lung Etiologies

Exercise-induced asthma is a common cause of chest pain in children. Children complain of deep, substernal chest pain and "tightness" that worsens 5–10 minutes into recovery, then lessens over the next 30 minutes or so. Children with chronic asthma are also at risk.

The "stitch" has become more common. Pain is felt in the right upper quadrant of the abdomen and right costal margin, with occasional radiation to the right shoulder. The pain is sharp with a cramp-like sensation. It occurs while running or walking and is relieved by rest.

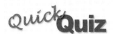

- What illicit drug is associated with acute MI in adolescents?

- An adolescent with Marfan syndrome presents with acute chest pain that is "tearing" and radiating to his back. What should you immediately be concerned about?

- What type of chest pain occurs over the rib/cartilage junction and is always reproducible with palpation over the area?

GI Causes of Chronic Chest Pain

GE reflux with esophagitis is seen more commonly today. The pain is retrosternal in nature and worsens with meals and lying down. Manometry and esophagoscopy are diagnostic. Most attempt a trial of antacids, histamine blockers, or proton pump inhibitors before proceeding with diagnostic testing because symptoms are fairly classic. Esophageal spasm, achalasia, and foreign body are less common in children.

Heart

Cardiac causes of chronic, recurring chest pain are uncommon. Ischemic pain is rare, but may result from known cardiomyopathy, obstruction (AS), or coronary disease. The most common coronary artery anomaly in children is anomalous origin of the left coronary artery; as discussed previously, this usually presents in infancy. Kawasaki disease is the most common acquired coronary disease, with resultant coronary aneurysms and/or stenosis.

Whether mitral valve prolapse (MVP) results in chest pain in children is controversial. Controlled studies do not indicate a correlation between MVP and chest pain in pediatric patients.

Psychogenic Etiologies

Depending on the cardiologist you talk to, psychogenic factors are probably responsible for at least some chronic chest pain in children and adolescents. Usually, a history of a particular, specific situation or stressful event can be associated with the onset of pain in these settings; e.g., death of parent, divorce, school failure, family member diagnosed with coronary artery disease, or abuse. Pain is generally vague and difficult to localize or describe. Tenderness may be found on palpation in unusual locations.

CARDIOVASCULAR PREPARTICIPATION SPORTS SCREENING

Sudden death in the young athlete is a rare but devastating event. Most recent estimates are that the incidence of sudden death in young athletes is approximately 100 cases per year.

Know that the most common cardiac cause of sudden death in the young athlete in the U.S. is hypertrophic cardiomyopathy. Other important causes include: coronary artery anomalies, *commotio cordis* (a blow to the chest resulting in V-fib), aortic rupture (Marfan syndrome), and "other" (long QT, WPW, aortic stenosis).

Strategies to reduce sudden death in high school and college athletes are geared toward identifying high-risk athletes, treating underlying conditions that can predispose them to sudden death, and/or excluding the athlete from participation in athletics, when appropriate.

There has been much debate on how best to identify at-risk athletes. Know that in the U.S., routine ECG or echo screening of all high school and college athletes is not recommended. Rather, the American Academy of Pediatrics and others recommend a screening approach to identify high-risk athletes. This includes a targeted history and cardiovascular-focused examination.

All athletes should be screened before participation in high school or college sports. Look for exertional syncope, near syncope, chest pain, excessive fatigue, or shortness of breath in the history. Also obtain a family history looking for premature death or disability from heart disease in young relatives (< 50 years of age), and, of course, a family history of Marfan's, hypertrophic cardiomyopathy, long QT.

On physical examination, look for stigmata of Marfan's, elevated blood pressure and absent or diminished femoral pulses, and pathologic murmurs. If any of the above is positive, refer to a pediatric cardiologist for further evaluation!

PREVENTIVE CARDIOLOGY

It is well established that adult cardiovascular disease (coronary artery disease, hypertension, stroke) has its origins many decades before the disease manifests in adulthood. Thus, landmark studies such as the Bogalusa Heart Study, the Muscatine Study, and others have documented that risk factors for adult heart disease can be identified in childhood (such as hyperlipidemia, hypertension, and obesity), that these risk factors "track" into adulthood, and that they are associated with an elevated risk for adult cardiovascular disease. Furthermore, autopsy studies have documented fatty streaks and even raised fatty lesions in the aorta of children, adolescents, and young adults. The extent of these fatty streaks and raised lesions correlates with risk factors, such as serum cholesterol and LDL (low-density lipoprotein—the "bad" cholesterol).

There is no question that promoting healthy lifestyles in all children is a very important strategy to reduce the burden of cardiovascular disease later in life. These strategies include proper diet (reduced saturated fats), regular exercise, and tobacco avoidance. In addition, identification of at-risk children and screening them for hyperlipidemia is recommended to supplement the overall healthy lifestyles strategy.

Know that for many years in the U.S., we have used a targeted screening method to identify hyperlipidemia in childhood—i.e., not all children required blood testing. Specifically, it was recommended that a fasting lipid profile be obtained in children in whom there is a family history of:

• Myocardial infarction
• Stroke
• Peripheral vascular disease
• Sudden cardiac death in a parent or grandparent < 55 years of age (or even the identification of coronary artery disease by diagnostic testing, such as a cardiac catheterization)
• A parent with a total cholesterol of > 240 mg/dL or a known history of familial hypercholesterolemia
    or
• If the family history is not known
• If there are other risk factors present, such as obesity or smoking

Recommendations vary and some say that lipid screening of such at-risk children should occur as early as 2 years of age—but all agree that certainly before 10 years of age. Note: Recent guidelines now recommend lipid profile screening of all children (even low-risk children) between 9 and 11 years of age.

If the lipid profile is normal, repeat in 3–5 years. For children found to have elevated triglycerides or low HDL (high-density lipoprotein—the "good" cholesterol), weight management should be the treatment of choice (nutritional intervention and increased physical activity).

For children with elevated LDL levels, intensive nutritional counseling should be provided. For those children > 8 years of age with LDL > 190 mg/dL (or > 160 mg/dL if there is a family history of early cardiovascular disease or 2 additional risk factors, or > 130 mg/dL if diabetic), drug therapy should be considered if lifestyle interventions alone fail to lower lipid levels.

Statins are increasingly recognized as the drugs of choice, particularly in children > 10 years of age. Needless to say, these children require expert monitoring.

ANTIBIOTIC PROPHYLAXIS FOR SBE

Antibiotic prophylaxis recommendations have changed quite a bit! In 2007, new guidelines came out, and now very few conditions require prophylaxis!

Give subacute bacterial endocarditis (SBE) prophylaxis for dental procedures, respiratory procedures, or infected skin procedures only in the presence of:

• Prosthetic cardiac valve
• Previous history of endocarditis
• Congenital heart disease in certain instances
• Unrepaired cyanotic heart disease
• Completely repaired congenital heart disease with prosthetic material or device for 6 months post-procedure
• Cardiac transplant recipients who develop cardiac valvulopathy

Other key points:

• Antibiotic prophylaxis is no longer recommended for any other form of congenital heart disease (other than those listed above).
• No antibiotic prophylaxis for GU or GI procedures!

[Know:] Table 12-3. If the patient is already on chronic amoxicillin/penicillin, the prophylaxis antibiotic should be of a different class.

Table 12-3: Prophylactic Regimens — Dental, Oral, and Respiratory Procedures		
Situation	**Antibiotic**	**Regimen (no post-procedure doses!)**
Standard general prophylaxis	Amoxicillin	50 mg/kg orally 1 hour before procedure (max 2 g)
Unable to take oral medications	Ampicillin	50 mg/kg IM/IV within 30 mins before procedure (max 2 g)
Allergic to penicillin	Clindamycin or Cephalexin or cefadroxil* or Azithromycin or clarithromycin	20 mg/kg orally 1 hour before procedure (max 600 mg) 50 mg/kg orally 1 hour before procedure (max 2 g) 15 mg/kg orally 1 hour before procedure (max 500 mg)
Both allergic to penicillin and unable to take oral meds	Clindamycin or Cefazolin**	20 mg/kg IV within 30 mins before procedure (max 600 mg) 25 mg/kg IM/IV within 30 mins before procedure (max 1 g)

*Note: Cephalosporins should not be used if the PCN allergy is an immediate-type hypersensitivity reaction.
**Note: The oral doses are given 1 hour before the procedure, whereas the IM/IV doses are given within 30 min.

Quick Quiz

- With which family history risk factors is it recommended that a fasting lipid profile be obtained at an early age in children?
- By what age should lipid screening for all children occur? If the lipid profile is normal, how often should it be repeated?
- What are the only instances in which antibiotics are recommended to prevent endocarditis?
- Know Table 12-3.
- Which heart valves are most commonly affected in rheumatic fever?
- List the major and minor Jones criteria for rheumatic fever.
- Describe the arthritis of rheumatic fever.
- Which 2 murmurs are most common in acute rheumatic fever?
- Describe chorea seen in rheumatic fever.

RHEUMATIC FEVER

CAUSES / SIGNS & SYMPTOMS

Rheumatic fever (RF) is a disease that follows infection with pharyngeal strains of group A streptococci (*Streptococcus pyogenes*). It occurs most commonly in children 5–15 years of age. Those with a previous history of RF have the highest risk of recurrence.

Aschoff bodies are pathognomonic for rheumatic fever. Histopathology shows palisading giant cells and swelling and fragmentation of collagen. RF affects the mitral and aortic valves most commonly. Joints develop reversible swelling with fluid accumulation of synovial membranes and in the joint space proper. Subcutaneous nodules are similar to Aschoff bodies and are granulomas with localized collagen infiltration.

There are 5 major manifestations of rheumatic fever known as the Jones criteria:

1) Polyarthritis (migratory)   4) Subcutaneous nodules
2) Carditis   5) Erythema marginatum
3) Chorea

There are also 5 minor manifestations:

1) Arthralgia   4) Fever
2) Increased ESR   5) Increased C-reactive protein
3) Prolonged PR interval

To make the diagnosis, you must have evidence of a recent or concurrent *Streptococcus pyogenes* infection and have either 2 major manifestations or 1 major and 2 minor manifestations.

MANIFESTATIONS

Arthritis

The RF arthritis is traditionally an acute, migratory polyarthritis with fever. The joints are red, hot, swollen, and very tender. It is painful to move them. Larger joints are more commonly affected. Typically, as pain and swelling subside in 1 joint, another will become painful and swell. The arthritis usually lasts < 1 month and is very effectively treated with aspirin. There is no permanent joint damage.

Carditis

Some patients with carditis are asymptomatic. The disease can affect the valves (endocardium), myocardium, or pericardium. Murmurs are the most common findings on examination. Most common is an apical pansystolic murmur of mitral regurgitation. Some patients with moderate-to-severe rheumatic mitral regurgitation have a soft, mid-diastolic murmur heard only at the apex. This is known as the Carey Coombs murmur. Aortic regurgitation is the 2nd most common murmur heard. If there is a mid-diastolic apical murmur with aortic insufficiency, it is called an Austin Flint murmur, which is due to impingement of the mitral valve opening by the jet of aortic insufficiency.

Myocarditis can manifest as tachycardia with cardiomegaly or arrhythmias. Prolongation of the PR interval occurs in 20% of cases, but it is too nonspecific to make the diagnosis of carditis itself.

Pericarditis can occur and has the classic symptoms of pericardial pain, friction rub, or marked increase in heart size, but most patients with rheumatic pericarditis are asymptomatic. Pericarditis rarely occurs without pancarditis (valvular and myocardial involvement, in addition to pericardial involvement).

Chorea

Chorea, formerly known as "Sydenham chorea," is characterized by sudden, aimless, irregular movements of the extremities associated with emotional instability and weakness. Some liken it to "a break dancer gone crazy." Since the symptoms typically do not occur with sleep, some children are viewed as "faking it." Chorea generally occurs by itself without any other major symptoms (though 18% do have associated heart disease!), and it may develop months after the inciting infection.

Subcutaneous Nodules

These are small (0.5- to 1-cm), painless swellings occurring over body prominences—usually over the extensor tendons of the hands, feet, elbows, scalp, scapulae, and vertebrae. They occur in crops and can last for months. These are rarely seen.

Erythema Marginatum

This is the least common major condition and occurs in only ~ 5–10% of patients. The rash is an evanescent, pink-to-red macule, often with a clear area in the center and a snake-like serpiginous course. The rash is short-lived, migratory, and does not itch. It blanches with pressure and is typically located on the trunk or proximal arms and legs. This rash is quite rare now.

PROOF OF GROUP A *STREPTOCOCCUS*

The ability to prove causality is important. Sometimes, though, rapid throat tests or cultures are either not done before antibiotics are given or are negative. Also, many children are carriers for group A *Streptococcus* and not necessarily infected with the organism. As such, the most specific and reliable proof of previous streptococcal infection is found in serum antibody levels. Consistently rising values are more significant than an isolated elevated value. The most widely used test is the antibody formation against streptolysin O (AS or ASO titer). In children, a titer > 333 U is considered elevated. Other tests available include antideoxyribonuclease B (anti-DNase B), antihyaluronidase, antistreptokinase, and antinicotinamide adenine dinucleotidase (anti-NADase). A 2-fold rise in titer to 1 or more of these is commonly confirmatory.

The bottom line is that you must have 1 of these:

1) Positive throat culture for group A beta-hemolytic streptococci or positive rapid streptococcal antigen test or
2) Elevated or rising streptococcal antibody titer

TREATMENT

In acute rheumatic fever, always give penicillin, even if cultures are negative for group A *Streptococcus*. Administer either oral or intramuscular penicillin therapy upon diagnosis of acute rheumatic fever regardless of culture results. Dosing for intramuscular injection is 600,000 units penicillin G benzathine for those < 27 kg (60 pounds) and 1.2 million units penicillin G benzathine for those ≥ 27 kg. Mixed dosing of procaine penicillin with benzathine penicillin is not recommended for adolescents and adult-sized patients because this does not administer the full benzathine dose and has not been shown to be equally effective. Intramuscular penicillin avoids the problem of compliance issues. Oral dosing consists of penicillin V 250 mg 2–3 times daily for 10 days for those < 27 kg and 500 mg 2–3 times daily for 10 days in those ≥ 27 kg. Give erythromycin orally x 10 days to the PCN-allergic child. Begin prophylaxis immediately after acute therapy to prevent future recurrences of rheumatic fever (see below in Prognosis).

Use salicylates and steroids to control acute symptoms. Aspirin is generally given in a dose of 80–100 mg/kg/day for a minimum of 6 weeks, with gradual tapering over 2–4 weeks. If HF develops, give patients prednisone 2 mg/kg/day. Chorea does not respond to these therapies, though other agents, such as haloperidol or benzodiazepines, can be helpful.

PROGNOSIS

Around 75% of children with acute rheumatic fever are well after 6 weeks. Beyond 6 months, < 5% are still symptomatic, typically with chorea or carditis. Most children with carditis recover without sequelae, except for those with HF and pericarditis, a majority of whom develop permanent cardiac damage. The most likely chronic, residual lesions in childhood are mitral insufficiency and aortic insufficiency. After childhood, the most likely chronic, residual lesion is mitral stenosis. Those with recurrent disease tend to have the same manifestations during recurrences.

Most recommend continuing prophylaxis for a minimum of 5 years, or until the age of 21, whichever is longer. Those with heart disease usually receive longer-duration prophylaxis well into adulthood, especially if they work around children. Give 1.2 million U of benzathine PCN every 4 weeks or 250 mg of PCN V-K orally twice daily. You can give sulfadiazine or sulfisoxazole 0.5 g orally on a daily basis for those weighing ≤ 27 kg; increase to 1 g orally and daily for those > 27 kg. (Remember: This is for prophylaxis only, not treatment.) You may give erythromycin 250 mg twice a day for those allergic to PCN and sulfa drugs.

KAWASAKI DISEASE

Kawasaki disease is an acute inflammatory vasculitis of unknown etiology. It probably represents an autoimmune inflammatory response to an as yet undefined infection. 85% of cases occur between 6 months and 5 years of age, and it is most common in the Asian population.

The diagnosis of Kawasaki disease is made clinically with fever for 5 days or more and 4 of the following 5 criteria:

1) Conjunctival injection without drainage
2) Cervical lymphadenopathy (unilateral > 1.5 cm)
3) Extremity changes with erythema and edema of the hands and feet and later desquamation
4) Mucous membrane changes with erythema, cracked and peeling lips, and strawberry tongue
5) Polymorphous exanthem—usually macular or maculopapular erythematous, but any rash except vesicles and bullae

Atypical Kawasaki's can be seen with < 4 criteria but with typical coronary findings.

Adjunctive laboratory findings include leukocytosis, elevated ESR and CRP, thrombocytosis often with very high platelet counts, elevated liver enzymes, sterile pyuria, aseptic meningitis, hydrops of the gallbladder, and lipid abnormalities.

Quick Quiz

- A child with rheumatic fever presents and is found to be culture-negative for *S. pyogenes*. Should he receive penicillin therapy?

- What cardiac residual lesions are most likely to occur after rheumatic fever in childhood? Which persists more often in adulthood?

- What drugs are used for monthly prophylaxis after acute rheumatic fever? What if the child is penicillin-allergic?

- What is the pathognomonic finding of Kawasaki disease?

The patients develop carditis and may have myocarditis, pericarditis, or valvulitis, but the pathognomonic finding is coronary artery aneurysms that develop in 20–25% of inadequately treated cases. These may be bilateral and have a predilection for the proximal vessels. They may be saccular, ectasia, or transient dilation. If > 8 mm in diameter, they are "giant" aneurysms and a much greater risk for complications. Aneurysms can occur in other arteries about 1% of the time. About 50% of the aneurysms will "resolve" in time to normal appearing coronaries. Long term, they (particularly giant aneurysms) can develop thrombosis, stenosis, and ischemia. This can lead to myocardial ischemia and infarction or death in less than 1% of cases.

Treatment is primarily with IVIG infusion of 2 g/kg over 12 hours. This improves the fever, inflammatory response, and clinical picture, but it mainly decreases the risk of coronary aneurysms to 5–8%. About 7–8% of children will get a 2nd dose of IVIG for persisting fever and inflammation. If still not responding, IV steroids or other antiinflammatory agents are an option. Give aspirin at antiinflammatory doses (80–100 mg/kg/day) initially and later decrease to antiplatelet doses (2–5 mg/kg/day) when the fever resolves. If there are no aneurysms by 6–8 weeks, then the aspirin can be discontinued.

The primary diagnostic modality for evaluating the coronary arteries is echocardiography. This is done initially with the diagnosis, or suspected diagnosis, and then followed at 2–8 weeks to look for aneurysms that mostly develop in the subacute phase. Catheterization is reserved for patients with complex or giant aneurysms or evidence of coronary insufficiency.

The long-term care and follow-up depend on the degree of coronary artery involvement. Those patients with persisting aneurysms are maintained on ASA (or warfarin with giant aneurysms) and followed regularly by cardiology with echocardiography and later stress testing when old enough.

HEART CATHETERIZATION

A classic exam question presents oxygen saturations from cardiac catheterizations and asks you to interpret them. So let's review these briefly, as well as possible questions.

Normally, there are no intracardiac shunts; therefore, saturations in the right and left heart remain constant as venous (pulmonary and systemic) return flows through the heart and out the great arteries. Normal mixed venous saturation is 75% (70–80%) in the superior vena cava, and this remains constant through the right atrium → right ventricle → pulmonary arteries. Venous blood is then oxygenated and returns to the pulmonary veins with a normal saturation of 95–100%. Again, in the absence of shunting, this should remain fairly constant to the left atrium → left ventricle → aorta (Figure 12-3 on page 12-42).

In the presence of a left-to-right shunt, there will be a "step up" in the right heart saturation at the level of the shunt and then beyond (Figure 12-4 on page 12-42). For example, in the presence of a VSD the left ventricular saturation would be normal (95–100%) while the right ventricular saturation would now be increased to 90% because of the flow of oxygenated blood to the right ventricle via the shunt. Structures beyond this "step up" would also retain elevated saturations; therefore, in our example of a VSD, you would also expect the pulmonary artery saturation to be high. So remember: In a left-to-right shunt, the left heart saturations will be normal, and the right heart saturations will be increased initially at the site of the shunt.

The opposite is true for right-to-left shunts. Here, the right heart saturations will remain in the normal range, and the left heart saturations will be decreased at the site of the shunt. For example, if you have a VSD and a right-to-left shunt, you would expect the normal right ventricular saturation, 75%; but now, with decreased left ventricle saturation, it is 85%. Don't forget that the distal structures, such as the aorta in our example, will also be desaturated.

To help you, there are a few figures on page 12-42 showing examples in the format that could be presented on an exam, including PDA (Figure 12-5), ASD (Figure 12-6), and partial anomalous venous return (Figure 12-7).

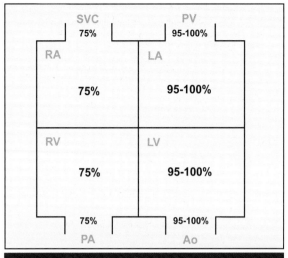

Figure 12-3: Normal Saturations

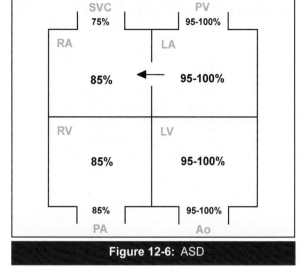

Figure 12-6: ASD

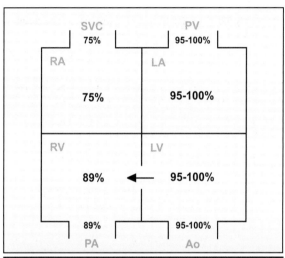

Figure 12-4: Left-to-Right Shunt

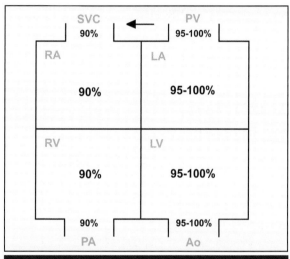

Figure 12-7: Partial Anomalous Venous Return

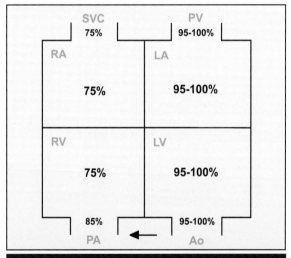

Figure 12-5: PDA

FOR FURTHER READING

[Guidelines in blue]

THE 15-LEAD ECG

O'Connor M, et al. The pediatric electrocardiogram part I: age-related interpretation. *Am J Emerg Med.* 2008 May;26(4):506–512.

O'Connor M, et al. The pediatric electrocardiogram part II: dysrhythmias. *Am J Emerg Med.* 2008 Mar;26(3):348–358.

O'Connor M, et al. The pediatric electrocardiogram part III: congenital heart disease and other cardiac syndromes. *Am J Emerg Med.* 2008 May;26(4):497–503.

RATES AND INTERVALS

Ray WA, et al. Azithromycin and the risk of cardiovascular death. *N Engl J Med.* 2012;366:1881–1890.

VENTRICULAR HYPERTROPHY

Harrigan RA, Jones K. ABC of clinical electrocardiography. Conditions affecting the right side of the heart. *BMJ.* 2002 May 18;324(7347):1201–1204.

Rijnbeek PR, et al. Electrocardiographic criteria for left ventricular hypertrophy in children. *Pediatr Cardiol.* 2008 Sep;29(5):923–928.

VENTRICULAR ARRYTHMIAS

Berul CI, et al. Indications and techniques of pediatric cardiac pacing. *Expert Rev Cardiovasc Ther.* 2003 Jul;1(2):165–176.

Sliz NB Jr, Johns JA. Cardiac pacing in infants and children. *Cardiol Rev.* 2000 Jul-Aug;8(4):223–239.

CONGENITAL HEART DISEASE

Dolbec K, Mick NW. Congenital heart disease. *Emerg Med Clin North Am.* 2011 Nov;29(4):811–827, vii.

Saenz RB, et al. Caring for infants with congenital heart disease and their families. *Am Fam Physician.* 1999 Apr 1;59(7):1857–1868.

Silberbach M, Hannon D. Presentation of congenital heart disease in the neonate and young infant. *Pediatr Rev.* 2007 Apr;28(4):123–131.

OBSTRUCTIVE LESIONS

Matsui H, et al. Anatomy of coarctation, hypoplastic and interrupted aortic arch: relevance to interventional/surgical treatment. *Expert Rev Cardiovasc Ther.* 2007 Sep;5(5):871–880.

HEART FAILURE

Hsu DT, Pearson GD. Heart failure in children: part I: history, etiology, and pathophysiology. *Circ Heart Fail.* 2009 Jan;2(1):63–70.

Hsu DT, Pearson GD. Heart failure in children: part II: diagnosis, treatment, and future directions. *Circ Heart Fail.* 2009 Sep;2(5):490–498.

Rossano JW, Shaddy RE. Update on pharmacological heart failure therapies in children: do adult medications work in children and if not, why not? *Circulation.* 2014 Feb 4;129(5):607–612.

O'Connor CM, et al. Effect of nesiritide in patients with acute decompensated heart failure. *NEJM.* 2011;365:32–43.

Topol EJ. The lost decade of nesiritide. *NEJM.* 2011;365:81–82.

CHEST PAIN

Cico SJ, et al. Miscellaneous causes of pediatric chest pain. *Pediatr Clin North Am.* 2010 Dec;57(6):1397–1406.

Ives A, et al. Recurrent chest pain in the well child. *Arch Dis Child.* 2010 Aug;95(8):649–654.

Jindal A, Singhi S. Acute chest pain. *Indian J Pediatr.* 2011 Oct;78(10):1262–1267.

McDonnell CJ, White KS. Assessment and treatment of psychological factors in pediatric chest pain. *Pediatr Clin North Am.* 2010 Dec;57(6):1235–1260.

Reddy SR, Singh HR. Chest pain in children and adolescents. *Pediatr Rev.* 2010 Jan;31(1):e1–e9.

Selbst SM. Approach to the child with chest pain. *Pediatr Clin North Am.* 2010 Dec;57(6):1221–1234.

Son MB, Sundel RP. Musculoskeletal causes of pediatric chest pain. *Pediatr Clin North Am.* 2010 Dec;57(6):1385–1395.

Yokitis J, Repeta R. Acute chest pain in an adolescent. *Am Fam Physician.* 2006 Aug 1;74(3):473–474.

CARDIOVASCULAR PREPARTICIPATION SPORTS SCREENING

Schoenbaum M, et al. Economic evaluation of strategies to reduce sudden cardiac death in young athletes. *Pediatrics.* 2012 Aug;130(2):e380–e389.

American Academy of Pediatrics. Section on Cardiology and Cardiac Surgery. Pediatric sudden cardiac arrest. *Pediatrics.* 2012 Apr;129(4):e1094–e1102.

Maron BJ, et al. Recommendations and considerations related to preparticipation screening for cardiovascular abnormalities in competitive athletes: 2007 update: a scientific statement from the American Heart Association Council on Nutrition, Physical Activity, and Metabolism: endorsed by the American College of Cardiology Foundation. *Circulation.* 2007 Mar 27;115(12):1643–1655.

PREVENTIVE CARDIOLOGY

American Academy of Pediatrics. Expert Panel on Integrated Guidelines for Cardiovascular Health and Risk Reduction in Children and Adolescents; National Heart, Lung, and Blood Institute. Expert panel on integrated guidelines for cardiovascular health and risk reduction in children and adolescents: summary report. *Pediatrics.* 2011 Dec;128 Suppl 5:S213–S256.

CARDIOLOGY

ANTIBIOTIC PROPHYLAXIS FOR SBE

Wilson W, et al. Prevention of infective endocarditis: guidelines from the American Heart Association: a guideline from the American Heart Association Rheumatic Fever, Endocarditis, and Kawasaki Disease Committee, Council on Cardiovascular Disease in the Young, and the Council on Clinical Cardiology, Council on Cardiovascular Surgery and Anesthesia, and the Quality of Care and Outcomes Research Interdisciplinary Working Group. *Circulation*. 2007 Oct 9; 116(15):1736–1754. Erratum in: *Circulation*. 2007 Oct 9; 116(15):e376–e377.

MedStudy®

Pediatrics Review
Core Curriculum

Seventh Edition 2016–2017

7

RESPIRATORY DISORDERS

Section Editor:

Kimberly Jones, MD
Associate Professor, Pediatrics/Medicine
Chief, Pediatrics Pulmonary
LSU Health Sciences Center
Shreveport, LA

Editor:

Mark Yoffe, MD
York Hospital
York, PA

Reviewers:

Marianna M. Sockrider, MD, DrPH
Associate Professor—Pediatric Pulmonology
Baylor College of Medicine
Chief of Pulmonary Clinics
Texas Children's Hospital
Houston, TX

Mary Cataletto MD, FAAP
Professor of Clinical Pediatrics
SUNY at Stony Brook
Stony Brook, NY

Table of Contents
Respiratory Disorders

CONGENITAL DISORDERS OF THE UPPER RESPIRATORY TRACT

CONGENITAL DISORDERS OF THE NOSE

Choanal Atresia

Choanal atresia is the most common congenital anomaly of the nose and occurs in ~ 1/7,000 newborns. It presents as a unilateral or bilateral, bony (90%) or membranous (10%) septum between the nose and the pharynx. Nearly half of these infants have other associated congenital anomalies. Look for **CHARGE** syndrome (**c**oloboma, **h**eart disease, **a**tresia choanae, **r**etarded growth and development, **g**enital anomalies, and **e**ar anomalies/deafness).

Symptoms are variable depending upon the infant's ability to breathe through the mouth and the severity of the atresia. These infants can appear normal with mouth breathing or crying, but, because infants are primarily nasal breathers, they typically show symptoms early. Infants with bilateral atresia frequently suck in their lips when they inspire, and they have respiratory distress and cyanosis. Infants who are able to breathe through their mouths still have difficulty with breathing when fed. Symptoms improve with crying. Infants with unilateral choanal atresia can be asymptomatic until the nonaffected nares become blocked, for example, with secretions.

Diagnosis is suggested by the inability to pass a firm catheter through each nostril past a depth of about 3–4 cm. CT scan is confirmatory.

Treatment initially involves providing an adequate oral airway that also allows the infant to feed. Usually, an orogastric tube is sufficient for infants who can breathe by mouth. Consider performing corrective neonatal surgery if the infant does not have other associated defects. Infants with severe bilateral involvement who cannot breathe effectively by mouth require a tracheotomy until reconstructive surgery can be safely performed. Unilateral correction can typically be delayed for several years. Restenosis after surgery is common.

For infants requiring surgical intervention, various techniques are available, including transnasal excision of the obstructing tissue with curettes, lasers, microdebriders, bone punchers, or drills. Less frequently, when the plate is very thick or there is an extremely narrow posterior nasal cavity, a transpalatal approach is more efficient.

Other Less Common Disorders

Congenital perforation and deviation of the nasal septum are rare. If they occur, most are due to birth trauma.

Pyriform aperture stenosis is an abnormality of the anterior nasal aperture that is rare and has symptoms that mimic choanal atresia.

Congenital midline nasal masses can include dermoids, gliomas, and encephaloceles. Nasal dermoids may have a dimple or pit on the nasal dorsum and sometimes contain hair.

Intracranial extension of any defect increases the risk of recurrent intracranial infections. A full workup, usually with high resolution CT and MRI, determines if there is intracranial extension. Resection is indicated if intracranial extension is found with any of these lesions.

CONGENITAL DISORDERS OF THE TONGUE AND PHARYNX

Cleft Lip and Palate

A cleft lip occurs because of the incomplete fusion of embryonic structures that surround the primitive oral cavity (Image 13-1). It can be unilateral or bilateral. Cleft palates involve the soft palate and sometimes include the hard palate as well (Image 13-2). Cleft palates can vary greatly and often connect to a cleft lip. This disorder can run in families; however, the majority of cases are not associated with any genetic syndrome.

Submucosal cleft palates are often not obvious until several years of age. The uvula is commonly bifid. Occasionally, you see a blue line in the midline of the soft palate due to a lack of musculature in the midline; this is known as a zona pellucida. A notch of the posterior hard palate is sometimes palpated.

Treatment requires a multifaceted approach and includes craniofacial teams, speech pathologists, and occupational therapists. You must first address feeding issues. Lip repair usually occurs around 10 weeks of age and palate repair between 9 and 12 months of age.

Lingual Ankyloglossia (Tongue-Tie)

Lingual ankyloglossia is a common disorder in which the lingual frenulum limits the movement of the anterior tongue tip. Infants have difficulty extending the tongue past the alveolar ridge, which can make breastfeeding difficult. Most newborns can adjust and do well, but some require a frenulectomy, which is done in the outpatient office setting by a dentist or oral surgeon.

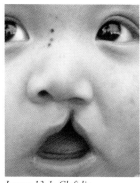

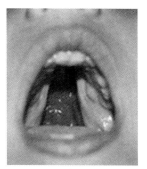

Image 13-1: Cleft lip   *Image 13-2: Cleft palate*

Speech difficulties are rare, especially with the English language. However, one very important social activity—licking an ice cream cone—may be impossible for a child to do, and some children proceed to frenulectomy.

Lingual Thyroid

A lingual thyroid is the most common ectopic location for the thyroid (90% of cases). It is more common in girls and occurs when thyroid tissue fails to descend into the neck from its site of origin in the tongue base. Usually, the lingual thyroid appears as a raised, violaceous mass that you see in the base of the tongue. Of those with lingual thyroid, > 70% do not have a normally located thyroid gland and ~ 30% present with hypothyroidism. The lingual thyroid can enlarge with upper respiratory infections during puberty or during pregnancy and can cause dysphagia or airway obstruction. Thyroid hormone is used to try and reduce the size of the thyroid remnant. Since this ectopic thyroid may be the only thyroid tissue, a thorough evaluation is required prior to surgical evaluation.

Thyroglossal Duct Cysts

Thyroglossal duct cysts, often seen with ectopic thyroid glands, are cystic masses in the midline of the neck. Generally, these cysts are asymptomatic unless they become infected. If infection occurs, the cyst can rapidly increase in size and cause respiratory compromise. Surgically remove thyroglossal duct cysts.

Cleft Tongue

Cleft tongue is part of **oral-facial-digital syndrome type I** (OFD1), which is inherited as an X-linked disorder. It presents with cleft tongue, hypoplasia of the nasal alar cartilages, medial cleft of the upper lip, asymmetric cleft of the palate, digital malformations, and mild intellectual disability. About 1/2 have hamartomas between the lobes of the divided tongue.

Mohr syndrome is an autosomal recessive disorder with lobulated nodular tongue, conductive hearing loss, cleft lip, high-arched palate, hypoplasia of the mandible, polydactyly, and syndactyly.

CONGENITAL DISORDERS OF THE LARYNX

Laryngomalacia

Laryngomalacia is the most common cause of stridor in the newborn. The laryngeal cartilage in some children is just not stiff enough, and inspiration causes significant luminal narrowing, resulting in inspiratory stridor. The stridor can occur at birth but is most commonly heard by 2 weeks of age. The stridor is more pronounced with agitation, feeding, and lying in a supine position. For most, close observation is sufficient, and the cartilage

becomes more rigid with age. Most children outgrow the disorder by 12–24 months of age. In severe cases, feeding is often affected, and/or nighttime obstructive hypoxia occurs; these symptoms are sometimes alleviated by trimming the supraglottis.

Confirm diagnosis by awake flexible laryngoscopy, which you can perform in the office setting. Consider complete bronchoscopy in infants with evidence of moderate-to-severe obstruction because up to 15–20% of these children demonstrate synchronous airway anomalies.

Vocal Cord Paralysis

Vocal cord paralysis occurs in one or both vocal cords. It may be seen in infants with neurologic abnormalities. It can also occur following birth trauma. Diagnose with awake fiberoptic nasopharyngoscopy.

Subglottic Stenosis

Subglottic stenosis can cause stridor and respiratory distress in the newborn or in the first few months of life. Infants with Down syndrome have an increased incidence of congenital subglottic stenosis. Diagnose by direct laryngoscopy or bronchoscopy. Treat only stenosis that produces symptoms, and treat those cases as early as possible. Some cases require tracheostomy before surgery can be performed. Cases that occur later in life are acquired and present with recurrent episodes of croup.

Laryngeal Atresia / Webs

Laryngeal atresia is a rare condition due to failure of the larynx to recanalize by the 10th week of gestation, which can lead to laryngeal web. The condition is usually incompatible with life, but with early prenatal diagnosis the fetus may be able to survive with airway intervention by fetal *ex utero* intrapartum treatment (EXIT). This type of anomaly and similar abnormalities (e.g., laryngeal cysts) have been given the label of congenital high airway obstruction syndrome (CHAOS).

Laryngeal webs can be partial or complete and occur with abnormal development of structures in and around the laryngeal inlet in the developing embryo. Webs can present with abnormal voice or with stridor and respiratory distress. Glottic webs are identified by direct laryngoscopy. Treatment options include incision or dilation in most cases. Tracheostomy is required for severe glottic webs. Webs can be seen in velocardiofacial syndrome. Order genetic testing for 22q11 gene deletions in these children.

Laryngeal Cysts

Cysts of the larynx develop from the mucus-secreting epithelium of the supraglottic region and, on occasion, from the subglottic region. They present with stridor

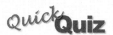

- What is the most common congenital anomaly of the nose?
- What is CHARGE syndrome?
- How is tongue-tie usually managed?
- What is the significance of thyroglossal duct cysts?
- What is the most common cause of stridor in the newborn?
- Which chromosomal abnormality is tested for in patients with glottic webs?
- How does tracheal stenosis present?

and hoarseness. Most subglottic cysts are not congenital but are due to secondary causes such as prolonged or traumatic intubation. Remove the cysts with an endoscopic CO_2 laser.

Laryngoceles

Laryngoceles are epithelium-lined diverticula that come from the laryngeal ventricle. They can present with laryngeal obstruction or as a neck mass. Excision or endoscopic marsupialization is the treatment of choice.

CONGENITAL DISORDERS OF THE LOWER RESPIRATORY TRACT

TRACHEAL DISORDERS

Tracheal Agenesis

Tracheal agenesis is very rare and presents as 1 of 3 different types:

- **Type 1**: The proximal trachea is closed off, and the distal part communicates with the esophagus.
- **Type 2**: The bronchi meet in the midline and communicate with the esophagus through a fistula.
- **Type 3**: The trachea is absent, and both main bronchi communicate directly with the esophagus separately.

In all 3 types, infants present at delivery in severe respiratory distress with absent cry. Affected infants die shortly thereafter. Suspect this condition if the trachea cannot be intubated even though the larynx is visualized.

Tracheal Stenosis

Tracheal stenosis presents most commonly as a segmental stenosis and usually involves complete cartilaginous rings. It can occur anywhere along the trachea. Infants present with severe retractions and dyspnea and have expiratory stridor. Also consider tracheal stenosis if a child presents with recurrent or prolonged croup. Perform bronchoscopy, CT, or MRI to confirm the diagnosis. Mild cases are usually observed and improve as the airway grows. Manage symptomatic cases by balloon dilatation, by resection of the stenotic portion, or with slide tracheoplasty.

Tracheomalacia and Bronchomalacia

Tracheomalacia produces collapse of the trachea severe enough to cause airway obstruction. It can be a generalized or localized weakness of the tracheal wall. Bronchomalacia is the same disorder in the bronchi. Tracheobronchomalacia is the condition in both the tracheal wall and bronchi. The airway cartilage does not have adequate tone and collapses with breathing, resulting in airway obstruction, and difficulty clearing secretions. Secondary malacia can occur from external compression from an aberrant vessel. The resulting airway obstruction produces an expiratory stridor as opposed to the inspiratory stridor heard with obstruction above the thoracic inlet, such as laryngomalacia.

Tracheobronchomalacia is usually mild and self-limited and does not require specific therapy. It can sometimes be found with other disorders, such as tracheoesophageal fistula, cardiac abnormalities, and cervical/mediastinal masses. More severe cases may require positive pressure ventilation to help stent the airways open. Severe tracheomalacia, particularly in infancy, sometimes requires tracheostomy.

LOBAR EMPHYSEMA AND OVERINFLATION

Congenital lobar emphysema can cause severe respiratory distress in the neonatal period, or onset of distress can be delayed up to 5–6 months. In this condition, 1 or more lobes are markedly enlarged with fluid or air. The left upper lobe is most commonly involved. The enlarged lobe pushes the diaphragm downward and the mediastinum to the opposite side. Lobar emphysema can be due to abnormalities of bronchial cartilage, with obstruction causing a ball-valve effect with resulting air trapping. Obstruction is usually intrinsic to the airway but can be caused by extrinsic vascular compression.

The condition is sometimes diagnosed antenatally. Infants can present with tachypnea or grunting soon after birth. Physical examination shows increased resonance, diminished breath sounds, and often expiratory wheezing. Because of the mediastinal shift, the heart sounds and trachea are also shifted on examination.

Manage mild symptoms conservatively with oxygen and a short course of mechanical ventilation (if needed). Severe cases require lobectomy.

RESPIRATORY DISORDERS

PULMONARY HYPOPLASIA

Pulmonary hypoplasia is a common cause of neonatal death. Infants present at birth with respiratory distress and have severe hypoxemia and hypercarbia. Lung development is a complicated multifactorial process, and, if something in this process is disturbed, development can be severely affected.

Pulmonary hypoplasia is commonly associated with oligohydramnios, as well as premature rupture of membranes, which leads to premature delivery. This causes delivery of an infant with variable lung function. The hypoplasia is due to a decrease in the number of alveoli with or without a decrease in the number of airway "generations."

It can be bilateral or unilateral (e.g., in association with congenital diaphragmatic hernia).

Prognosis depends on the severity of the pulmonary hypoplasia and the associated anomalies that typically coexist with or induce pulmonary hypoplasia. In severe cases, the lungs are too small and the infant dies. In less severe cases, the neonate is kept alive on mechanical ventilation or extracorporeal membrane oxygenation (ECMO) until adequate lung growth occurs. Interestingly, some infants who appear to have markedly severe pulmonary hypoplasia improve dramatically within hours of being placed on mechanical ventilation.

CONGENITAL PULMONARY VENOLOBAR SYNDROME ("SCIMITAR SYNDROME")

Congenital pulmonary venolobar syndrome is a rare disorder in which the pulmonary venous blood from all or part of the right lung returns to the inferior vena cava (IVC) just above or below the diaphragm. It is a left (oxygenated blood) to right (deoxygenated blood) shunt. In the infantile form, abnormalities of venous drainage (hemianomalous pulmonary venous drainage to the inferior caval vein) can present as heart failure and/or pulmonary hypertension in the newborn period. A chest x-ray may show the shadow of these veins as they course, giving a "scimitar-like" (Turkish sword) appearance. Infants with this condition presenting with heart failure have a worse prognosis, often because of associated abnormalities, including malformations in the left side of the heart.

Occlude aortopulmonary collaterals. Other treatment options include re-implantation of the vein or pneumonectomy. Mortality is high.

PULMONARY ARTERIOVENOUS MALFORMATIONS

Pulmonary arteriovenous malformations ([PAVM]; including pulmonary arteriovenous fistulas, aneurysms, and telangiectases) occur with several distinct congenital disorders. The most common cause (70%) is autosomal dominant hereditary hemorrhagic telangiectasia (HHT), also known as Osler-Weber-Rendu syndrome. It can present at any age. By age 20 years, 50% of patients have had episodes of epistaxis. PAVM in HHT is uncommon in childhood and increases in incidence with age. Many patients with PAVM are asymptomatic and are not aware of their risk of complications.

Large PAVMs cause problems due to right-to-left shunting of systemic venous blood directly into the pulmonary veins and left heart, leading to hypoxemia. Those with large-volume shunts present with dyspnea, bleeding with hemoptysis, and exercise intolerance. Congestive heart failure (CHF) is very uncommon though because the blood flow is a "low-pressure" system. In those with persistent hypoxemia, polycythemia is common. Patients with PAVM are at increased risk of cerebral events, such as stroke, transient ischemic attacks, and brain abscesses from paradoxical embolism.

Both contrast echocardiograms and lung perfusion scans can be employed to confirm the abnormal right-to-left shunt at the level of the pulmonary vasculature in these patients.

Treat symptomatic patients with pulmonary angiography and occlusion of the feeding arteries. Surgically remove the fistulas if they are large or if ablation is unsuccessful. Pulmonary AVMs can recur, and/or previously unrecognized PAVMs may enlarge.

PULMONARY SEQUESTRATIONS

Pulmonary sequestration is a mass of abnormal, nonfunctioning lung tissue isolated from the normal, functioning lung tissue and fed by systemic arteries. Pulmonary sequestrations can be either intralobar (contained within the normal visceral pleura) or extralobar (outside the normal lung with its own visceral pleura and venous drainage).

The **intralobar** form generally occurs in the lower lobes of each lung, most commonly in the posterior basal section of the left lower lobe. Anomalous vessels off the aorta supply the intralobar sequestrations with drainage through the pulmonary veins. The intralobar form is usually isolated and is typically identified during childhood or adolescence.

The **extralobar** form occurs most commonly in males and is located just above or below the diaphragm, with almost all cases being on the left side. These sequestrations are supplied by pulmonary or systemic artery branches and drain into a systemic vein. The sequestration communicates frequently with the foregut, and other anomalies are common, including colon duplication, vertebrae abnormalities, and diaphragmatic defects. Most extralobar forms are diagnosed in infancy because of associated malformations.

Pulmonary sequestration may also be identified prenatally on ultrasound and often partially or completely resolves before delivery.

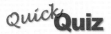

- What is scimitar syndrome?
- Why is bronchoscopy not useful in diagnosing pulmonary sequestrations?
- What do you suspect in a child who presents with a unilateral, foul-smelling nasal discharge?
- What is the most common etiology for epistaxis?
- Ask an adolescent with epistaxis about what type of illicit drug usage?

Besides respiratory distress in infants, it is possible to see recurrent pneumonia, hemoptysis, or signs of infection. Older children complain of severe pleuritic chest pain out of proportion to other findings. Some are asymptomatic and discovered as incidental findings on a CXR.

CXR or CT scan shows a dense mass in the lung or thorax representing recurrent infection, cystic changes, or air-fluid levels. A Doppler ultrasound can help demonstrate the arterial supply and venous drainage. Bronchoscopy is not helpful because the sequestration is not connected to the normal airways. Surgical removal of the sequestered lobe is the treatment of choice.

BRONCHOGENIC CYSTS

Bronchogenic cysts result from abnormal budding of the tracheal diverticulum of the foregut before 16 weeks of gestation. They are the most common cysts in infancy and are typically single, unilocular, and usually on the right. The cysts can present as an isolated incidental finding of a posterior mediastinal mass on a CXR or as significant symptoms because of compression of surrounding tissues. They may also be prone to infection.

Fever, chest pain, and productive cough are the most common presenting symptoms. Most bronchogenic cysts present as solitary and are filled with mucus. They can occur in the paratracheal, carinal, hilar, or paraesophageal area. They do not communicate with the tracheobronchial tree. The paraesophageal cyst sometimes communicates with the esophagus.

If the cyst ruptures, pneumothorax or hemoptysis can occur. Order a CT or an MRI to define the diagnosis. Cyst excision is curative in symptomatic cases. Excision is also the preferred treatment in asymptomatic patients because of a high likelihood of future symptoms and the potential for serious illness, including rarely malignant degeneration.

DIAPHRAGM MALFORMATIONS

Eventration

Eventration is a marked elevation of the diaphragm. It is almost always congenital but can be acquired with an injury to the phrenic nerve (acquired during difficult instrumental delivery, insertion of a chest tube for pneumothorax, or cardiac surgery). It is more common in males, typically affects the left diaphragm, and can be partial or diffuse. Some children who have lung hypoplasia and compression of the lung bases are at risk for atelectasis—which increases risk of pneumonia. Infants can be asymptomatic or have tachypnea, dyspnea, retractions, and cyanosis.

Physical examination shows unilateral decrease in breath sounds. CXR shows elevation of the hemidiaphragm. Ultrasound or fluoroscopy confirms and shows minimal or paradoxical movement of the affected diaphragm. Usually, no treatment is needed, and the condition may improve with time. Surgical plication is done in cases that have significant respiratory compromise.

Accessory Diaphragm

Accessory diaphragm is rare and occurs when a fibromuscular band divides a hemithorax into 2 parts. (The right side is more commonly affected.) In most patients, it results in hypoplasia of the lung on the affected side, with resulting respiratory distress in the neonate. Older children tend to have recurrent infections. Lateral x-ray shows the accessory diaphragm. If it is symptomatic, surgically remove the accessory diaphragm.

ACQUIRED DISORDERS OF THE NOSE

FOREIGN BODY

The nose is the toddler's playground. Various items can end up there without anyone's knowledge as to how they got there. These include crayons, various foods, toys, erasers, paper, beads, beans, stones, and pencils. Suspect a foreign body when a child presents with a unilateral prurient nasal discharge. Over time, the drainage (and the child) becomes foul smelling.

Frequently, you can see the foreign material with good lighting and an otoscope or nasal speculum. Do not push the foreign body further into the nose.

Outpatient treatment includes topical anesthetics and forceps or nasal suction. In some cases, general anesthesia is required.

EPISTAXIS

Epistaxis (nose bleed) is common in children. The most common cause is "nose picking." Nose bleeds typically occur during the dry, winter months. Besides nose picking, other causes include trauma (during sports, particularly), foreign bodies, and neoplasms (nasopharyngeal carcinoma, rhabdomyosarcomas, and lymphomas) of the nose. Question any adolescent with epistaxis about drug use. Cocaine abuse is a common mucosal irritant in those who use it and can result in epistaxis. Coagulopathies can obviously predispose to prolonged epistaxis. HHT can also present with recurrent epistaxis.

Most bleeding originates from the Kiesselbach plexus, and therapy involves putting pressure on this area by pinching the nose for 5–10 minutes to compress the nasal alae. If bleeding does not stop, try other therapies, including vasoconstrictor nose sprays or cautery of the bleeding site with silver nitrate. If bleeding still persists, refer the patient to an ENT specialist for nasal packing and observation.

Search for other underlying conditions if epistaxis continues to recur or is difficult to correct. In these cases, you need to order coagulation and hematologic studies. Also, fully evaluate the nasal passages and look for nasal masses or other causes of epistaxis.

NASAL POLYPS

Nasal polyps are benign tumors that form in the nasal passages and are usually due to chronically inflamed nasal mucosa. The most common cause in children is cystic fibrosis (CF). With any child < 12 years of age who has nasal polyps, evaluate for cystic fibrosis—even in the absence of other findings for cystic fibrosis. Other predisposing conditions include chronic sinusitis and allergic rhinitis. Note: There is also a condition called aspirin-exacerbated respiratory disease (AERD), which is diagnosed in patients who have (1) nasal polyposis and (2) acute respiratory tract reactions to ingestion of aspirin and other cyclooxygenase-1 (COX-1) inhibitors.

Kids with nasal polyps present with mouth breathing and a nasal-sounding voice. Polyps are sometimes visible using an otoscope or nasal speculum (Image 13-3). However, diagnosis may require nasal endoscopy or CT scan. The polyps look like gray, grape-like masses found between the nasal turbinates and septum.

Nasal decongestants are not effective in decreasing polyp size. Nasal steroids, however, have been shown to be quite effective for many polyps, especially in children with CF. Surgically remove polyps if they do not respond to steroids and cause symptomatic obstruction, recurrent sinus infection, or nasal deformity. Nasal polyps can recur after surgery.

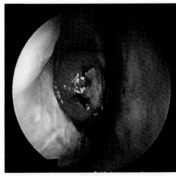

Image 13-3: Nasal polyp

CHEST WALL AND RESPIRATORY MUSCLE DISEASES

CHEST WALL MALFORMATIONS

Kyphosis and Scoliosis

Kyphosis refers to how the spine is angled in the anterior-posterior direction, while scoliosis refers to how the spine is angled in the lateral direction. Kyphosis usually affects the upper spine and does not cause respiratory compromise. Most cases of scoliosis are idiopathic, with the remainder due to neuromuscular diseases or congenital rib/vertebral anomalies. Scoliosis results in abnormal positioning of the ribs, which in turn results in abnormal configuration of the chest cavity. If scoliosis is severe, respiratory abnormalities can occur, including restrictive lung disease and/or distortion of the airways or large pulmonary vessels. Cardiopulmonary compromise generally occurs if scoliosis exceeds 90° or more.

Idiopathic scoliosis makes up 80–85% of all scoliosis and is divided into 3 categories (Table 13-1). About 3% of the general school population has a scoliotic curve of 10° or more and 0.5% has a curve of 20° or more. Scoliosis doubles death rates, sometimes occurring in the 4th or 5th decade due to cardiopulmonary insufficiency.

Mild scoliosis is asymptomatic, but when the thoracic curve exceeds 50°, you may find pulmonary function abnormalities. Alveolar hypoventilation is common. Respiratory symptoms sometimes occur with lesser curves in association with other respiratory compromise with neuromuscular disease from weakness, poor secretion control, or dysphagia.

Ideally, congenital forms of scoliosis are diagnosed early in childhood. If found, bracing usually corrects or limits progression of the curve. Surgical intervention is often required when the cause for scoliosis is congenital or neuromuscular weakness.

Pectus Excavatum

Pectus excavatum (hollowed chest; a.k.a. funnel chest) is a depression of the midsternum (Image 13-4). It can occur as a congenital condition and be familial or acquired. Pectus excavatum is sometimes seen with connective tissue disorders and other genetic conditions. It can occur in response to underlying pulmonary

Table 13-1: Idiopathic Scoliosis Divided into 3 Categories		
Age	**Type**	**Sex Predilection**
0–3 years	Infantile	Boys > girls
3–9 years	Juvenile	Girls > boys
9 years and older	Adolescent	Girls > boys

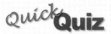

Quick Quiz

- What studies do you do for a child with recurrent or severe epistaxis?
- If you find nasal polyps in a child < 12 years of age, what diagnosis do you consider first?
- What is an effective treatment of nasal polyps?
- What degree of thoracic curvature in scoliosis may result in respiratory symptoms?
- What is pectus excavatum?
- What is pectus carinatum?
- What is the classic presentation of Werdnig-Hoffmann syndrome?

conditions. By itself, pectus excavatum rarely causes respiratory or cardiac problems, though some complain of exercise intolerance. More severe pectus excavatum can shift the heart leftward. Spirometry is usually normal but can show mild restriction in severe cases. Normal spirometry does not exclude the possibility of cardiopulmonary limitation with exercise. A CT scan can help define the severity, and exercise testing can help identify impairment in those with severe pectus excavatum.

Consider surgery on those who also have an associated thoracic scoliosis or who have significant cardiopulmonary limitation. Many have elective surgery to improve the aesthetic appearance of the chest.

Pectus Carinatum

Pectus carinatum (pigeon chest; a.k.a. pigeon breast) is the "sticking out" of the sternum with the lateral depression of the costal cartilages (Image 13-5). Pectus carinatum is rarely symptomatic. Surgical repair is done mainly for cosmetic effect.

Asphyxiating Thoracic Dystrophy (Jeune Syndrome)

Jeune syndrome is an autosomal recessive disorder that presents with short ribs, a small rib cage, and renal disease. Some children also have short-limb dwarfism, pelvic anomalies, polydactyly, and hepatic involvement. Because of the short rib cage, restrictive lung disease is common. Respiratory failure results in death after birth if ventilatory support is not provided. Some improvement in bone abnormalities can occur with age, which supports the approach to provide long-term ventilation early in life. Rib expansion procedures have improved survival rates, but their effect on lung function is unclear.

NEUROMUSCULAR DISEASES

Spinal Muscular Atrophy

Spinal muscular atrophy (SMA) is the 2nd most common lethal autosomal recessive disorder! (CF is #1.) The gene is located on chromosome 5q. Patients with spinal muscular atrophy present with hypotonia, muscle atrophy and fasciculations, and weakness of the intracostal muscles. The cause is the degeneration of the anterior horn cell and, sometimes, the bulbar nuclei. Muscle weakness is symmetric, with the proximal muscles affected to a greater degree. The legs are more commonly affected than the arms. Because this affects only the motor anterior horn cell, you do not see sensory or intellectual deficits.

There are 4 types of SMA (but only 3 are diagnosed in pediatric patients):

- **Type 1**: Werdnig-Hoffmann, or severe infantile SMA, is the most severe type and presents before 6 months of age with hypotonia and weakness, difficulty feeding, and tongue fasciculations. Most patients die by 2 years of age due to respiratory failure unless supported with tracheostomy and chronic ventilation.

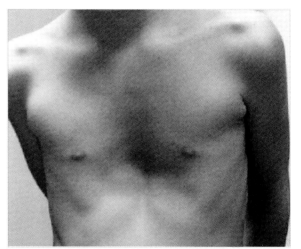
Image 13-4: Pectus excavatum

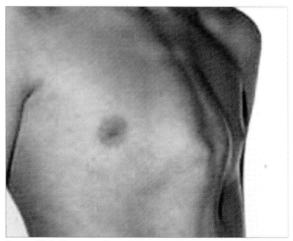
Image 13-5: Pectus carinatum

• **Type 2**: Intermediate or chronic infantile SMA occurs in up to 1/15,000 live births and represents the largest group of SMA patients. Children are "normal" at birth and achieve initial normal milestones, but these are lost by 2 years of age. With adequate respiratory management some can live into adulthood. Weakness can be static for long periods and then progress with intercurrent illness.

• **Type 3**: Kugelberg-Welander or mild SMA presents between 2 and 17 years of age. With this type, the child becomes unable to walk or stand unaided, but a normal lifespan is expected.

• **Type 4**: This presents later in the 2nd or 3rd decade, and is otherwise like type 3.

Outcomes in type 3 and type 4 depend more on severity at presentation rather than age of presentation.

Today, 95% of cases can be diagnosed with gene mutation screening. The defect is the *SMN1* gene found on 5q13. CPK is normal. Management is supportive with aggressive respiratory, nutritional, and orthopedic interventions. Before respiratory failure occurs, discuss the options of tracheostomy and lifelong mechanical ventilation with the family, in consultation with experts in the field.

Duchenne Muscular Dystrophy

Duchenne muscular dystrophy is an X-linked recessive disorder. Duchenne's is caused by a mutation in the dystrophin gene and results in absent or deficient dystrophin protein. It is the most common muscular dystrophy in childhood. It occurs in ~ 1/3,000 male births.

Boys present between 2 and 6 years of age with frequent falling, a "waddling" gait, and toe walking. Classic things to look for in exam questions: a child with calf muscle pseudohypertrophy and the Gowers sign—"climbing up the legs" using the hands when rising from a seated position on the floor (pushing against the shins, then knees, and finally the thighs). CPK is elevated. Affected boys generally lose the ability to walk by 12 years of age. Respiratory muscle weakness corresponds to gross motor weakness. Eventually, swallowing is impaired and secretions cannot be handled, and aspiration/infection commonly occurs. Cardiomyopathy is also seen in patients with Duchenne's.

Diagnosis is made by muscle biopsy, which shows atrophic muscle fibers and, on immunohistochemical staining, deficient dystrophin. Genetic testing is also available.

Management is supportive. Scoliosis begins before loss of muscle function and progresses rapidly once the child is wheelchair-bound. Early surgical intervention is indicated for scoliosis to preserve some lung function. Long-term care is an important issue, and respiratory failure is a common cause of death. Ventilatory support may improve survival. Even in the absence of symptoms, screen with serial tests for progressive respiratory insufficiency, such as negative inspiratory force or NIF and sleep apnea, via polysomnography. There is evidence to support the use of corticosteroid (prednisone) to improve muscle strength and respiratory function. Boys with Duchenne's are prone to obesity, which further worsens lung function. Proactive weight management is therefore important.

Myasthenia Gravis

Myasthenia gravis is rare in children but is still the most common primary disorder of neuromuscular transmission. In this disease, the postsynaptic receptors for acetylcholine are reduced in number, resulting in the postjunctional membrane being less sensitive to acetylcholine. Almost all adolescents who develop myasthenia gravis have autoantibodies that attack the acetylcholine receptor (AChR), thereby reducing the number of AChRs over time. These autoantibodies also fix complement. They probably originate in the thymus where there are clusters of myoid cells expressing AChR.

Neonatal myasthenia gravis occurs when the newborn is exposed, transplacentally, to maternal acetylcholine receptor antibodies. The neonate usually presents within a few hours of birth (72 hours at the latest) with hypotonia, weak cry, difficulty feeding, facial weakness, and ptosis. Respiratory compromise occurs due to aspiration and progressive respiratory muscle weakness. Neonatal myasthenia resolves in 2–12 weeks after the maternal antibodies have cleared.

Congenital myasthenia gravis is an autosomal recessive disorder with variable age of onset. Those affected do not have circulating antibodies to the acetylcholine receptor.

Juvenile myasthenia gravis is an acquired autoimmune disorder and more often affects girls, usually after the age of 10 years, but can present at any age during childhood. Circulating autoantibodies to acetylcholine receptors are in 80–90% of affected children. The disease progresses gradually, with worsening muscle weakness and respiratory compromise. Muscle weakness is exacerbated by repetitive muscle use. Ocular muscles are involved. Myasthenia gravis crises can lead to life-threatening respiratory failure. Possible triggers include infection, fever, stress, or medications.

Classically diagnose myasthenia gravis by testing for specific autoantibodies directed at the acetylcholine receptor (AChR-Ab) or against a receptor-associated protein, muscle-specific tyrosine kinase (MuSK-Ab). One of these autoantibodies is found in 88–94% of those with myasthenia gravis.

Treat with an oral anticholinesterase, most commonly pyridostigmine; these increase the concentration of acetylcholine at the receptor site. Immunosuppression can be beneficial as well. Thymectomy induces remission in as many as 50–60% of cases. Finally, plasmapheresis is beneficial for short-term amelioration of worsening symptoms.

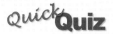

• What genetic testing do you order to diagnose spinal muscular atrophy syndrome?

• What is the pattern of inheritance seen in Duchenne muscular dystrophy?

• What is the mutation in Duchenne muscular dystrophy?

• What is Gowers sign?

• Is the CPK elevated in patients with Duchenne muscular dystrophy?

• How does juvenile myasthenia gravis differ from congenital myasthenia gravis? From neonatal?

• With which receptors do the circulating autoantibodies react in children with juvenile myasthenia gravis?

• Removal of which tissue may result in remission in myasthenia gravis?

• Does secondhand smoke increase the risk of having a URI?

• Which viruses most commonly cause URIs?

• Is routine viral testing appropriate in children with URIs?

• Does green nasal discharge in the first few days of a URI indicate that bacterial sinusitis is likely?

• Are antihistamines recommended in the therapy for URIs in children?

INFECTIONS OF THE NOSE, PHARYNX, AND UPPER RESPIRATORY TRACT

THE COMMON COLD

Upper respiratory infections (URIs) are the most commonly occurring illnesses in children. Most children have between 3 and 8 "colds" a year, most often in the fall and winter months. Certain factors increase a child's risk for developing a cold: attending day care, inhaling secondhand smoke (or actively smoking), lower socioeconomic status, and conditions that result in overcrowding.

Viruses cause the majority of URIs. Rhinoviruses make up nearly 33% of cases, followed by coronaviruses, adenoviruses, and coxsackieviruses. Once a child gets a virus and develops immunity, it is a lifelong immunity to that serotype. The problem is that each virus has potentially hundreds of other serotypes to which immunity is not conferred. Some viruses that cause URIs can spread to the lower respiratory tract, most notably the parainfluenza viruses, human metapneumovirus, and respiratory syncytial virus (RSV). Viruses that

cause URIs rarely cause acute bloodstream infection or viremia.

URI viruses clinically present with low-grade fever and malaise, with upper respiratory symptoms of runny nose, cough, and congestion. Shedding of virus peaks at 2–7 days after initial symptoms and can last as long as 2 weeks.

Viruses that cause URIs can be transmitted in 3 ways:

1) Large-particle droplets, which can travel through coughing or sneezing and spread to another person

2) Small-particle aerosols, which travel longer distances and can directly enter the alveoli

3) Secretions on hands or other surfaces (fomites), which can transmit the virus by direct physical contact (The recipients inoculate themselves by touching their nose or other mucous membranes with their contaminated hands/fingers.)

Do not order laboratory tests in children with URIs unless the diagnosis is unclear or if history/physical is incompatible with a diagnosis of URI.

The most common complication of a typical cold is acute otitis media. Other complications can include sinusitis, asthma exacerbation, and pneumonia. Thick, "green" nasal discharge by itself in the first few days of a URI does not mean the patient has bacterial sinusitis; it usually signifies an increase in the number of inflammatory cells.

Treat symptoms as needed, most often with acetaminophen. No pharmacologic therapy has shown to reduce the duration of a URI. Additionally, for children younger than 2 years, certain medications (pseudoephedrine, carbinoxamine, and dextromethorphan) have been associated with deaths. Thus, do not use antitussives and decongestants for relief of cold symptoms in children younger than 2 years of age. Instead use saline nose drops with a gentle bulb syringe to loosen secretions. Antihistamines are also not recommended for most children because they decrease cilia movement and can delay mucus clearance. Some recommend guaifenesin, a mucolytic agent, to thin secretions and improve ciliary function. Topical decongestants can relieve nasal congestion in older children; however, limit them to short time periods because of the risks of rebound congestion (rhinitis medicamentosa).

ACUTE SINUSITIS

Almost all cases of rhinitis are viral in origin. The common bacterial causes of acute sinusitis are *Streptococcus pneumoniae*, *Moraxella catarrhalis*, and nontypeable *Haemophilus influenzae*. With chronic sinusitis (symptoms more than 30 days), you sometimes find *Staphylococcus aureus*, α-hemolytic streptococci, and anaerobes.

RESPIRATORY DISORDERS

Children with sinusitis typically present clinically with cough, nasal discharge, and halitosis. The more "adult-like" presentation is seen in adolescents and includes facial pain, tenderness, and facial edema. In children, cough is bad in the daytime and worsens with supine position. Nasal discharge can be clear or green. Sore throat is common from postnasal drainage. Fever occurs more commonly in older children.

Clinically, viral sinusitis is almost indistinguishable from bacterial sinusitis. One clue is the duration of symptoms. Most URIs improve in 7–10 days. Suspect bacterial sinusitis if sinus symptoms last longer than 10 days or when sinus symptoms worsen during the course of a resolving URI. Occasionally, severe sinusitis occurs in the initial 7 days of the illness, but these children typically have high fever and headache.

Sinus x-rays and CT scans are unreliable in most situations. Obtain valid bacterial cultures by aspirating the sinus by direct maxillary antral puncture or endoscopic middle meatal aspiration; however, reserve this only for those who have life-threatening illness, are immunocompromised, or have illness that is unresponsive to empiric therapy.

Treatment is aimed at the most common etiologies. Most centers still recommend amoxicillin; however, many use amoxicillin with clavulanic acid, extended-spectrum macrolides, or 2nd and 3rd generation cephalosporins due to the increasing rate of β-lactamase production by *H. influenzae* and *M. catarrhalis*. *S. pneumoniae* resistance rates to amoxicillin and trimethoprim/sulfamethoxazole have risen dramatically, leading many to use high-dose amoxicillin (80–100 mg/kg/day) for therapy. Treatment duration is 10–21 days. Saline nose drops and/or saline nasal sprays are recommended. Decongestants, antihistamines, or nasal corticosteroids are not recommended.

Complications of sinusitis include:

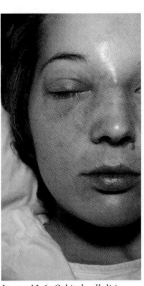

Image 13-6: Orbital cellulitis

- Preseptal (periorbital) cellulitis: mild complication characterized by swelling and erythema of the lids and periorbital area; no proptosis or limitation of eye movement
- Orbital cellulitis (Image 13-6): pain with eye movement, conjunctival swelling (chemosis), proptosis, limitation of eye movements (ophthalmoplegia), diplopia, vision loss

- Septic cavernous sinus thrombosis: bilateral ptosis, proptosis, ophthalmoplegia, periorbital edema, headache, change in mental status
- Meningitis: fever, headache, nuchal rigidity, change in mental status
- Osteomyelitis of the frontal bone associated with a subperiosteal abscess (Potts puffy tumor): forehead or scalp swelling and tenderness, headache, photophobia, fever, vomiting, lethargy
- Epidural abscess: papilledema, focal neurologic signs, headache, lethargy, nausea, vomiting
- Subdural abscess: fever, severe headache, meningeal irritation, progressive neurologic deficits, seizures, signs of increased intracranial pressure (papilledema, vomiting)
- Brain abscess: headache, neck stiffness, changes in mental status, vomiting, focal neurologic deficits, seizures, 3rd and 6th cranial nerve deficits, papilledema

For any of these complications, order a CT scan and hospital admission for IV antibiotics.

Unusual organisms can cause sinusitis, depending on underlying conditions. In children with prolonged neutropenia due to chemotherapy, the risk of *Aspergillus* or *Candida* sinusitis is increased. Mucormycosis is another fungal disease that can be life-threatening. It occurs in poorly controlled diabetes and may present as a black eschar on the nasal turbinate. It is dangerous because it frequently "grows backward" into the bone and brain.

ACUTE PHARYNGITIS ("SORE THROAT")

Acute pharyngitis peaks between the ages of 4 and 7 years in children; it is rare in children < 1 year of age. The most common cause of acute pharyngitis is viruses. Clinical features suggestive of viral etiology include concurrent conjunctivitis, coryza, cough, hoarseness, anterior stomatitis, discrete ulcerative lesions, viral exanthems, and/or diarrhea. You can culture other bacteria during a viral infection, but rarely, if ever, are they the etiology of the pharyngitis.

Streptococcus pyogenes (a.k.a. group A β-hemolytic *Streptococcus* [GAS]) is the most common bacterial cause but makes up only 15% of cases of acute pharyngitis! Other, less common causes include *Mycoplasma* and *Arcanobacterium haemolyticum*. Remember: In the case of sexually active adolescents, also consider *Neisseria gonorrhea*. *Corynebacterium diphtheriae*, which also causes acute pharyngitis, is discussed in Infectious Disease, Book 2.

Streptococcal pharyngitis frequently begins with nonspecific complaints of headache, abdominal pain, or vomiting. Fever is usually quite high. After these initial symptoms, children develop a sore throat. Children can have exudates, pharyngeal redness, enlarged tonsils, and petechiae of the soft palate. Tender, enlarged anterior cervical lymph nodes are common. Fever can last 1–4 days.

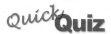
Quick**Quiz**

- If a child presents at day 9 of a URI with new fever, worsening nighttime cough, and increased sinus drainage, what do you suspect?

- A child with severe immunosuppression presents with suspected sinus infection. What is the best way to diagnose the infection and treat appropriately?

- What is Potts puffy tumor?

- In a diabetic adolescent with uncontrolled serum glucose and the finding of a black eschar in the nose, what infection do you suspect?

- What is the most common cause of acute pharyngitis in children?

- In an older child, is a sore throat accompanied by conjunctivitis, runny nose, or hoarseness likely to be due to *S. pyogenes*?

- Same question as previous, but now in a 1-year-old, and add the findings of cervical lymphadenitis and poor appetite.

- Does treatment with penicillin shorten the disease course in group A strep throat infections?

- How soon may a child return to school after being treated for group A strep pharyngitis?

- In retropharyngeal abscess, what does the lateral x-ray show?

For *Streptococcus pyogenes*, the most helpful clues are finding diffuse erythema of the tonsils and tonsillar pillars, petechiae of the soft palate, and absence of URI symptoms.

In children < 2 years of age, be familiar with this clinical presentation: coryza with postnasal discharge, fever (can last up to 8 weeks), pharyngitis, poor appetite, and tender cervical lymphadenitis. This is called streptococcosis and is a persistent illness in these younger children.

Diagnose with rapid detection methods of optical immunoassay and chemiluminescent DNA probes. The AAP recommends following up with a throat culture if the rapid test is negative.

Be most concerned with the 2 complications of *S. pyogenes* infection:

1) Rheumatic fever, which can be prevented if antibiotic treatment is given within 9 days after onset of symptoms. (Remember that rheumatic fever occurs only after pharyngitis—not skin infections!)

2) Post-streptococcal glomerulonephritis, which can occur regardless of therapy—and the infection can be pharyngeal, skin, or other locations for this to occur.

Treat with penicillin V 250 mg 2–3x/day orally for children < 27 kg, and 500 mg 2–3x/day for children ≥ 27 kg. Use IM injections (penicillin G benzathine 600,000 U for children < 27 kg, and 1.2 million U for children ≥ 27 kg) when adherence is a concern or if the child is vomiting. Children respond with defervescence within 24 hours of therapy, and penicillin shortens the disease course by 1.5 days on average. Amoxicillin 1x/day (750 mg x 10 days) has also been shown to be effective. Use erythromycin, clindamycin, or azithromycin for those allergic to penicillin.

A common question: How soon can children go back to school? In other words, when are they no longer infectious? The answer is: The child becomes noninfectious within a few hours after penicillin therapy; so, many allow the child to return to school or day care the next day if clinically improved.

Recurrence can occur and be retreated with the same antimicrobial agent, an alternative oral drug, or an IM dose of penicillin G (especially if nonadherence to oral therapy was likely). The 2015 Red Book® does not recommend any 1 of these agents as more appropriate than the other in this setting.

RETROPHARYNGEAL ABSCESS

Retropharyngeal abscess occurs as a complication in children with bacterial pharyngitis or can occur as an extension from a wound infection following a penetrating injury (e.g., pencil injury to the posterior pharynx). The most common causes are *S. pyogenes* (a.k.a. group A β-hemolytic *Streptococcus* [GAS]), oral anaerobes (most commonly *Fusobacteria* or *Prevotella*), and *S. aureus*.

Toddlers and children (most typically affected are 2–4 years of age) present with an abrupt onset of high fever and difficulty swallowing. This occurs during their "acute pharyngitis," and they develop the following symptoms in the midst of the infection: refusal to eat, severe throat pain, hyperextension of the head, and gurgling respirations. Drooling soon develops. Patients might not want to open their mouth because of pain (trismus); however, if they do, an erythematous, angry looking "bulge" is sometimes visible in the posterior pharyngeal wall. A lateral x-ray of the nasopharynx and neck with mild extension shows a widened retropharyngeal space with anterior displacement of the airway; in addition, the retropharyngeal soft tissue is more than 50% of the width of the adjacent vertebral body.

A retropharyngeal abscess is a medical emergency. Without prompt treatment, pus can extend into fascial planes or rupture into the pharynx, which can lead to aspiration. Stridor can also occur and simulate croup. You can order a CT scan to delineate the pathology.

In the pre-fluctuant phase, treatment with nafcillin for *S. aureus* and clindamycin for anaerobes may prevent suppuration. Some use single-agent therapy with ampicillin-sulbactam instead. Admit to the hospital and monitor closely. Continue IV antibiotic therapy until the patient is afebrile and clinically improved, and then complete therapy with oral amoxicillin-clavulanate or clindamycin to provide a total of 14 days of therapy. If the abscess is fluctuant, drainage is necessary.

PERITONSILLAR ABSCESS

Peritonsillar abscesses (PTAs) are often polymicrobial. The predominant bacterial species are *Streptococcus pyogenes* (a.k.a. group A β-hemolytic *Streptococcus* [GAS]), *Staphylococcus aureus* (including methicillin-resistant *S. aureus* [MRSA]), and respiratory anaerobes (including *Fusobacteria*, *Prevotella*, and *Veillonella* species). The abscess occurs after or with an acute pharyngotonsillitis. Fever can abate for several days and then recur or be continuous. The temperature can be as high as 105° F. The patient, often an adolescent, presents with severe pain and trismus and refuses to speak or swallow. A "hot potato" voice is described. The uvula is often displaced to the opposite side.

Imaging is not necessary to make the diagnosis of PTA, but it is sometimes necessary to differentiate PTA from peritonsillar cellulitis and other deep neck space infections and to look for complications. CT scan with IV contrast is the preferred imaging modality. It distinguishes peritonsillar abscess from cellulitis and also demonstrates the spread of infection to contiguous deep neck spaces. Careful monitoring during transportation and CT scanning is important; mild airway distress can be exacerbated by sedation and positioning. Do not do CT scanning in children with moderate-to-severe respiratory distress, particularly when sedation is necessary; evaluate these children in the operating room, where an artificial airway can be established when needed.

Management is dependent on age and the cooperativeness of the child. For most without a history of sore throat or recurrent pharyngitis, simple incision and drainage is best done in the operating room. If there is a history of previous recurrent pharyngitis or a prior PTA, then a tonsillectomy is recommended. Treat with the same antibiotics as used for retropharyngeal abscess (see above). Surgery can be postponed for 12–24 hours pending response to antibiotics if there is no evidence of airway compromise, septicemia, severe trismus, or other complications. For those patients < 6 years of age, antibiotic therapy alone was shown to be effective in one series.

CHRONIC TONSILLITIS

Indications for tonsillectomy:

- Recurrent pharyngitis (7 episodes in the past year, 5 in each of the last 2 years, or 3 in each of the past 3 years)

- Marked/Severe adenotonsillar hypertrophy (exclude tumor)
- Severe sleep apnea (Adenotonsillectomy is the 1st line treatment in children with obstructive sleep apnea.)

Tonsillectomy does not help prevent or treat acute or chronic sinusitis or chronic otitis media. Tonsillectomy does not help prevent URIs! Perform surgery 2–3 weeks after any uncomplicated infection has resolved. Assess for risk factors of persistent sleep apnea, and consider overnight postoperative observation for cases with significant sleep-related hypoxemia.

CHRONIC ADENOIDAL HYPERTROPHY

Indications for adenoidectomy:

- Persistent mouth breathing
- Repeated or chronic otitis media with effusion
- Hyponasal speech
- Adenoid facies
- Persistent or recurrent nasopharyngitis when it seems to be temporally related to hypertrophied adenoid tissue

Do not perform a tonsillectomy for these problems.

LARYNGOTRACHEOBRONCHITIS (CROUP)

Croup is predominantly a clinical diagnosis in which the child presents with a high-pitched, barking cough and inspiratory stridor. It typically occurs between the ages of 3 months and 3 years, with a peak around 2 years of age. Boys are more often affected than girls. Most episodes occur in fall and early winter. Most cases are due to parainfluenza virus, Types I and II. Sporadic cases can occur with other parainfluenza virus types, influenza virus, RSV, measles, and other viruses.

The virus usually causes subglottic airway narrowing at the cricoid cartilage, which results in the barking cough and stridor. Neck x-ray frequently shows subglottic narrowing (steeple sign, Image 13-7).

Croup is commonly managed supportively with cool-mist vaporizers, using a shower to steam up the bathroom, or taking a child outside in the cool night air. If the child presents to the emergency department, most centers give a single 0.6 mg/kg (max 10 mg) dose of oral (if possible, if not then IM/IV)

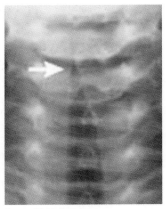

Image 13-7: Steeple sign

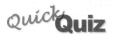

Quick Quiz

- What type of voice is described with peritonsillar abscess?
- What are the indications for tonsillectomy?
- Does tonsillectomy help with chronic otitis media? Does adenoidectomy help?
- What virus causes most cases of croup?
- What is the treatment for croup?
- What are the common causes of epiglottitis?
- If you visualize a cherry-red epiglottis, what is your diagnosis?
- What is the treatment of epiglottitis?
- What organism most commonly causes bacterial tracheitis?

dexamethasone, which decreases the length and severity of the illness.

For moderate stridor at rest, moderate retractions, or more severe symptoms, add aerosolized racemic epinephrine as 0.05 mL/kg/dose (max 0.5 mL) of a 2.25% solution diluted to 3 mL total volume normal saline via nebulizer with 100% oxygen. The main problem with this therapy is the "rebound phenomenon," with symptom recurrence after the medication has worn off, approximately after 2 hours. Therefore, observe children in the emergency department for at least 3–4 hours after therapy has begun.

Spasmodic croup is typically a noninfectious croup in which the child wakes up in the middle of the night with symptoms of barking cough and mild-to-moderate stridor. The next day the child is healthy, but the cycle repeats itself that night and possibly again over 2–3 nights. Spasmodic croup may or may not respond to cool mist or night air. Gastrointestinal reflux can be an important component. There can be mild signs of acute respiratory tract infection (coryza) but no fever; the child usually appears well otherwise.

Recurrent croup sometimes indicates a variant of asthma, in which case there is a positive bronchodilator response.

EPIGLOTTITIS

Epiglottitis is an infection of the larynx with rapid swelling of the epiglottis and increasing respiratory distress. It is now rare in developed countries because of widespread use of *Haemophilus influenzae* type b vaccine. Currently in the U.S., *H. influenzae* (nontypeable) is the most common cause of epiglottitis, followed by *Streptococcus pneumoniae*, *Streptococcus pyogenes* (a.k.a. group A β-hemolytic *Streptococcus* [GAS]), and *Staphylococcus aureus*.

Epiglottitis affects children between 2 and 5 years of age. Patients present with abrupt onset of fever, sore throat, drooling, and stridor. Frequently, the child is very ill appearing, sitting forward in a tripod position with the chin extended.

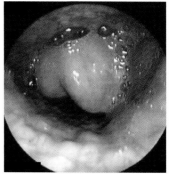
Image 13-8: Epiglottitis

Never use a tongue depressor on a symptomatic child; it may provoke airway spasm. Provide oxygen supplementation if necessary. Stay calm and keep the child calm. If respiratory failure is not imminent, the best next step is to seek the immediate help of an experienced pediatric anesthesiologist or otolaryngologist. The finding of a cherry-red epiglottis on laryngoscopy is diagnostic (Image 13-8).

Besides airway management, treatment must include prompt antibiotic therapy, which typically includes an antistaphylococcal drug (oxacillin, cefazolin, or clindamycin) and either ceftriaxone or cefotaxime. Most of these children are bacteremic. When MRSA (methicillin-resistant *Staphylococcus aureus*) carriage is high in the community, many use vancomycin as the antistaphylococcal agent.

Admit patients with epiglottitis to a closely monitored hospital bed. The risk of invasive *Haemophilus influenzae* type b disease is increased among unimmunized household contacts < 4 years of age.

Prophylaxis with rifampin eradicates *Haemophilus influenzae* type b from the pharynx in approximately 95% of carriers, and it decreases the risk of secondary invasive illness in exposed household contacts. Nursery and child-care center contacts may also be at increased risk of secondary disease. Secondary disease in child-care contacts is rare when all contacts are > 2 years of age.

BACTERIAL TRACHEITIS

Bacterial tracheitis is most commonly due to *Staphylococcus aureus*. It can also be caused by parainfluenza virus Type I, *Moraxella catarrhalis*, nontypeable *H. influenzae*, and anaerobes. Bacterial tracheitis usually follows a viral URI, such as croup, and does not involve the epiglottis. Because of the *H. influenzae* vaccine, bacterial tracheitis is more common than epiglottitis.

A child with tracheitis is typically < 3 years of age and presents with high fever and a brassy, productive cough; however, the stridor/croup does not respond to usual treatment measures for croup, and the child deteriorates rapidly. Intubation or tracheostomy is frequently required.

The majority of cases of bacterial tracheitis occur in previously healthy children in the setting of a viral respiratory tract infection. There is a slight male predominance (male-to-female ratio of 1.3:1). Most cases occur in the fall and winter, coinciding with the typical seasonal epidemics of parainfluenza, respiratory syncytial virus (RSV), and seasonal influenza.

Treatment includes antibiotics, particularly nafcillin, aimed at *Staphylococcus aureus*. Patients respond to therapy within 2–3 days; however, due to the continued edema from the tracheitis, most patients require an average of 10–14 days of hospitalization. Vancomycin is used if MRSA is common in the community.

INFECTIONS OF THE LOWER RESPIRATORY TRACT

BRONCHIOLITIS

Bronchiolitis is very common in infants and young children, especially during the winter and spring. It is most commonly due to respiratory syncytial virus (RSV), which is ubiquitous. Risk factors for severe RSV infection include secondhand smoke exposure, family history of asthma, crowded living conditions, and low birth weight. RSV can be spread by large-particle dispersion as well as through contact with fomites. Other etiologies include parainfluenza, human metapneumovirus, influenza, rhinovirus, coronavirus, and human bocavirus.

Those affected frequently have a prodrome of low-grade fever, runny nose, and poor feeding before progressing to cough and wheezing. On physical examination, look for wheezing, crackles, stridor, retractions, or cough. CXR shows hyperinflation and is nonspecific. Rapid immunofluorescent and enzyme immunoassays for detection of viral antigen in nasopharyngeal specimens are available commercially and are generally reliable in infants and young children.

Treatment is supportive; hospitalization is reserved for patients who are hypoxic, unable to feed, dehydrated, and/or toxic-appearing. β-agonist therapy possibly benefits selected children but is not recommended for routine care in first-time wheezing. Inhaled hypertonic saline (3%) has been used as a mucolytic. Corticosteroids are not recommended. Use ribavirin primarily in critically ill children and in those who are immunocompromised.

Infants can be severely affected and sometimes require intubation with mechanical ventilation, especially if they are premature.

Most infants are infectious for about 7 days, but some can have persistent shedding for months.

RESPIRATORY SYNCYTIAL VIRUS IMMUNOPROPHYLAXIS

Respiratory syncytial virus (RSV) can affect the lower respiratory tract, causing bronchiolitis, bronchospasm, pneumonia, and respiratory failure—especially in infants and small children.

In August 2014, the AAP revised the guidelines on RSV immunoprophylaxis to include monthly palivizumab for high-risk infants and children during the active season. Consider it for:

- Infants and children < 24 months of age with chronic lung disease of prematurity who require medical therapy (e.g., diuretics, oxygen, systemic corticosteroids) within 6 months before the start of RSV season (Chronic lung disease of prematurity is defined as the requirement of oxygen for > 28 days in infants born at < 32 weeks of gestation.)
- Infants born at < 29 weeks of gestation
- Infants born at < 28 weeks of gestation in their 1st winter
- Children < 24 months of age with hemodynamically significant cyanotic and acyanotic congenital heart disease (but not secundum ASD, small VSD, pulmonic stenosis, uncomplicated aortic stenosis, PDA, mild coarctation, or those with more severe disease who have been corrected and no longer require medication)

Consideration of infants who are immunocompromised or have significant pulmonary or neurologic problems that interfere with the ability to clear upper airway secretions is made on a case-by-case basis. Once a child "qualifies" for initiation of prophylaxis at the start of the RSV season, continue prophylaxis based on month of birth and gestational age for up to 5 doses. Discontinue prophylaxis if an infant has an RSV infection.

PNEUMONIA—GENERAL CONSIDERATIONS

Clinical markers of pneumonia are not the same in infants and children as in adults, and the younger patients do not present with the typical fever, cough, and productive sputum. Thus, various clinical guidelines have been developed to help us sort this all out. The following information on diagnosing pneumonia refers to children > 2 months of age. Infants < 2 months of age with pneumonia are discussed in The Fetus & Newborn, Book 3.

First, consider whether the child has signs of respiratory distress:

- Tachypnea
- Subcostal retractions
- Cough
- Crackles
- Decreased breath sounds

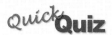

Quiz

- Which pathogen most commonly causes acute bronchiolitis?
- In children, the absence of which vital sign abnormality makes the diagnosis of pneumonia unlikely?
- When do you get a CXR in a child with fever?
- Are blood cultures routinely recommended in the management of outpatient pneumonia in children?
- Which serologic tests are routinely ecommended in the management of outpatient pneumonia in children?

Note: The positive predictive values of these signs are best if the child has fever or cyanosis, in addition to 2 or more of these signs.

Tachypnea alone, in association with cough, has a sensitivity of about 70% and a specificity of only 40–70%. Furthermore, the positive predictive value of tachypnea falls to 20% in children ≤ 2 years of age. Just what "number" defines tachypnea? The World Health Organization (WHO) has set up thresholds based on the child's age (Table 13-2). So, using the guidelines, a 4-year-old with cough and respiratory rate of 50 is at risk for pneumonia.

Note that without the presence of fever, the negative predictive value of tachypnea is 97%. In other words, without fever, pneumonia is unlikely.

What about CXR?

CXR is recommended in the following:

- Children < 5 years of age with fever and high WBCs of unknown source.
- There is clinical evidence of possible pneumonia, but the clinical findings are not clear-cut.
- Pleural effusion is suspected.
- Pneumonia is unresponsive to antibiotics.

Most studies have shown that CXR cannot distinguish between viral and bacterial pneumonia, and many studies have failed to show that CXR actually alters management decisions. (See Image 13-9, left lower lobe pneumonia.)

Table 13-2: WHO Tachypnea Thresholds for Diagnosing Pneumonia in the Presence of Cough

Age	Normal (breaths/min)	Tachypnea (breaths/min)
< 2 months	35–55	60
2–12 months	25–40	50
1–5 years	20–30	40

What about WBC count and differential?

Most data show that the likelihood of a bacterial cause increases as the WBC count increases above 15,000–20,000, and a bacterial etiology is especially likely with WBCs this high and a fever > 39° C (102.2° F). But when do you order a WBC count? Consider a WBC count when the information available to you is insufficient to determine if antibiotics should be used.

Sputum Gram stain and cultures are very controversial, primarily because of the difficulty getting a high quality sample. If possible, in a child with severe disease, obtain a high-quality specimen (< 10 squamous epithelial cells and > 25 PMNs/low-power field suggests a purulent specimen). Sputum can be induced with a 3% hypertonic saline treatment. For mild or moderate disease, sputum studies are generally not necessary.

Blood cultures are not recommended as routine studies in the outpatient setting (the chance of a positive blood culture in this setting is < 5%), but they are recommended for inpatients with more severe pneumonia.

What about serologic testing, cultures, and PCR testing?

Testing for specific pathogens, such as *Mycoplasma pneumoniae* or *Chlamydophila pneumoniae*, is not routinely recommended. Use other tests, such as viral cultures, viral antigens, and cold agglutinins, only when the result would alter therapy.

Use of ESR and C-reactive protein (CRP) is not recommended to diagnose pneumonia.

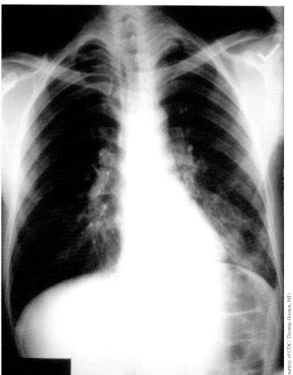

Image 13-9: Left lower lobe pneumonia

RESPIRATORY DISORDERS

VIRAL PNEUMONIA

Pneumonia in children is most likely due to viruses. These include RSV, parainfluenza viruses, adenoviruses, rhinoviruses, influenza viruses, varicella virus, and rubeola (measles) virus. Clinically, children have a prodrome of URI-type symptoms, which is followed by a sudden onset of tachypnea, nonproductive and frequently paroxysmal cough, and low-grade fever. Physical findings consistent with pneumonia include dullness or decreased breath sounds, wheezing and crackles, or, in other cases, the lung examination can be normal except for tachypnea. CXR usually shows perihilar and parenchymal infiltrates.

Treatment is supportive, with fluids and oxygen if necessary. Specific viruses are discussed in Infectious Disease, Book 2.

ACUTE BACTERIAL PNEUMONIA

Streptococcus pneumoniae

Streptococcus pneumoniae classically presents as an abrupt infection with fever, chills, chest pain, and dyspnea, as well as blood-tinged sputum. (Remember, pneumococci are gram-positive diplococci.) Children with pneumococcal pneumonia appear clinically ill and have tachypnea and tachycardia.

Physical examination shows dullness to percussion over the affected lung segment and diminished breath sounds. A pleural friction rub may be detected. Frank crackles may not be heard until later in the course of the illness.

Pleural effusions occur in 60%. These are usually uncomplicated, sterile, and exudative. Empyema is a late complication. See Image 13-10, an AP CXR showing right-sided pneumonia, and Image 13-11, a lateral decubitus x-ray of a different patient showing layering from a large pleural effusion.

Poor prognostic findings are leukopenia and shock; if both are present, mortality can approach 50%.

Of major concern is the emergence of penicillin-resistant pneumococci; in some centers, it approaches 40–50% of cases. For outpatient therapy, use high-dose amoxicillin (80–100 mg/kg/day) for 7–10 days. For children with vomiting who are still well enough to return home, give IM ceftriaxone; then follow up the next day with oral outpatient therapy. For inpatient therapy, use a 2nd or 3rd generation cephalosporin. For those penicillin-allergic in either setting, consider a macrolide or cephalosporin (if no anaphylaxis to penicillin). Vancomycin can be used if macrolide resistance is high or if cephalosporins cannot be used.

Pleural effusions often persist for weeks and resolve without specific therapy. Later, if the child has recurrence of fever or symptoms with a persistent pleural effusion, perform appropriate studies (thoracentesis with cell count, pH, protein, glucose, and bacterial culture) on the fluid to determine if empyema has occurred. If empyema has occurred, closed suction drainage is often required.

Streptococcus pyogenes (Group A β-hemolytic Streptococcus [GAS])

Streptococcus pyogenes causes pneumonia usually after a rash disease, such as rubeola, varicella, or scarlet fever. It can also occur sporadically without prior illness. *S. pyogenes* pneumonia presents abruptly with fever, chest pain, cough, and leukocytosis. Physical findings are similar to pneumococcal pneumonia. Pneumatoceles are common and disappear spontaneously, but often take weeks to resolve. The most common complications from *S. pyogenes* pneumonia are abscesses and empyema.

Treat outpatients with oral penicillin/amoxicillin for 10–14 days. For hospitalized children, treat with IV penicillin. If empyema has occurred, closed suction drainage is usually necessary.

Haemophilus influenzae

Since *Haemophilus influenzae* vaccine use has become widespread, the incidence of this bacterium as a cause of pneumonia has decreased markedly. Findings are similar to pneumococcus, although it usually has a

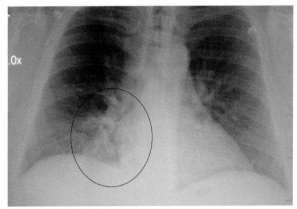
Image 13-10: Right lower lobe pneumonia

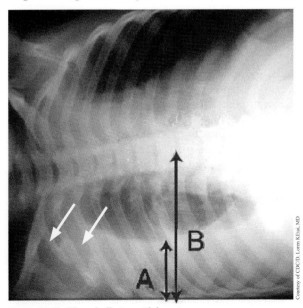
Image 13-11: Pleural effusion with layering

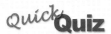

Quick Quiz

- Gram-positive diplococci seen in a sputum sample with a large number of PMNs and few epithelial cells most likely indicate which organism?

- What do you do about a persistent (1 week out) pleural effusion in a child with recent pneumococcal pneumonia who clinically is responding to therapy?

- What do you do about pneumatoceles if they occur in *S. pyogenes* pneumonia?

- A patient with influenza develops a secondary bacterial pneumonia. Besides pneumococcus, what bacterial pathogen do you especially consider?

- Which antibiotic is commonly used for presumed anaerobic pneumonia?

- Name the geographical areas for histoplasmosis, coccidioidomycosis, and blastomycosis.

more insidious course. Outpatient therapy includes amoxicillin-clavulanate acid. Inpatient therapy is generally ceftriaxone or cefotaxime.

Staphylococcus aureus

Staphylococcus aureus is much less common than pneumococcus and *S. pyogenes*, but it is very serious and frequently a fulminant cause of pneumonia. Infants with *S. aureus* pneumonia frequently develop pneumatoceles, pneumothoraces, abscesses, and empyema. The right lung is affected more often than the left.

Suspect *Staphylococcus aureus* pneumonia in a patient with recent URI, chicken pox, or influenza who presents with abrupt onset of fever, tachypnea, tachycardia, and cyanosis. CXR showing distinct pneumatoceles is classic. Blood cultures are frequently positive.

Patients with suspected staphylococcal pneumonia require prompt hospitalization treatment with nafcillin or vancomycin (if there is high prevalence of MRSA in the community or if the patient has had recent hospitalization, indwelling catheter, or tracheostomy).

Pneumothoraces require decompression. Pneumatoceles are very common and appear 3–4 days into therapy. They require no specific therapy and usually resolve over time. Empyema requires closed suction drainage.

Klebsiella pneumoniae

Klebsiella pneumoniae is a rare cause of pneumonia in children. When it occurs, it is typically in children with underlying immunosuppression or those who have had prolonged endotracheal intubation. Treatment consists

of piperacillin-tazobactam 300 mg/kg per day IV in 4 divided doses or meropenem 60 mg/kg per day IV in 3 divided doses.

Anaerobes

Anaerobes are rare causes of pneumonia in children and occur mainly in those who are prone to aspirate oral secretions. Strong putrid sputum is characteristic; many times just walking into the room gives the diagnosis away! Clindamycin is commonly used for anaerobic pneumonia.

FUNGAL INFECTIONS

Note

Fungal infections occur less commonly than bacterial or viral infections. Unlike bacterial or viral infections, endemic fungal infections occur in geographically distinct regions. See Figure 13-1.

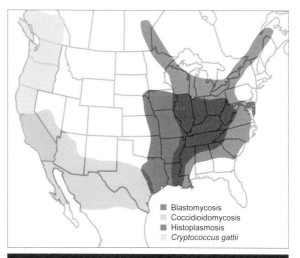

Figure 13-1: Map of Endemic Fungal Infection Areas

Histoplasmosis

Histoplasmosis is common in endemic areas—the southern and midwestern U.S. Histoplasmosis is especially seen in the Mississippi and Ohio River valleys. (Do not confuse this with "[San Joaquin] valley fever"; next.) Think of histoplas**MO**sis (**M**ississippi, **O**hio). It is transmitted through soil contaminated with bird (including chickens) and bat droppings. Most cases are asymptomatic, and a majority of residents in endemic areas have serologic evidence of past exposure.

With acute disease, the chest x-ray shows hilar adenopathy and focal alveolar infiltrates. Heavy exposure ("epidemic," disseminating form) is suggested by a chest x-ray revealing multiple nodules in addition to the hilar adenopathy. No treatment is indicated for acute pulmonary disease without complications. Use itraconazole for persistent disease > 4 months or if hypoxia occurs in the acute setting.

Disseminating disease requires amphotericin B. Urinary and serum antigen testing is useful in disseminated *H. capsulatum* disease.

Coccidioidomycosis ("Valley Fever")

Coccidioides immitis infection (**c**occidioidomycosis) is endemic in the southwestern U.S. (**C**alifornia)—the term comes from the San Joaquin Valley. Spores grow best in arid, desert-like climates. Erythema nodosum and erythema multiforme commonly occur in infected people. A typical presentation is a person with erythema multiforme and a history of travel to the Southwest.

Diagnose with complement fixation titers.

The self-limited form generally does not require treatment and can leave thin-walled lung cavities. Treat with fluconazole and/or amphotericin B if there is severe disease, symptoms last > 2 months, or there is high risk of disseminated disease.

Disseminated coccidioidomycosis is seen in immuno-compromised and HIV patients. Individuals of African or Filipino descent are also at higher risk. This is a fulminant disease with meningitis and with skin and bone involvement. Even with treatment (amphotericin B), it is frequently fatal.

Blastomycosis

Blastomycosis is uncommon. It is usually acquired in the central, southeastern, and mid-Atlantic seaboard states. M:F ratio is 10:1! Progression can be indolent to severe. No reliable skin test is available. Chest x-ray shows infiltrates that appear mass-like. Sputum shows large, single, broad-based budding yeasts (Image 13-12). Blastomycosis is more pyogenic than the other fungal infections—patients can have purulent sputum. In children, it likes to disseminate to bone and skin.

Treatment of blastomycosis:

• Indolent: Observe or prescribe oral itraconazole.
• Severe: Prescribe amphotericin B. HIV patients require chronic suppression with itraconazole.

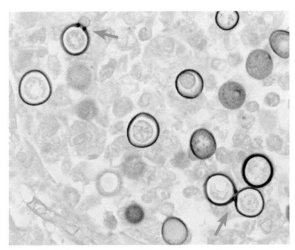

Image 13-12: Blastomycosis with budding yeast cells

Allergic Bronchopulmonary Aspergillosis

Allergic bronchopulmonary aspergillosis (ABPA) is caused by an allergic reaction to *Aspergillus* in which there is immune complex deposition. There is usually a very high serum IgE. This allergy causes Type I (immediate wheal and flare; IgE-mediated) and Type III (> 4 hours out), but not Type IV (delayed) reactions. Suspect it in patients with asthma who have difficult-to-control or worsening asthma symptoms, are coughing up brownish mucous plugs, have recurrent infiltrates, and have peripheral eosinophilia. ABPA may also occur in patients with cystic fibrosis.

Chest x-ray and CT show central mucus impaction and central bronchiectasis causing a "fingers in glove"-appearing central infiltrate. Sputum may show branching hyphae (nonspecific). If there is only lung eosinophilia (no peripheral eosinophils), consider instead a chronic eosinophilic pneumonia. If the patient has immediate skin reactivity to *Aspergillus*, then an ABPA panel confirms the diagnosis with *Aspergillus*-specific IgE and IgG titers.

Treat ABPA with oral corticosteroids and itraconazole.

ATYPICAL PNEUMONIAS

Overview

Atypical pneumonias usually occur in children older than 5 years of age. Patients typically have no sputum production, a nontoxic appearance, and a normal or slightly elevated WBC count. Atypical pneumonia often follows an upper respiratory infection and can be caused by *Mycoplasma, Chlamydophila pneumoniae* (TWAR), *Chlamydia psittaci* (bird farmers), *Legionella, Histoplasma, Coccidioides,* and viruses. Other causes include Q fever and tularemia. Consider tularemia in patients who hunt or skin animals and are from Arkansas or Missouri. Think of Q fever if the patient lives around cattle or sheep—these animals are naturally infected; the causative organism, *Coxiella burnetii*, is not transmitted between humans.

Mycoplasma pneumoniae

Mycoplasma pneumoniae is a common cause of community-acquired pneumonias in children > 5 years of age and in adolescents, occurring year round. Having a 2- to 3-week incubation period, it spreads slowly (person to person). A prodrome of headache, fever, and pharyngitis is classic. It usually has an insidious onset, with the chest x-ray often appearing worse than the symptoms suggest. Occasionally, it has a more acute onset and can mimic a pneumococcal pneumonia.

Extrapulmonary manifestations of *Mycoplasma* pneumonia include hemolytic anemia, splenomegaly, erythema multiforme (and Stevens-Johnson syndrome), arthritis, myringitis bullosa, pharyngitis, tonsillitis, and neurologic changes—especially confusion. Diagnosis: **Definitive** is with an IgM antibody (think

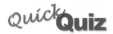

- If you see the words "San Joaquin Valley" in a test question, you need to look for which fungus on the exam?
- A patient presents with worsening control of their asthma and an extremely high IgE level. What do you suspect as an etiology?
- How do you treat ABPA?
- What are the extrapulmonary manifestations of *Mycoplasma* infection?
- Does having an abnormal sinus x-ray indicate bacterial infection in a child with asthma?

IgM-M-*Mycoplasma*), and **suggestive** is with a positive cold agglutinin titer (seen in up to 50% of cases with pneumonia).

Treat with a macrolide or doxycycline. Patients sometimes take a long time (> 6 months) to fully recover!

Chlamydophila pneumoniae (formerly *Chlamydia pneumoniae*)

Chlamydophila pneumoniae, formerly known as the Taiwan acute respiratory agent (TWAR), is increasingly recognized as a respiratory pathogen in children and adults. It causes epidemic pneumonia in older children and adolescents. It is the cause of up to 10% of community-acquired pneumonias. Symptoms are similar to *Mycoplasma* pneumonia. Often there is a biphasic illness: The patient presents with a sore throat negative for group A strep, and, 2–3 weeks later, pneumonia develops. Treat with tetracycline/doxycycline or a macrolide.

ASTHMA

OVERVIEW

Asthma is the most common chronic disease of childhood. Prevalence data shows increasing rates of asthma since the 1980s. Asthma is more common in African Americans of all ages and in boys of all races. Asthma is quite variable in its presentation and course. Airway obstruction is the most common pathologic problem, which is due to bronchial smooth muscle spasm, airway mucosa edema, mucus impaction of bronchi, airway inflammation, and/or airway hyperresponsiveness.

Diagnosis begins with the history and physical examination. Common symptoms include recurrent wheezing, shortness of breath, chest tightness, exercise intolerance, mucoid vomiting, and chronic cough (common in patients with cough-variant asthma). Various factors seem to trigger an asthma attack, including

viruses. As many as 85% of exacerbations coincide with viral infection in school-aged children. Viral infection is the biggest risk factor for hospitalization. Other factors that can trigger asthma exacerbation include smoke; exercise; allergen exposure; breathing cold, dry air; aspirin; aspiration; and acid reflux. Physical examination during "normal" times may not show anything or can show only a prolonged expiratory phase; wheezing, respiratory distress, tachypnea, and use of accessory muscles can be present during attacks.

Children who have recurrent wheeze during infancy continue to wheeze after the age of 6 years approximately 15% of the time. Also, about 15% of children develop their 1st "wheezing" episode of asthma after the age of 6 years.

CLASSIFICATION OF ASTHMA

Asthma is classified by severity as well as level of control. The latest guidelines issued by the National Asthma Education and Prevention Program (NAEPP) Expert Panel Review 3 established 3 age groups (0–4 years, 5–11 years, and ≥ 12 years of age). With increasing age, additional factors play a role in the classifications of severity and control. Symptom patterns define whether the asthma is intermittent or persistent, and they also define the severity. Based on this classification, treatment regimens can be determined. See Figure 13-2 to Figure 13-10 at the end of this section for details. Know this stepwise approach!

COMORBIDITIES AND TRIGGERS

Sinusitis

It is known that children with asthma have a high incidence of abnormal sinus x-rays. However, we know that a majority of these children likely do not have clinical bacterial sinusitis but rather simple acute rhinitis with an abnormal sinus x-ray. Therefore, having an abnormal sinus x-ray and asthma does not equate to needing antibiotic therapy. Pursue clinical diagnosis of sinusitis before initiating antibiotic therapy.

GE Reflux

Gastroesophageal (GE) reflux is sometimes a significant problem in the child with asthma. First, in the neonate, significant GE reflux can imitate asthma and lead to an incorrect diagnosis. Second, in older children, significant GE reflux can exacerbate underlying asthma and initiate an acute attack. However, indiscriminate use of acid blockers in children with asthma without symptoms of reflux is of no benefit. Theophylline, which is used in some asthma therapy, can reduce the lower esophageal sphincter (LES) tone, resulting in increased risk of GE reflux.

Exercise

Exercise causes bronchodilatation and an increase in expiratory flow rates in otherwise normal as well as asthmatic children. Exercise-induced asthma is seen most commonly in adolescents who have no other signs or symptoms of asthma. They develop cough or difficulty breathing after 6–10 minutes of exercise, especially in cold, dry air. Pretreatment with montelukast (requires days or even weeks to start working) or a short-acting β-adrenergic agent (10–20 minutes before exercise) usually prevents or reduces the severity of symptoms. People with poorly controlled asthma are likely to have increased symptoms with activity due to limited lung function, which is seen with inadequate asthma control.

The Difficult, Refractory Patient

Think of **ICE** when you are presented with a patient who does not respond to routine therapies for asthma:

- **I**nhalation technique: problems with inhaled drug delivery
- **C**ompliance: poor adherence to the treatment plan
- **E**xacerbating factors: e.g., tobacco smoke exposure, GE reflux, and sinusitis

Also consider pathologic causes of poor response: CF, allergic bronchopulmonary aspergillosis, vocal cord dysfunction, hypersensitivity pneumonia, and sleep apnea.

Note: ~ 5% of children do not respond to standard therapy and require prolonged courses of corticosteroids to maintain a symptom-free period.

TREATMENT

Overview

The NHLBI published a comprehensive guideline for asthma management, last updated in late 2007. The complete compendium is available online. See the reference in For Further Reading on page 13-32.

We've included the important figures from the guideline in Figure 13-2 through Figure 13-10 at the end of this section. Be sure you know these perfectly! Treatment varies by age and is based on the symptoms the patient is having.

Let's review a few key points.

For intermittent or mild persistent asthma, treatment is straightforward:

- Note that for **intermittent** asthma, no daily medication is recommended for any age group.
- For **mild persistent** asthma (symptoms occurring > 2x/week but not daily), use low-dose inhaled corticosteroid as the preferred initial treatment for all age groups.

If a low-dose inhaled corticosteroid does not control symptoms, then the age of the child factors into treatment. For a child:

- ≤ 4 years of age, use a medium-dose inhaled corticosteroid.
- 5–11 years of age, use either a medium-dose inhaled corticosteroid or a low-dose inhaled corticosteroid combined with an inhaled long-acting β$_2$-agonist, a leukotriene receptor antagonist, or theophylline.
- ≥ 12 years of age, use a low-dose inhaled corticosteroid plus a long-acting inhaled β$_2$-agonist or a medium-dose inhaled corticosteroid.

Know that in all patients who have an exacerbation, quick relief includes using a short-acting inhaled β$_2$-agonist (peak effect in 15 minutes, with duration of 4 hours); oral or parenteral corticosteroids also are recommended, depending on response.

See Figure 13-10 on page 13-42 for management of asthma exacerbations in the hospital or emergency department setting.

Home peak flow monitoring can be a helpful adjunct to symptom monitoring in some patients to identify a change in control and to monitor response to therapy. It requires skill and effort to get reliable readings and can typically be done by children ≥ 6 years of age. Consider use of peak flow for children with persistent asthma, and observe the child doing the maneuver. Education is the key to preventing exacerbations as well as to getting exacerbations under control quickly. Families need to have a clear understanding of how and when to use asthma medicines, the skills to correctly deliver inhaled medication, and the knowledge of how to avoid or eliminate asthma triggers. A written home asthma management (action) plan can help guide self-management.

The goal is to get and keep the asthma under good control, which includes minimal or no daily (including nighttime) symptoms; minimal or no exacerbations; no limitations on daily activities; no missed school or work; minimal use of short-acting β$_2$-agonists, such as albuterol; and minimal-to-no adverse effects from therapy. If these goals are met, reassess in 3 months and determine if you can "step down" to a less intense treatment regimen. If the symptoms are not being controlled, "step up" to a higher level of management and determine if the asthma can be better controlled.

Drug dosages are listed (Figure 13-8 on page 13-40), but for exams, you won't have to memorize specific dosages for most of the agents; in particular, you won't be responsible for remembering the "comparative" daily dosages for inhaled steroids.

Corticosteroids

Corticosteroids are the most effective antiinflammatory agents available for the treatment of asthma. They are formulated in oral, inhaled, and intravenous forms.

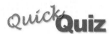
Quiz

- What is the preferred treatment for the prevention of exercise-induced bronchospasm?
- What do asthma action plans provide for the families of children with asthma?
- When do you consider stepping down controller therapy in a child with asthma?
- What are some long-term complications of prolonged use of systemic corticosteroids?
- What are some complications of prolonged use of inhaled steroids?
- Should long-acting beta-agonists be used for rescue therapy in acute asthma attacks?
- What does adding erythromycin to a patient's regimen that already includes theophylline potentially do to the theophylline level?

Unfortunately, long-term use of systemic (oral, IV) corticosteroids has many adverse effects.

Side effects of systemic corticosteroids include:

- Suppression of the hypothalamic-pituitary-adrenal axis (See below for clinical significance.)
- Immunosuppression
- Osteoporosis
- Cataracts
- Hyperglycemia
- Weight gain
- Thinning of the skin, easy bruisability
- Abdominal striae
- Growth retardation

You must closely monitor patients on chronic oral steroids and be prepared to give stress corticosteroid (hydrocortisone) with fever, acute infection, surgery, or other significant physiologic stressors. These patients are not able to mount an appropriate adrenal response due to suppression of the hypothalamic-pituitary-adrenal axis.

Prolonged use of inhaled steroids can cause some of these particular problems:

- Growth velocity changes.
- Dermal thinning and increased ease of skin bruising.
- Rarely, cataracts form and hypothalamic-pituitary-adrenal axis function is affected.
- Oral candidiasis (thrush) is common and can be prevented by using a spacer (valved holding chamber) with metered-dose inhalers and rinsing the mouth after inhalation.

Cromolyn Sodium

Cromolyn sodium is an antiinflammatory medication that stabilizes mast cell membranes, but its mechanism of action is not well understood. It is no longer available as an MDI (metered-dose inhaler) but continues to be available for nebulization. It has a very good safety profile, with only occasional side effects of cough, dermatitis, myositis, and gastroenteritis. It is listed as an alternative but is not preferred.

Salmeterol and Formoterol (Long-Acting Inhaled β_2-Agonists)

These 2 inhaled agents provide bronchodilatation for up to 12 hours. The caveat for these agents is that you do not use them to treat an acute exacerbation; their onset of action is much slower than albuterol or levalbuterol. In addition, do not use them as monotherapy. Formoterol has a faster onset of action than salmeterol.

Combination Therapy

Three drug combinations work synergistically against inflammation and muscle dysfunction. These include an inhaled corticosteroid and a long-acting β_2-agonist, which are available for use as asthma controllers:

- Fluticasone + salmeterol (Advair®)
- Budesonide + formoterol (Symbicort®)
- Mometasone + formoterol (Dulera®)

They are not indicated for treatment of acute bronchospasm.

Leukotriene Modifiers

The available leukotriene modifiers are montelukast and zafirlukast. They are biologically active fatty acids derived from the oxidative metabolism of arachidonic acid. They work by inhibiting leukotriene binding to receptors. Montelukast has efficacy in preventing exercise-induced asthma. Neurobehavioral side effects have been reported with montelukast.

Theophylline

Theophylline is a methylxanthine and requires serum monitoring of levels. (Serum concentrations of 5–15 mcg/mL are considered optimal.) It has a slow onset of action and is not recommended for acute therapy.

Theophylline has a narrow therapeutic range and significant toxicity beyond that range. Toxicity usually presents with tachycardia, GI symptoms, and behavioral effects. Drug-drug interactions can affect dosing: Oral contraceptives, erythromycin, ciprofloxacin, and cimetidine can increase serum blood levels, while phenobarbital and phenytoin can decrease serum theophylline levels.

Omalizumab

Omalizumab is an anti-IgE monoclonal antibody given intramuscularly to patients ≥ 12 years of age who have severe, difficult-to-control, allergic asthma. The dose is based on weight and serum IgE level. Omalizumab works by blocking IgE receptors and reducing allergic reactivity. It takes time to work but, in some patients, allows weaning of chronic systemic or high-dose inhaled corticosteroids.

NON-ASTHMA CAUSES OF WHEEZING AND / OR CHRONIC COUGH

FOREIGN BODY ASPIRATION

Toddlers frequently place objects in their mouths. Fortunately, aspiration is infrequent. The most commonly aspirated objects are seeds, nuts, and peanuts. Other common items include coins, hot dogs, small toys, balloons, jewelry, batteries, and firm vegetables. Materials most typically lodge in the right main or left main bronchi, but objects can pretty much go anywhere. The child presents with a sudden onset of choking or coughing followed by expiratory wheezing, dyspnea, or stridor—often with asymptomatic intervals. For unwitnessed aspiration, there is a delay of the diagnosis for more than a month in as many as 20% of cases.

Chest x-ray is very helpful even though most of these items are radiolucent. You see obstructive asymmetric hyperinflation in nearly 66% of children who have bronchial foreign bodies; however, note that 10–25% have a normal x-ray.

For children who are cyanotic, cannot breathe, and cannot get the foreign body up, consider a variety of techniques. For infants < 1 year of age, most recommend turning the infant over (face down) and forcefully giving 5 back blows. For children > 1 year of age, the Heimlich maneuver (subdiaphragmatic abdominal thrusts) is the 1st intervention. Never do a blind finger sweep. This can cause the object to go further back (as well as put you at risk for the "bite the doctor's finger off" scenario in the uncooperative child).

If the initial maneuvers are unsuccessful, perform a "jaw thrust." If the foreign body can be visualized, attempt to remove it with a Magill or other large forceps. If this fails and the child is unconscious or not breathing, establish a surgical airway distal to the obstruction.

Finally, if all the previous maneuvers fail, rigid endoscopy is performed by an experienced endoscopist to remove the foreign body.

BRONCHIOLITIS OBLITERANS / CRYPTOGENIC ORGANIZING PNEUMONIA

Bronchiolitis Obliterans

Bronchiolitis obliterans (BO) occurs when small bronchi and bronchioles are obstructed by intraluminal masses of fibrous tissue. This can be caused by a variety of disorders, but in children, it commonly occurs following a lower respiratory tract infection, particularly with adenovirus serotypes 3, 7, or 21. Children can become infected *in utero* or throughout childhood, but the highest incidence occurs between 6 months and 2 years of age. Children who have adenovirus pneumonitis have nearly a 33% risk of developing chronic lung disease; this increases to nearly 66% in some Native American populations! The incidence of BO has increased due to lung transplantation and also due to graft-versus-host disease that is seen in bone marrow transplant.

Typically, the infant recovers from the acute viral illness, only to have persistent (> 60 days) respiratory symptoms. Signs and symptoms include tachypnea, chronic cough, wheezing, and/or crackles and can coincide with failure to thrive. Bronchiolitis obliterans results in hypoxemia and hypercarbia because of poor gas exchange. Pulmonary edema becomes common over time. You must perform a lung biopsy to confirm the diagnosis.

Treatment is supportive, with oxygen and avoidance of another lung injury. Treat pulmonary edema with diuretics. Some advocate corticosteroids based on adult data showing improvement. If bronchiectasis is also present, airway clearance and secretion mobilization are useful.

Prognosis varies because some children improve by 8–10 years of age, while others develop debilitating chronic lung disease with the potential for respiratory failure and death.

Cryptogenic Organizing Pneumonia (COP)

In patients with COP (formerly known as bronchiolitis obliterans with organizing pneumonia or BOOP), the alveolar septa are thickened by a chronic inflammatory cell infiltrate, as well as the alveolar septa having Type II cell hyperplasia. In children, the cause is idiopathic, AIDS-related, or due to chemotherapy or post-BMT complications. Patients frequently present with numerous episodes of "bronchitis" that respond to antibiotics and then recur. There are usually multiple cycles of bronchitis followed by antibiotics before you make a diagnosis. Corticosteroids are beneficial and a positive response helps distinguish it from bronchiolitis obliterans. Diagnosis is confirmed by lung biopsy.

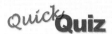

- Is omalizumab an appropriate therapy for a 6-year-old asthmatic child with mild disease?
- Is the CXR abnormal in all cases of foreign body aspiration?
- Which viruses most commonly cause bronchiolitis obliterans?
- How do you diagnose bronchiolitis obliterans?
- An adolescent presents with multiple episodes of "bronchitis" that clear with antibiotics and then recur in a month or two. He has had 6 episodes now. What diagnosis do you entertain?
- Is apnea of prematurity a risk factor for SIDS?
- Is prematurity itself a risk factor for SIDS?
- Which strategy has had the greatest impact on reducing incidences of SIDS?
- Does maternal smoking increase the risk of SIDS?

BRONCHIECTASIS

Bronchiectasis refers to "dilatation of the bronchi." The bronchi become damaged during an infection or inflammation and become distorted. Etiologies of bronchiectasis include cystic fibrosis, chronic aspiration, α_1-antitrypsin deficiency, dysmotile cilia syndromes, immune deficiencies, and allergic bronchopulmonary aspergillosis. Focal bronchiectasis can occur with retained foreign body or with severe infections, such as tuberculosis, pertussis, measles, *Mycoplasma*, or adenovirus. It is usually irreversible. The diagnostic criteria for bronchiectasis are based on radiographic features of chest high-resolution computerized tomography (c-HRCT), which is the gold standard for the diagnosis.

Bronchiectasis can be focal or generalized. Children present with a chronic productive cough and wheezing, and have recurrent infections. Clubbing of the fingers is very common (Image 13-13). Affected children have an obstructive pattern on spirometry and a pattern of air trapping on lung volumes with a normal or increased total lung capacity, increased functional residual capacity, and a reduced vital capacity. Areas of ventilation-perfusion mismatch are common.

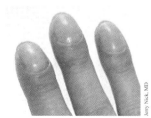
Image 13-13: Clubbing

Treatment includes bronchodilators with airway clearance. Sometimes chronic antibiotic therapy is required to control colonization or prevent recurrent infections.

SUDDEN INFANT DEATH SYNDROME (SIDS)

SIDS is defined as the sudden death of an infant < 1 year of age that remains unexplained after an intensive review, including a thorough autopsy, examination of the death scene, and review of the clinical history. In the U.S., SIDS is the 3rd leading cause of death in infants. (1st is congenital anomalies, and 2nd is prematurity-associated conditions.)

Note: Neither apnea of infancy nor apnea of prematurity is an independent risk factor for SIDS, but prematurity itself is a risk factor for SIDS. Make sure that all caregivers know basic CPR.

The SIDS death rate has decreased markedly since implementation of the "Back to Sleep" campaign, now known as the Safe to Sleep® campaign, which emphasizes placing infants on their backs to sleep. SIDS is a diagnosis of exclusion, and no specific etiology has been determined.

SIDS usually occurs between 1 and 6 months of life with a peak between 2 and 4 months of age. Boys are more commonly affected than girls. Evidence suggests that deaths can also occur while the infant is awake.

A higher incidence of SIDS is seen with:
- Prematurity
- Intrauterine growth restriction (IUGR)
- Winter months
- Hours between midnight and 8 a.m.
- Native American or African American ethnicity

Other higher risk factors include:
- Low socioeconomic status
- Young maternal age
- High parity
- Short interval between pregnancies
- Absent or late prenatal care
- Maternal UTI or STI
- Intrauterine cocaine or opiate exposure
- Smoking during pregnancy
- Secondhand smoke exposure after birth

There appears to be a slightly higher risk of SIDS in future siblings of SIDS infants.

Breastfed infants have a lower risk, as do children who have received their immunizations.

DROWNING AND SUBMERSION EVENTS

Drowning is the 2nd major cause of unintentional death in children in the U.S., and it is the leading cause of death in children < 5 years of age in the sun-drenched states of California, Florida, and Arizona. Drowning occurs in all age groups and is responsible for approximately

4,000 deaths per year in the U.S., with a mortality frequency of 12–18 deaths per million person-years.

Two peaks of submersion injury occur: < 5 years of age (related to bathtubs and unsupervised swimming pools) and 15–25-year-old males at lakes, beaches, and streams.

Hypoxia results in hypoxemia leading to tissue hypoxia and end-organ damage. Aspiration of fluid causes loss of surfactant and can produce pulmonary edema and acute respiratory distress syndrome (ARDS) with an often-normal initial chest x-ray. Sequelae depend on the degree of organ dysfunction, including neurologic, cardiovascular, metabolic, and renal.

Administer CPR, when indicated, with the knowledge that a cervical spinal cord injury may be present. Implement rescue breathing as soon as possible. Postural drainage has no role. Pulses are commonly weak and difficult to find in a hypothermic patient who has sinus bradycardia or atrial fibrillation. In general, chest compressions can be delayed for up to a minute to be sure a pulse is not present. If the victim is breathing, give oxygen; if not breathing, intubate. Rewarm all hypothermic patients with a core temperature of < 32° C (90° F). Remove wet clothing. Because hypothermia is neuroprotective, continue all efforts of resuscitation until the patient's core body temperature is 32–35° C (90–95° F); this can take up to several hours!

Some risk factors for poor prognosis include:

- Submersion > 10 minutes
- > 10 minutes elapsed before life support is begun at the scene
- Resuscitation takes > 25 minutes
- Age < 3 years
- Water temperature > 10° C (50° F)

There are no good early predictors of poor outcomes that can help determine when to discontinue resuscitation—normal neurologic recovery has occurred following prolonged submersion and hypoxia, especially in cold water. In contrast, 1 study shows that if there is no spontaneous, purposeful movements at 24 hours, then the outcome is very poor, with severe neurologic damage or death.

CYSTIC FIBROSIS

OVERVIEW

Cystic fibrosis (CF) is an autosomal recessive disorder involving a mutation of *CFTR* (CF transmembrane receptor, or the "CF gene") on the long arm of chromosome 7. The CF gene spans 256 Kb. The most common mutation (ΔF508) in the CF gene is a 3-base pair deletion that leads to the loss of a single phenylalanine at position 508. The ΔF508 mutation is present in nearly 80% of all CF cases, but homozygosity for this mutation is only about 50%. There are more than 1,000 other mutations identified at the CF locus! The resulting mutations cause abnormal ion transport across epithelial surfaces, including impermeable chloride channels and overactive sodium pumps. This results in viscid secretions in affected tissues and organs and further leads to blockage of ducts and air passages. The tissues most affected are the lungs, pancreas, intestinal mucous glands, liver, reproductive tracts, and sweat glands.

Median survival has increased from 10.6 years in 1966 to more than 37 years today, and almost 1/2 of all CF patients in the U.S. now are adults. In addition to aggressive therapy and good nutritional status, exercise appears to be an important factor. The patient's level of fitness, even more than pulmonary function, correlates with longer survival.

CLINICAL MANIFESTATIONS

Respiratory Tract

CF patients universally have pansinusitis, which is a helpful clue in a young child with persistent disease. Nasal polyps can occur in about 25% of patients with CF, and the finding of nasal polyps in a child under the age of 12 guides you toward CF as a possible diagnosis. Eventually, clubbing of the digits occurs in almost every patient with lung disease.

The lower respiratory tract is normal at birth. However, over time—with recurrent airway inflammation, chronic viscid mucus production, and recurrent infection—the child develops obstructive pulmonary disease. Initially, you may diagnose the child as having recurrent cough and wheezing with recurrent bronchiolitis, asthma, or pneumonia. Eventually, hyperinflation and crackles occur with the development of chronic diffuse bronchiectasis (Image 13-14). Finding decreased FEF_{25-75} can indicate early obstructive disease. The obstructive component can later be evidenced by finding

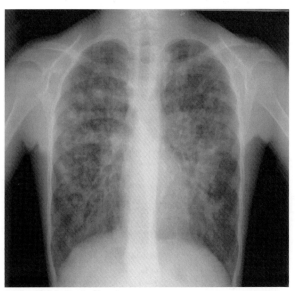

Image 13-14: Cystic fibrosis

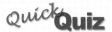

- What is the mode of inheritance for CF?
- Which gene is responsible for CF?
- Which factor correlates best with survival in CF patients?
- What sinus and nasal findings commonly occur in CF patients?
- Early in CF, which bacterial organisms are most likely to cause infection? What about later in CF?
- When does pancreatic insufficiency occur in CF?
- What GI findings are more common in CF?
- What is the abnormality of the sweat glands in patients with CF?
- What is the abnormality of the reproductive tract in males with CF?
- What is the laboratory test for diagnosing CF?

decreased FEV_1, decreased peak expiratory flow, and increased residual volume. Lung function testing is very helpful in following progression of the disease in the older child and adolescent.

Most patients with CF have chronic pulmonary infections with acute exacerbations. Early in the disease, the bacteria most commonly responsible for exacerbations are *Staphylococcus aureus*, *Haemophilus influenzae*, and common gram-negative organisms such as *Klebsiella*. Later, *Pseudomonas aeruginosa* becomes the predominant organism. The *Pseudomonas* in CF is characterized as being a more "mucoid" strain. Today, new pathogens have emerged as important in progressive pulmonary disease; these include *Aspergillus fumigatus*, *Burkholderia cepacia* species, *Alcaligenes xylosoxidans*, and *Stenotrophomonas maltophilia*. MRSA also has become an increasingly prominent pathogen; nationwide incidence has increased to nearly 20%. Interestingly, infection outside the respiratory tract is unusual.

The rate of progression of lung disease is variable for each child. Worse prognosis results from secondhand cigarette smoke and recurrent viral infections. Pulmonary complications can include pneumothorax, hemoptysis, atelectasis, pulmonary hypertension, cor pulmonale, and respiratory failure.

GI Tract

Pancreatic insufficiency is present at birth in 50% of children with CF. Although 90% have signs/symptoms of pancreatic insufficiency by 9 years of age, diagnosis is delayed in about 10% with CF who do not have GI disease. Exocrine pancreatic insufficiency manifests with maldigestion of fats and proteins, which results in malabsorption, steatorrhea, and FTT.

Patients with CF who present at birth (about 10–20%) frequently do so with bowel obstruction, which is manifested by meconium ileus. In childhood, an additional 20–25% have distal intestinal obstruction syndrome ([DIOS]; a.k.a. meconium ileus equivalent). About 20% have rectal prolapse during early childhood. Intussusception is much less common than the above manifestations in CF, but CF is 1 of the more common causes of intussusception in children > 1 year of age. Other GI disorders found with increased frequency in CF patients are GE reflux, cholelithiasis, focal biliary cirrhosis, and nonspecific steatosis of the liver. Frank cirrhosis with liver failure is rare in CF, as is portal hypertension and its complications, affecting 5–15% of patients.

Sweat Glands

Sweat glands in CF patients produce a very high salt content, which is a hallmark of the diagnosis. Sodium and chloride concentrations in a CF patient's sweat are > 60 mEq/L (normal is < 40 mEq/L). Infants can develop severe hyponatremia. Because of these findings, the sweat test is very helpful in diagnosing CF, even today with molecular genetics.

Reproductive Tract

Males with CF have atresia of the vas deferens, which results in obstructive azoospermia and sterility. Males can have children by using *in vitro* methods. Females have thick cervical mucus, which also results in decreased fertility. Because of poor nutrition and/or chronic illness, many children with CF have delayed puberty.

Other Tissues

Knee and other joint pain can occur in CF due to hypertrophic pulmonary osteoarthropathy. It appears on x-ray as periosteal thickening of the long bones and adjacent joints. A rare systemic vasculitis is described in CF with arthritis and a skin rash.

DIAGNOSIS

Diagnosis is 2-pronged:

1) At least 1 of the following is required:
   - Typical features of CF (pulmonary disease, exocrine pancreas deficiency, sweat salt loss syndrome, and/or male infertility)
   - CF in a sibling
   - Positive newborn screening test
2) Plus, 1 of the following is required:
   - Positive sweat test
   - Identification of 2 CF mutations known to cause CF
   - Abnormal nasal potential difference measurement

Because there are more than 1,000 mutations, it is still common for CF to be diagnosed with the sweat test. Sweat tests using quantitative iontophoresis done in "CF centers" are reliable. Typically, an infant > 36 weeks of gestation, 2 weeks of age, and > 2 kg are able to get adequate sweat. Those tests done outside a reliable testing center have a high risk for false-positive and false-negative results! There are numerous reasons for false-positive results (> 60 mEq/L) but only 3 for false-negative (< 40 mEq/L): laboratory error (most common), edema due to hypoproteinemia, and rare CF mutations that do not result in sweat gland abnormalities. Who should have a sweat test? Obviously, if FTT, steatorrhea, and chronic pulmonary disease are present, it is an easy decision. However, be suspicious of certain other findings; these are listed in Table 13-3. Many of these findings are "key word" clues to get you looking for CF! Be suspicious!

You can identify CF mutations by using blood, buccal brushings, or chorionic villous sampling. Most commercial labs look for 25–100 of the most common mutations, which can account for about 95% of all patients with CF. However, we know that 4% of the Caucasian population is heterozygous for the CF mutation, so finding one mutation does not rule in or rule out CF.

Table 13-3: Reasons to Consider Sweat Testing

GI pearls for testing:

Meconium ileus

Rectal prolapse

Prolonged neonatal jaundice

Chronic diarrhea

Steatorrhea

Respiratory pearls for testing:

Nasal polyps

Pansinusitis

Chronic cough

Recurrent wheezing

Staphylococcus aureus pneumonia

Finding *Pseudomonas* in throat, sputum, or bronchus cultures

Miscellaneous pearls for testing:

Digital clubbing

Family history of CF

FTT

"My baby tastes salty"

Male infertility

The nasal potential difference test measures the bioelectric voltage difference across nasal epithelium and is done only in a few CF centers.

Newborn screening for elevated blood immunoreactive trypsinogen (IRT) has become routine in all states. It has few false negatives but > 90% false positives. Depending on the state, if the IRT is abnormal, it is repeated or sent for mutation analysis. PCR testing for the most common mutations (ΔF508 in particular) has also been used.

TREATMENT OF CYSTIC FIBROSIS

Cystic Fibrosis Centers

Survival is greatest in children followed in a Cystic Fibrosis Foundation accredited CF care center.

Therapy for Pulmonary Disease

Airway clearance is a core therapy to manage and prevent airway obstruction. It is done using postural drainage and percussion and/or a percussive vest. In older children, devices generating positive expiratory pressure can also be used. Airway clearance is directed at all pulmonary segments at least 1–4 times/day routinely and is increased during exacerbations.

Exercise, particularly aerobic activities such as swimming and jogging, is beneficial. This can also help stimulate appetite.

Inhalational therapy can include bronchodilators, mucolytic agents (N-acetylcysteine, 7% hypertonic saline, recombinant human DNase), and antibiotics. Each of these may benefit the individual patient or may actually worsen the patient's symptoms; thus, each must be taken on a case-by-case basis.

The use of **prophylactic macrolide therapy** (azithromycin 1x/day, 3x/week) to reduce inflammation has shown to decrease exacerbations, decrease hospitalizations, improve pulmonary function, and result in small increases in weight. Additionally, high-dose ibuprofen is being used by some because of its antiinflammatory effects.

Corticosteroids have been shown to be beneficial in some trials but have obvious side effects and drawbacks. While inhaled corticosteroids benefit those who have asthma as well, they are not recommended for routine use in all CF patients.

Antibiotics have probably provided the greatest benefit in prognosis. Treatment of exacerbations with anti-staphylococcal and anti-pseudomonal drugs is paramount. Once *Pseudomonas* is established, it is almost impossible to get rid of it. However, there is some success in temporary eradication of newly acquired *Pseudomonas* using inhaled tobramycin. It is particularly bad if a mucoid form establishes itself. Quinolone use in CF is widespread, and data to date has not shown significant bony or cartilage abnormalities.

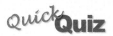

COMPLICATIONS

Pneumothorax

Pneumothorax (Image 13-15) occurs in about 10% of CF patients and can be a common cause of chest pain. Many small pneumothoraces resolve with bedrest and oxygen therapy, but some require chest tube placement; a majority of patients have recurrence. Having a pneumothorax is typically a poor prognostic sign of severe lung disease. Prevention of recurrences is aided by the use of open thoracotomy through a small subaxillary incision, excision of apical blebs, stripping the apical pleura, and manual abrasion of the remaining accessible pleura. A caveat is that some transplant centers view surgical or chemical ablation of pleura as a relative contraindication for lung transplant.

Hemoptysis

Hemoptysis involving blood-streaked sputum is quite common with bronchiectasis associated with CF, particularly during pulmonary exacerbations. Massive hemoptysis is defined as acute bleeding of > 240 mL within 24 hours or recurrent bleeding of > 100 mL daily for several days. The guidelines recommend suspension of all chest physiotherapy in the event of massive hemoptysis. Massive hemoptysis occurs in only about 5–10% of patients and is rarely significant enough to require transfusions or other interventions. If hemoptysis occurs, it is usually due to infection, so treatment of the exacerbation with IV antibiotics and other routine management of the current exacerbation is the best therapy.

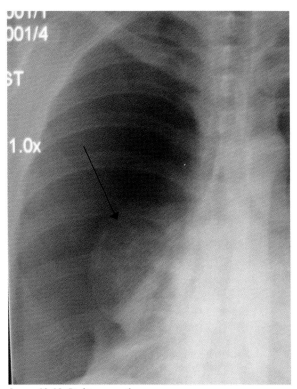

Image 13-15: Right pneumothorax

Quick Quiz

- Who should get a sweat test?
- Is ceftriaxone acceptable therapy for *Pseudomonas*?
- Does the finding of a pneumothorax suggest more severe lung disease in a CF patient?

Use of antibiotics varies from center to center and patient to patient, but 3 general categories emerge:

1) Use of continuous (often cycled) **prophylactic antibiotics** (inhaled or oral) with addition of IV antibiotics for acute exacerbations
2) **No antibiotics** except with exacerbations
3) **Aggressive antibiotics** (oral, aerosol, or IV) based on sputum cultures, for 2–3 weeks every 1–2 months for patients with any evidence of pulmonary disease

In many centers, oral antibiotics are given at the 1st sign of pulmonary exacerbation. Aerosolized antibiotics, typically tobramycin or aztreonam, can be useful as therapy to keep *Pseudomonas* colonization from causing an exacerbation or to treat in the midst of an acute exacerbation. IV antibiotics are indicated when the patient either does not respond to outpatient therapy or else presents with a moderate-to-severe exacerbation. Antibiotic choices include the aminoglycosides (frequently tobramycin is used followed by gentamicin or amikacin), semisynthetic antipseudomonal penicillins (ticarcillin, ticarcillin-clavulanate, piperacillin-tazobactam), imipenem or meropenem, ceftazidime, aztreonam, quinolones, and (rarely) colistin. Note: Do not use ceftriaxone for *Pseudomonas*. Intravenous therapy is continued until the patient has clinically improved or reached a new plateau of functioning. This commonly takes 2–3 weeks but can take longer.

The 1st therapy targeting the basic cellular defect, ivacaftor (Kalydeco®), is available. It is a targeted *CFTR* function potentiator for individuals with *G551D* and several other similar gating-type mutations. In July 2015, the FDA approved Orkambi®, a combination of ivacaftor and lumacaftor (*CFTR* corrector), to treat the most common cause of *CFTR* mutation, which is 2 copies of *F508del*. It is approved for patients ≥ 12 years of age. It works by correcting the misfolded CFTR protein. Patients have demonstrated improved lung function with the drug. The dosage is 2 tablets every 12 hours taken with fatty foods.

End-stage lung disease is the most common cause of death in CF and is an indication for bilateral lung transplantation. CF is the most common reason for lung transplantation in children.

CF patients can have malabsorption of fat-soluble vitamins, so consider vitamin K deficiency if there is hemoptysis (often with other signs of abnormal blood loss such as melena, mucosal bleeding, and easy bruisability). This can be seen with CF-related liver disease and in those with pancreatic insufficiency not taking vitamin K supplement.

Pulmonary Hypertension

Pulmonary hypertension with the development of cor pulmonale and enlargement of the right ventricle is seen in late CF. Heart failure with peripheral edema and hepatomegaly are poor prognostic signs and usually indicate survival of < 8 months. Standard therapy of oxygen, fluid restriction, and diuretics is beneficial; do not use digitalis unless there is accompanying left ventricular dysfunction. Combined heart-lung transplant is sometimes used in CF patients with cor pulmonale and severe lung disease.

Nutritional Abnormalities

Growth with normal weight-to-height ratio has been shown to be an important prognostic factor in keeping CF patients' lung function healthy. Thus, nutritional efforts are aggressive in helping these patients gain weight and encouraging them with sound nutritional guidance. Use of pancreatic enzyme replacement is a cornerstone of therapy for pancreatic insufficiency (PI). Dosages of enzymes must be titrated to the individual patient. H_2 blockers may enhance the bioavailability of the enzymes. Supplementation with fat soluble vitamins, A, D, E, and K are necessary for those with PI. Most patients with CF require 100–150% of the RDA for their age, even with control of malabsorption. For those patients who have difficulty gaining weight, a high-fat diet and oral nutritional supplements can be beneficial. Some patients cannot keep up with the daily intake needed to gain weight and require nighttime enteral feeds to provide enough calories.

Abdominal complaints are common in patients with CF. Constipation is a recurrent complaint. Chronic constipation can lead to distal intestinal obstruction syndrome (DIOS), so institute active therapy to relieve constipation. Lactulose and polyethylene glycol 3350 (MiraLAX®, GlycoLax®) are used to prevent chronic constipation. If DIOS occurs, treat with polyethylene glycol with added electrolytes (GoLYTELY®, CoLyte®) orally (if obstruction has not yet occurred), or hyperosmolar enemas, such as meglumine diatrizoate. Rectal prolapse can typically be reversed with gentle manual pressure and control of malabsorption.

Another complication of CF that is more common with age is CF-related glucose impairment and diabetes mellitus. While patients do not develop acute ketoacidosis, their inability to use glucose well contributes to malnutrition and increased infection risk. Insulin, rather than carbohydrate restriction, is indicated for those with significant hyperglycemia given the high calorie demands and concurrent pancreatic insufficiency. The Cystic Fibrosis Foundation recommends annual oral glucose tolerance testing for CF patients $\geq$ 10 years of age.

PRIMARY CILIARY DYSKINESIA

OVERVIEW

The prevalence of primary ciliary dyskinesia (PCD) is approximately 1:15,000–20,000. Most cases of PCD have an autosomal recessive inheritance pattern. Normally, cilia beat synchronously at 7–22 times per second. Any impairment with the beat or the synchrony can result in poor mucociliary clearance and subsequent recurrent episodes of upper and lower respiratory tract infections. Half of the patients with PCD have Kartagener syndrome (see next). Definitive diagnosis of PCD can be challenging and requires referral to specialized centers with expertise on this disease. There are different tests to assess ciliary motility, ciliary ultrastructure (sample is obtained from nasal or bronchial brush biopsy), nasal nitric oxide measurement, mucociliary clearance, and genetic defects. Genetic studies are recommended.

Treatment of these syndromes is the same as for bronchiectasis, consisting of chest physiotherapy and occasionally requiring antimicrobial treatment in the presence of bacterial overgrowth.

Prognosis is good for those with cilia-related symptoms; most have a normal lifespan.

KARTAGENER SYNDROME

Kartagener syndrome occurs when one or both dynein arms of the cilia are absent. It presents with recurrent infections (i.e., sinusitis, otitis, pneumonia), bronchiectasis, situs inversus, and reduced male fertility. It can be sporadic or familial in character and is autosomal recessive.

α_1-ANTITRYPSIN DEFICIENCY

OVERVIEW

α_1-antitrypsin deficiency (AATD) rarely causes pulmonary symptoms in children, and it typically does not manifest until the 5th decade of life. Like most enzyme deficiency disorders, α_1-antitrypsin deficiency is autosomal recessive; parents are frequently asymptomatic carriers, and the family history is often negative for the disease.

Suspect homozygous α_1-antitrypsin deficiency in nonsmokers with early-onset emphysema with lower lobe predominance. Know that about 15% of persons with the homozygote Pi^{ZZ} phenotype also get progressive liver fibrosis and cirrhosis—the manifestation most likely to be seen in children. With this type of cirrhosis,

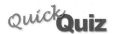

- Which vitamin deficiency do you consider in a CF patient who has hemoptysis with heavy bleeding and a history of easy bruisability?
- What is Kartagener syndrome?
- What pulmonary abnormalities are seen with α$_1$-antitrypsin deficiency?
- What liver abnormalities are seen in children with α$_1$-antitrypsin deficiency?

as with cirrhosis of any cause, there is an increased incidence of hepatoma.

Heterozygotes have no increase in pulmonary disease unless they smoke—in which case it can present similarly to homozygotes.

DIAGNOSIS

Test patients with persistent airflow obstruction on spirometry. Additional features that lead clinicians to test for severe α$_1$-antitrypsin deficiency include:

- Emphysema in a young individual (age ≤ 45 years)
- Emphysema in a nonsmoker or very light smoker
- Emphysema characterized by predominant basilar changes on the chest radiograph
- A family history of emphysema and/or liver disease
- Clinical findings or history of panniculitis
- Clinical findings or history of unexplained chronic liver disease

Testing includes measurement of AAT levels by rocket immunoelectrophoresis, radial immunodiffusion, or nephelometry. Those with lower levels of serum or plasma AAT levels should undergo genetic testing.

TREATMENT

Treatment is with IV α$_1$-antitrypsin. When the emphysema is severe, refer for lung transplantation.

HEMOPTYSIS

OVERVIEW

Hemoptysis is the presence of blood in the sputum or the spitting up of blood; it is rare in children ≤ 6 years of age because they generally swallow their sputum.

The most common causes in children are infection, foreign bodies, and bronchiectasis (sometimes from cystic fibrosis). Rarer causes include vasculitides such as HSP, granulomatosis with polyangiitis ([GPA]; formerly Wegener's), Goodpasture syndrome, SLE, congenital heart and lung defects, neoplasm, AV malformation, hemangioma, trauma, pulmonary embolism, and idiopathic pulmonary hemosiderosis (IPH).

Evaluate by localizing the bleeding source if possible. Is it gastrointestinal in origin? (Look for coffee-ground appearance or food.) Or, is it respiratory tract in origin? (Is it bright red or rust colored, "frothy," or mixed with sputum?) Check the mouth and nasal passages for any lacerations or lesions.

Other signs/symptoms that are helpful in determining the etiology:

- Fever or chills: pneumonia, lung abscess
- Illicit drug use: cocaine smoking
- Microscopic hematuria: GPA or Goodpasture's
- Skin telangiectasia: pulmonary AV malformation (with hereditary hemorrhagic telangiectasia [HHT])
- Recurrent nose bleeds: HHT or GPA
- Clubbing: chronic lung disease or congenital heart disease

Do a chest radiograph in the initial evaluation; however, up to 33% of patients have a normal CXR. Bronchoscopy with bronchoalveolar lavage (BAL) is the next step after bleeding is controlled; the finding of hemosiderin-laden macrophages is diagnostic for a pulmonary source of bleeding—they usually appear 3 days after bleeding. If the BAL is positive or there are suspicious findings on CXR, proceed to chest CT with contrast (or CTA) if the diagnosis is not clear. An echocardiogram is recommended in cases of pulmonary hemorrhage. If the echocardiogram is normal, look for pulmonary-renal syndromes, bleeding abnormalities, or suspect idiopathic pulmonary hemosiderosis (see next). Lung biopsy is done in most children with diffuse alveolar hemorrhage.

Management of most cases of hemoptysis is supportive because a majority of cases with mild hemoptysis resolve spontaneously and do not recur. Treat major hemoptysis with hemostasis and embolotherapy. This requires specialist intervention. Other therapy depends on the underlying cause.

IDIOPATHIC PULMONARY HEMOSIDEROSIS (IPH)

Hemosiderosis is rare, but it appears in the content specifications of the ABP; so we cover it here briefly. Recurrent pulmonary bleeding (alveolar hemorrhage in particular) can eventually cause pulmonary hemosiderosis. When no underlying etiology for repeated hemorrhages occurs, it is called idiopathic pulmonary hemosiderosis (IPH).

Children usually present before the age of 10 years with either abrupt hemoptysis or a progressive course of anemia, dyspnea, fatigue, and recurrent cough. Most patients present with iron deficiency anemia. There can be a restrictive pattern on lung function testing with the development of pulmonary fibrosis.

Sputum or bronchoalveolar lavage show hemosiderin-laden macrophages.

Confirm diagnosis with lung biopsy and to exclude other specific pathology. Other conditions to be excluded include vasculitis, granulomatous lung disease, or autoimmune disease.

Use corticosteroids in acute episodes, as well as chronically for patients with regular symptoms, but the response varies. If there is not a good response, use other immunosuppressants. Children generally have a more rapid course and poorer prognosis than adults.

INTERSTITIAL LUNG DISEASES (ILDs)

LYMPHOCYTIC INTERSTITIAL PNEUMONIA

Lymphocytic interstitial pneumonitis ([LIP]; a.k.a. lymphoid interstitial pneumonia) is the most commonly described ILD in children. Pathogenesis is unknown, but it appears to have 2 general causes:

1) An exaggerated response to inhaled antigens in a child with another autoimmune dysfunction

2) As a result of a primary infection with a virus such as HIV or EBV

LIP, as an exaggerated immune response, is seen in many autoimmune diseases.

LIP is commonly seen in children with a perinatally acquired HIV infection—with over 25% of these children developing it, usually at 2–3 years of age. LIP is considered an AIDS-defining illness in children. It is also associated with EBV and HTLV-1.

Patients with LIP present with dyspnea, cough, and fever. Chest x-ray shows a bibasilar infiltrate.

Treatment is supportive with oxygen, immunosuppressives (typically corticosteroids), and cytotoxic drugs as necessary.

SARCOIDOSIS

Sarcoidosis is a chronic multisystem disorder of unknown origin that affects young adults and, rarely, children. It is characterized by noncaseating epithelioid cell granulomas, which have a predilection for thoracic lymph nodes and lung tissue.

Chest x-ray findings are variable. Usually, there is bilateral hilar and/or mediastinal adenopathy +/– reticulonodular or alveolar infiltrates. Hilar adenopathy alone or in combination with parenchymal infiltrates is found in 40–60% of children with sarcoidosis. The radiographic staging of sarcoidosis (Table 13-4) illustrates the interesting point that hilar adenopathy disappears as the disease progresses. Pulmonary function tests (PFTs) are either normal or

show restrictive +/– obstructive mechanics. Serum angiotensin-converting enzyme (SACE) level is nonspecific and is considered of no use in diagnosis, but is sometimes useful for monitoring progression of disease (controversial). If the SACE level was previously elevated when the disease was active and low when inactive, it may be useful in determining if the disease is once again active. Hypercalcemia, hypercalciuria, and hypergammaglobulinemia are seen.

Sarcoidosis is a diagnosis of exclusion. It is imperative to exclude the other granulomatous diseases, including hypersensitivity pneumonitis, berylliosis, and infectious diseases caused by mycobacteria and fungi. Do a biopsy and obtain material for histological examination and culture. The best method for diagnosing sarcoidosis is by fiberoptic bronchoscopy with transbronchial or bronchial wall biopsies showing noncaseating granuloma.

Erythema nodosum is an associated skin lesion that denotes a good prognosis! Perform a slit-lamp exam on all patients with sarcoidosis to look for asymptomatic uveitis, which can lead to blindness.

Overall, 75% of sarcoid patients recover without treatment. It rarely progresses to pulmonary fibrosis or pulmonary hypertension. Treat severe disease with corticosteroids. Corticosteroids do not induce remissions in sarcoidosis, although they do decrease the symptoms and PFTs improve. Inhaled corticosteroids decrease the respiratory symptoms and are an alternative to systemic corticosteroids if the disease is primarily in the bronchi.

Indications for systemic corticosteroids:

- Involvement of eyes
- Heart conduction abnormalities
- CNS involvement
- Severe pulmonary symptoms
- Severe skin lesions
- Persistent hypercalcemia

Other medications include methotrexate and hydroxychloroquine. Consider those with end-stage lung disease for lung transplant.

PULMONARY ALVEOLAR PROTEINOSIS

In children, most cases of pulmonary alveolar proteinosis (PAP) result from a genetic or acquired defect in surfactant metabolism (including surfactant

Table 13-4: Radiographic Staging of Sarcoidosis	
Stage	**Chest X-Ray Findings**
0	Clear lung fields, no adenopathy
I	Bilateral hilar adenopathy
II	Adenopathy + parenchymal infiltrates
III	Diffuse parenchymal infiltrates
IV	Fibrosis, bullae, cavities

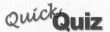

- What does the CXR characteristically show in sarcoidosis?
- What does the biopsy of an affected bronchial wall in sarcoidosis show?
- What collagen vascular disease causes pulmonary hypertension out of proportion to the pulmonary disease noted?
- Which laboratory test is positive in many patients with GPA?

protein mutations, lysinuric protein intolerance, and GM-CSF receptor mutations), leading to a buildup of proteinaceous material in the airways. Similar to cases in adults, acquired causes include infections, malignancies, immunodeficiencies, or exposure to inhaled chemicals or minerals, such as in silicosis.

Severity of cases can range from severe respiratory failure in neonatal forms to chronic interstitial lung disease in older children. Poor weight gain, fatigue, chronic cough with gelatinous sputum, and exercise intolerance are common. Often, patients are hypoxemic from a large right-to-left shunt because gas exchange is impaired secondary to clogged alveoli.

Diagnosis is usually confirmed with open lung biopsy, which shows intact alveolar walls and alveoli that are filled with fatty material.

Treatment depends on the underlying cause: If severe, a whole lung lavage is done under general anesthesia to remove proteinaceous material. Some patients experience long-term resolution, while others have recurrent problems. GM-CSF is a treatment that may restore proper alveolar macrophage function.

THE LUNGS IN AUTOIMMUNE DISEASES

OVERVIEW

Clinically significant pulmonary involvement due to systemic inflammatory disease is rare in the pediatrics setting. However, when present, it can indicate high morbidity and mortality in this population, and pulmonary disease is the predominant initial clinical presentation in some patients.

Systemic lupus erythematosus (SLE) causes painful pleuritis +/– effusion, but additionally, it causes diffuse atelectasis and sometimes diaphragmatic weakness—and, therefore, orthopneic dyspnea out of proportion to the chest x-ray findings, although the chest x-ray sometimes shows elevated diaphragms. SLE also occasionally causes hemoptysis similar to that in idiopathic pulmonary hemosiderosis (IPH). SLE affects

both lung and pleura more frequently than any other collagen vascular disease (60%), while scleroderma affects the lung alone more than any other collagen vascular disease (100%! but no pleural changes). So, not much in the way of ILD with SLE!

Scleroderma has 2 lung effects:

1) Interstitial fibrosis (as just mentioned)

2) Intimal proliferation

Intimal proliferation in the pulmonary artery causes pulmonary hypertension out of proportion to the pulmonary disease. So, it is not the ILD but the intimal proliferation that causes the real pulmonary problem in scleroderma patients. Scleroderma is often associated with pneumonia.

Sjögren's causes desiccation of the airways and is also associated with lymphocytic interstitial pneumonia (LIP).

GRANULOMATOSIS WITH POLYANGIITIS

Granulomatosis with polyangiitis ([GPA]; formerly Wegener's), is a systemic vasculitis with necrotizing granulomas, which affects both the upper respiratory tract (nose and sinuses) and the lower respiratory tract (with pulmonary vasculitis).

GPA can also cause necrotizing glomerulonephritis, although the disease is sometimes limited to the lungs.

Remember: sinus, lungs, kidneys. Consider GPA in any exam question scenario focusing on a patient with purulent nasal discharge, epistaxis, and/or signs of a glomerulonephritis with hematuria. The patient is typically not dyspneic and may or may not have a nonproductive cough or hemoptysis.

c-ANCA (**c**ytoplasmic **a**nti**n**eutrophil **c**ytoplasmic **a**ntibody—thought to be a destructive autoantibody) is often used as an adjunctive test. It is about 90% sensitive and 90% specific. When positive in a patient with GPA, it is virtually always c-ANCA (96%), whereas polyarteritis is usually p-ANCA positive.

You can confirm diagnosis from either a biopsy of the nasal membrane or an open lung biopsy. A kidney biopsy is not part of the diagnostic workup because it does not always show the granulomas and is much more invasive. Treatment of GPA: cyclophosphamide with or without corticosteroids.

ANTIGLOMERULAR BASEMENT MEMBRANE ANTIBODY DISEASE (GOODPASTURE SYNDROME)

Antiglomerular basement membrane antibody disease is an autoimmune disease. It tends to present in young adult males with a male-to-female ratio of 3:1. Lung disease is the same as IPH (see IPH on page 13-29), but Goodpasture syndrome also affects the kidneys. Typically, there is no frank hemorrhage, but often there is hemoptysis that precedes renal abnormalities. Think of this disease if the patient presents with dyspnea, hemoptysis, iron deficiency anemia, and glomerulonephritis, but without the upper airway signs that are seen in GPA.

Symptoms are due to antiglomerular basement membrane antibodies, which result in linear deposition of IgG and C3 on alveolar and glomerular basement membranes.

Like patients with IPH, patients with Goodpasture syndrome can also have iron deficiency anemia. These patients are usually ANCA negative.

Treat with immunosuppressives and plasmapheresis. If the patient does have severe pulmonary hemorrhages, nephrectomy may help.

FOR FURTHER READING

[Guidelines in blue]

CONGENITAL DISORDERS OF THE UPPER AND LOWER RESPIRATORY TRACT

Abel RM, et al (eds.). *Kendig & Chernick's Disorders of the Respiratory Tract in Children*, 8th edition. Chapter 21, 317–357. Philadelphia, PA: Elsevier Saunders. 2012.

Ahmad SM, Soliman AM. Congenital anomalies of the larynx. *Otolaryngol Clin North Am.* 2007 Feb;40(1):177–191, viii.

Arens C, et al. Clinical and morphological aspects of laryngeal cysts. *Eur Arch Otorhinolaryngol.* 1997;254(9–10):430–436.

Barthod G, Teissier N, et al. Fetal airway management on placental support: limitations and ethical considerations in seven cases. *J Obstet Gynaecol.* 2013 Nov;33(8):787–794.

Coran, AG, et al (eds.). *Pediatric Surgery*, 7th Ed. Chapter 55. Philadelphia, PA: Elsevier Saunders. 2012.

Coran, AG, et al (eds.). *Pediatric Surgery*, 7th Ed. Chapter 58. Philadelphia, PA: Elsevier Saunders. 2012.

Corbett HJ, Humphrey GM. Pulmonary sequestration. *Paediatr Respir Rev.* 2004 Mar;5(1):59–68.

Gupta M, Motwani G. Lingual thyroid. *Ear Nose Throat J.* 2009 Jun;88(6):e1.

Ida JB, Thompson DM. Pediatric stridor. *Otolaryngol Clin North Am.* 2014 Oct;47(5):795–819.

Miyamoto RC, et al. Association of anterior glottic webs with velocardiofacial syndrome (chromosome 22q11.2 deletion). *Otolaryngol Head Neck Surg.* 2004 Apr;130(4):415–417.

Sakai N, et al. Oral-facial-digital syndrome type II (Mohr syndrome): clinical and genetic manifestations. *J Craniofac Surg.* 2002 Mar;13(2):321–326.

Sameer KS, et al. Lingual thyroglossal duct cysts—a review. *Int J Pediatr Otorhinolaryngol.* 2012 Feb;76(2):165–168.

Segal LM, et al. Prevalence, diagnosis, and treatment of ankyloglossia: methodologic review. *Can Fam Physician.* 2007 Jun;53(6):1027–1033.

Kliegman RM, et al (eds.). *Nelson's Textbook of Pediatrics*, 19th Ed. Chapter 302, 1252–1253. Philadelphia, PA: Elsevier Saunders. 2012.

Toriello HV, Franco B. Oral-facial-digital syndrome type I. 2002 Jul 24 [Updated 2010 Oct 14]. In: Pagon RA, Bird TD, et al., editors. *GeneReviews™* [Internet]. Seattle (WA): University of Washington, Seattle; 1993–2015.

Vasileiadis I, et al. Internal laryngopyocele as a cause of acute airway obstruction: an extremely rare case and review of the literature. *Acta Otorhinolaryngol Ital.* 2012 Feb;32(1):58–62.

CHEST WALL AND RESPIRATORY MUSCLE DISEASES

Baxter P. Diagnosis and management of Duchenne muscular dystrophy. *Dev Med Child Neurol.* 2010 Apr;52(4):313.

Birnkrant DJ, Bushby KM, et al. The respiratory management of patients with duchenne muscular dystrophy: a DMD care considerations working group specialty article. *Pediatr Pulmonol.* 2010 Aug;45(8):739–748.

Chavhan GB, et al. Multimodality imaging of the pediatric diaphragm: anatomy and pathologic conditions. *Radiographics.* 2010 Nov;30(7):1797–1817.

Koumbourlis AC. Chest Wall Abnormalities and their Clinical Significance in Childhood. *Paediatr Respir Rev.* 2014 Sep;15(3):246–255.

Poyner SE, Bradshaw WT. Jeune syndrome: considerations for management of asphyxiating thoracic dystrophy. *Neonatal Netw.* 2013 Sep–Oct;32(5):342–352.

INFECTIONS OF THE NOSE, PHARYNX, AND UPPER RESPIRATORY TRACT

Choi J, Lee GL. Common pediatric respiratory emergencies. *Emerg Med Clin North Am.* 2012 May;30(2):529–563, x.

Hsin CH, Chen TH, et al. Aspiration technique improves reliability of endoscopically directed middle meatal cultures in pediatric rhinosinusitis. *Am J Rhinol Allergy.* 2010 May–Jun;24(3):205–209.

Magit, A. Pediatric Rhinosinusitis, *Otolaryngol Clin N Am.* 47(2014): 733–746.

Oomen KP, Modi VK, et al. Evidence-based practice: pediatric tonsillectomy. *Otolaryngol Clin North Am.* 2012 Oct;45(5):1071–1081.

Kimberlin DW, et al. *Red Book®: 2015 Report of the Committee on Infectious Diseases*, 30th Ed. American Academy of Pediatrics, 2015.

Baugh RF, et al. Clinical practice guideline: tonsillectomy in children. *Otolaryngol Head Neck Surg.* 2011 Jan;144 (1 Suppl):S1–S30.

Karmazyn B, Coley BD, et al, ACR Appropriateness Criteria® sinusitis–child. [online publication]. American College of Radiology (ACR). 2012.

Wald ER, Applegate KE, et al; American Academy of Pediatrics. Clinical practice guideline for the diagnosis and management of acute bacterial sinusitis in children aged 1 to 18 years. Pediatrics. 2013 Jul;132(1):e262–280.

INFECTIONS OF THE LOWER RESPIRATORY TRACT

Agarwal R. Allergic bronchopulmonary aspergillosis. *Chest.* 2009 Mar;135(3):805–826.

Iroh Tam PY. Approach to common bacterial infections: community-acquired pneumonia. *Pediatr Clin North Am*. 2013 Apr;60(2):437–453.

Ledford DK, Lockey RF. Asthma and comorbidities. *Curr Opin allergy Clin Immunol*. 2013 Feb;13(1):78–86.

Abel RM, et al (eds.). *Kendig & Chernick's Disorders of the Respiratory Tract in Children*, 8th Ed. Chapter 34, 531–544. Philadelphia, PA: Elsevier Saunders. 2012.

American Academy of Pediatrics Committee On Infectious Diseases And Bronchiolitis Guidelines Committee, Updated Guidance for Palivizumab Prophylaxis Among Infants and Young Children at Increased Risk of Hospitalization for Respiratory Syncytial Virus Infection. *Pediatrics*. 2014 Aug 1;134(2):415–420.

American Academy of Pediatrics. Management of community-acquired pneumonia (CAP) in infants and children older than 3 months of age. *Pediatrics*. 2011;128:e1677.

Bradley JS, et al. Executive summary: the management of community-acquired pneumonia in infants and children older than 3 months of age: clinical practice guidelines by the Pediatric Infectious Diseases Society and the Infectious Diseases Society of America. *Clin Infect Dis*. 2011 Oct;53(7):617–630.

ASTHMA

National Heart, Lung, and Blood Institute; National Asthma Education and Prevention Program. Expert panel report 3: guidelines for the diagnosis and management of asthma, 2007.

NON-ASTHMA CAUSES OF WHEEZING AND / OR CHRONIC COUGH

Al-Ghanem S, et al. Bronchiolitis obliterans organizing pneumonia: pathogenesis, clinical features, imaging and therapy review. *Ann Thorac Med*. 2008 Apr–Jun;3(2):67–75.

Campos MA, Lascano J. α1 Antitrypsin deficiency: current best practice in testing and augmentation therapy. *Ther Adv Respir Dis*. 2014 Oct;8(5):150–161.

Cordier JF. Cryptogenic organising pneumonia. *Eur Respir J*. 2006 Aug;28(2):422–446.

Knowles MR, Daniels LA, et al. Primary ciliary dyskinesia. Recent advances in diagnostics, genetics, and characterization of clinical disease. Am *J Respir Crit Care Med*. 2013 Oct 15;188(8):913–922.

Popatia R, Haver K, et al. Primary Ciliary Dyskinesia: An Update on New Diagnostic Modalities and Review of the Literature. *Pediatr Allergy Immunol Pulmonol*. 2014 Jun 1;27(2):51–59.

Stockley RA. Alpha1-antitrypsin review. *Clin Chest Med*. 2014 Mar;35(1):39–50.

CYSTIC FIBROSIS

Comeau AM, Accurso FJ, et al; Cystic Fibrosis Foundation. Guidelines for implementation of cystic fibrosis newborn screening programs: Cystic Fibrosis Foundation workshop report. *Pediatrics*. 2007 Feb;119(2):e495–518.

Flume PA, Mogayzel PJ Jr, et al, and the Clinical Practice Guidelines for Pulmonary Therapies Committee. Cystic Fibrosis Pulmonary Guidelines: Treatment of Pulmonary Exacerbations. *Am. J. Respir. Crit. Care Med*. 2009 Nov;180(9):802–808.

Flume PA, Mogayzel PJ Jr, et al; Clinical Practice Guidelines for Pulmonary Therapies Committee; Cystic Fibrosis Foundation Pulmonary Therapies Committee. Cystic fibrosis pulmonary guidelines: pulmonary complications: hemoptysis and pneumothorax. *Am J Respir Crit Care Med*. 2010 Aug 1;182(3):298–306.

LeGrys VA, Yankaskas JR, et al; Cystic Fibrosis Foundation. Diagnostic sweat testing: the Cystic Fibrosis Foundation guidelines. *J Pediatr*. 2007 Jul;151(1):85–89.

Mogayzel PJ Jr, Naureckas ET, et al; Pulmonary Clinical Practice Guidelines Committee. Cystic fibrosis pulmonary guidelines. Chronic medications for maintenance of lung health. *Am J Respir Crit Care Med*. 2013 Apr 1;187(7): 680–689.

INTERSTITIAL LUNG DISEASES (ILDs)

Antoniou KM, et al. Pivotal clinical dilemmas in collagen vascular diseases associated with interstitial lung involvement. *Eur Respir J*. 2009 Apr;33(4):882–896.

de Blic J. Pulmonary alveolar proteinosis in children. *Paediatr Respir Rev*. 2004 Dec;5(4):316–322.

Kurland G, Deterding RR, et al; American Thoracic Society Committee on Childhood Interstitial Lung Disease (chILD) and the chILD Research Network. An official American Thoracic Society clinical practice guideline: classification, evaluation, and management of childhood interstitial lung disease in infancy. *Am J Respir Crit Care Med*. 2013 Aug 1;188(3):376–394.

RESPIRATORY DISORDERS

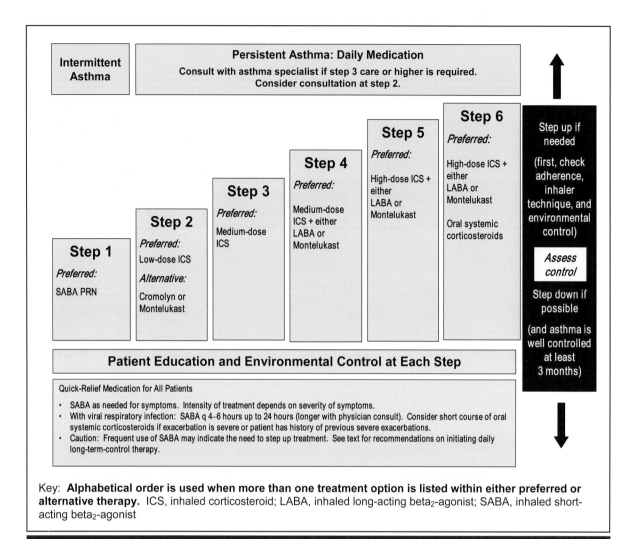

Figure 13-2: Stepwise Approach for Managing Asthma in Children 0–4 Years of Age

Source for Figures 13-2 through 13-10: Expert Panel Report 3: Guidelines for Diagnosis and Management of Asthma, by National Asthma Education and Prevention Program (NAEPP) Coordinating Committee/National Heart, Lung, and Blood Institute (NHLBI) of the National Institutes of Health (NIH) (Updated 2007).

Intermittent Asthma	**Persistent Asthma: Daily Medication** Consult with asthma specialist if step 4 care or higher is required. Consider consultation at step 3.

Step 1

Preferred:

SABA PRN

Step 2

Preferred:

Low-dose ICS

Alternative:

Cromolyn, LTRA, Nedocromil, or Theophylline

Step 3

Preferred:

EITHER:

Low-dose ICS + either LABA, LTRA, or Theophylline

OR

Medium-dose ICS

Step 4

Preferred:

Medium-dose ICS + LABA

Alternative:

Medium-dose ICS + either LTRA or Theophylline

Step 5

Preferred:

High-dose ICS + LABA

Alternative:

High-dose ICS + either LTRA or Theophylline

Step 6

Preferred:

High-dose ICS + LABA + oral systemic corticosteroid

Alternative:

High-dose ICS + either LTRA or Theophylline + oral systemic corticosteroid

Step up if needed

(first, check adherence, inhaler technique, environmental control, and comorbid conditions)

Assess control

Step down if possible

(and asthma is well controlled at least 3 months)

Each step: Patient education, environmental control, and management of comorbidities.

Steps 2–4: Consider subcutaneous allergen immunotherapy for patients who have allergic asthma (see notes).

Quick-Relief Medication for All Patients

- SABA as needed for symptoms. Intensity of treatment depends on severity of symptoms: up to 3 treatments at 20-minute intervals as needed. Short course of oral systemic corticosteroids may be needed.
- Caution: Increasing use of SABA or use >2 days a week for symptom relief (not prevention of EIB) generally indicates inadequate control and the need to step up treatment.

Key: **Alphabetical order is used when more than one treatment option is listed within either preferred or alternative therapy.** ICS, inhaled corticosteroid; LABA, inhaled long-acting beta₂-agonist, LTRA, leukotriene receptor antagonist; SABA, inhaled short-acting beta₂-agonist

RESPIRATORY DISORDERS

Figure 13-3: Stepwise Approach for Managing Asthma in Children 5–11 Years of Age

Assessing severity and initiating therapy in children who are not currently taking long-term control medication

Components of Severity		Classification of Asthma Severity (0–4 years of age)			
			Persistent		
		Intermittent	**Mild**	**Moderate**	**Severe**
Impairment	Symptoms	≤2 days/week	>2 days/week but not daily	Daily	Throughout the day
	Nighttime awakenings	0	1–2x/month	3–4x/month	>1x/week
	Short-acting beta₂-agonist use for symptom control (not prevention of EIB)	≤2 days/week	>2 days/week but not daily	Daily	Several times per day
	Interference with normal activity	None	Minor limitation	Some limitation	Extremely limited
Risk	Exacerbations requiring oral systemic corticosteroids	0–1/year	≥2 exacerbations in 6 months requiring oral systemic corticosteroids, or ≥4 wheezing episodes/1 year lasting >1 day AND risk factors for persistent asthma		
		← Consider severity and interval since last exacerbation. Frequency and severity may fluctuate over time. →			
		Exacerbations of any severity may occur in patients in any severity category.			
Recommended Step for Initiating Therapy **(See figure 4–1a for treatment steps.)**		Step 1	Step 2	Step 3 and consider short course of oral systemic corticosteroids	
		In 2–6 weeks, depending on severity, evaluate level of asthma control that is achieved. If no clear benefit is observed in 4–6 weeks, consider adjusting therapy or alternative diagnoses.			

Key: EIB, exercise-induced bronchospasm

Figure 13-4: Classifying Asthma Severity and Initiating Treatment in Children 0–4 Years of Age

Note: Figure 4-1a referred to in this table (treatment steps) is the same as MedStudy Figure 13-2 on page 13-34.

Assessing severity and initiating therapy in children who are not currently taking long-term control medication

Components of Severity		Classification of Asthma Severity (5–11 years of age): Intermittent	Persistent: Mild	Persistent: Moderate	Persistent: Severe
Impairment	Symptoms	≤2 days/week	>2 days/week but not daily	Daily	Throughout the day
	Nighttime awakenings	≤2x/month	3–4x/month	>1x/week but not nightly	Often 7x/week
	Short-acting $beta_2$-agonist use for symptom control (not prevention of EIB)	≤2 days/week	>2 days/week but not daily	Daily	Several times per day
	Interference with normal activity	None	Minor limitation	Some limitation	Extremely limited
	Lung function	• Normal FEV_1 between exacerbations • FEV_1 >80% predicted • FEV_1/FVC >85%	• FEV_1 = >80% predicted • FEV_1/FVC >80%	• FEV_1 = 60–80% predicted • FEV_1/FVC = 75–80%	• FEV_1 <60% predicted • FEV_1/FVC <75%
Risk	Exacerbations requiring oral systemic corticosteroids	0–1/year (see note)	≥2/year (see note) →		
		← Consider severity and interval since last exacerbation. → Frequency and severity may fluctuate over time for patients in any severity category.			
		Relative annual risk of exacerbations may be related to FEV_1.			
Recommended Step for Initiating Therapy (See figure 4–1b for treatment steps.)		Step 1	Step 2	Step 3, medium-dose ICS option and consider short course of oral systemic corticosteroids	Step 3, medium-dose ICS option, or step 4 and consider short course of oral systemic corticosteroids
		In 2–6 weeks, evaluate level of asthma control that is achieved, and adjust therapy accordingly.			

Key: EIB, exercise-induced bronchospasm; FEV_1, forced expiratory volume in 1 second; FVC, forced vital capacity; ICS, inhaled corticosteroids

Figure 13-5: Classifying Asthma Severity and Initiating Treatment in Children 5–11 Years of Age

Note: Figure 4-1b referred to in this table (treatment steps) is the same as MedStudy Figure 13-3 on page 13-35.

Components of Control		Classification of Asthma Control (0–4 years of age)		
		Well Controlled	**Not Well Controlled**	**Very Poorly Controlled**
Impairment	Symptoms	≤2 days/week	>2 days/week	Throughout the day
	Nighttime awakenings	≤1x/month	>1x/month	>1x/week
	Interference with normal activity	None	Some limitation	Extremely limited
	Short-acting beta₂-agonist use for symptom control (not prevention of EIB)	≤2 days/week	>2 days/week	Several times per day
Risk	Exacerbations requiring oral systemic corticosteroids	0–1/year	2–3/year	>3/year
	Treatment-related adverse effects	Medication side effects can vary in intensity from none to very troublesome and worrisome. The level of intensity does not correlate to specific levels of control but should be considered in the overall assessment of risk.		
Recommended Action for Treatment **(See figure 4–1a for treatment steps.)**		• Maintain current treatment. • Regular followup every 1–6 months. • Consider step down if well controlled for at least 3 months.	• Step up (1 step) and • Reevaluate in 2–6 weeks. • If no clear benefit in 4–6 weeks, consider alternative diagnoses or adjusting therapy. • For side effects, consider alternative treatment options.	• Consider short course of oral systemic corticosteroids, • Step up (1–2 steps), and • Reevaluate in 2 weeks. • If no clear benefit in 4–6 weeks, consider alternative diagnoses or adjusting therapy. • For side effects, consider alternative treatment options.

Key: EIB, exercise-induced bronchospasm

Figure 13-6: Assessing Asthma Control and Adjusting Therapy in Children 0–4 Years of Age

Note: Figure 4-1a referred to in this table (treatment steps) is the same as MedStudy Figure 13-2 on page 13-34.

Components of Control		Classification of Asthma Control (5–11 years of age)		
		Well Controlled	**Not Well Controlled**	**Very Poorly Controlled**
Impairment	Symptoms	≤2 days/week but not more than once on each day	>2 days/week or multiple times on ≤2 days/week	Throughout the day
	Nighttime awakenings	≤1x/month	≥2x/month	≥2x/week
	Interference with normal activity	None	Some limitation	Extremely limited
	Short-acting beta$_2$-agonist use for symptom control (not prevention of EIB)	≤2 days/week	>2 days/week	Several times per day
	Lung function • FEV$_1$ or peak flow	>80% predicted/ personal best	60–80% predicted/ personal best	<60% predicted/ personal best
	• FEV$_1$/FVC	>80%	75–80%	<75%
Risk	Exacerbations requiring oral systemic corticosteroids	0–1/year	≥2/year (see note)	
		Consider severity and interval since last exacerbation		
	Reduction in lung growth	Evaluation requires long-term followup.		
	Treatment-related adverse effects	Medication side effects can vary in intensity from none to very troublesome and worrisome. The level of intensity does not correlate to specific levels of control but should be considered in the overall assessment of risk.		
Recommended Action for Treatment (See figure 4–1b for treatment steps.)		• Maintain current step. • Regular followup every 1–6 months. • Consider step down if well controlled for at least 3 months.	• Step up at least 1 step and • Reevaluate in 2–6 weeks. • For side effects: consider alternative treatment options.	• Consider short course of oral systemic corticosteroids, • Step up 1–2 steps, and • Reevaluate in 2 weeks. • For side effects, consider alternative treatment options.

Key: EIB, exercise-induced bronchospasm; FEV$_1$, forced expiratory volume in 1 second; FVC, forced vital capacity

Figure 13-7: Assessing Asthma Control and Adjusting Therapy in Children 5–11 Years of Age

RESPIRATORY DISORDERS

Note: Figure 4-1b referred to in this table (treatment steps) is the same as MedStudy Figure 13-3 on page 13-35.

Medication	Dosage Form	0–4 years	5–11 years	Comments
Systemic Corticosteroids				***(Applies to all three corticosteroids)***
Methylprednisolone	2, 4, 8, 16, 32 mg tablets	0.25–2 mg/kg daily in single dose in a.m. or qod as needed for control	0.25–2 mg/kg daily in single dose in a.m. or qod as needed for control	■ For long-term treatment of severe persistent asthma, administer single dose in a.m. either daily or on alternate days (alternate-day therapy may produce less adrenal suppression).
Prednisolone	5 mg tablets, 5 mg/5 cc, 15 mg/5 cc	Short-course "burst": 1–2 mg/kg/day, maximum 60 mg/day for 3–10 days	Short-course "burst": 1–2 mg/kg/day, maximum 60 mg/day for 3–10 days	■ Short courses or "bursts" are effective for establishing control when initiating therapy or during a period of gradual deterioration.
Prednisone	1, 2.5, 5, 10, 20, 50 mg tablets; 5 mg/cc, 5 mg/5 cc			■ There is no evidence that tapering the dose following improvement in symptom control and pulmonary function prevents relapse. ■ Patients receiving the lower dose (1 mg/kg/day) experience fewer behavioral side effects (Kayani and Shannon 2002), and it appears to be equally efficacious (Rachelefsky 2003). ■ For patients unable to tolerate the liquid preparations, dexamethasone syrup at 0.4 mg/kg/day may be an alternative. Studies are limited, however, and the longer duration of activity increases the risk of adrenal suppression (Hendeles 2003).
Long-Acting Beta$_2$-Agonists (LABAs)				■ **Should not be used for symptom relief or exacerbations. Use only with ICSs.**
Salmeterol	DPI 50 mcg/blister	Safety and efficacy not established in children <4 years	1 blister q 12 hours	■ Decreased duration of protection against EIB may occur with regular use. ■ Most children <4 years of age cannot provide sufficient inspiratory flow for adequate lung delivery. ■ Do not blow into inhaler after dose is activated.
Formoterol	DPI 12 mcg/single-use capsule	Safety and efficacy not established in children <5 years	1 capsule q 12 hours	■ Most children <4 years of age cannot provide sufficient inspiratory flow for adequate lung delivery. ■ Each capsule is for single use only; additional doses should not be administered for at least 12 hours. ■ Capsules should be used only with the inhaler and should not be taken orally.

*Dosages are provided for those products that have been approved by the U.S. Food and Drug Administration or have sufficient clinical trial safety and efficacy data in the appropriate age ranges to support their use.

Figure 13-8: Usual Dosages for Long-Term Control Medications in Children

Medication	Dosage Form	0–4 years	5–11 years	Comments
Combined Medication				
Fluticasone/ Salmeterol	DPI 100 mcg/ 50 mcg	Safety and efficacy not established in children <4 years	1 inhalation bid	▪ There have been no clinical trials in children <4 years of age. ▪ Most children <4 years of age cannot provide sufficient inspiratory flow for adequate lung delivery. ▪ Do not blow into inhaler after dose is activated.
Budesonide/ Formoterol	HFA MDI 80 mcg/4.5 mcg	Safety and efficacy not established	2 puffs bid	▪ There have been no clinical trials in children <4 years of age. ▪ Currently approved for use in youths ≥12. Dose for children 5–12 years of age based on clinical trials using DPI with slightly different delivery characteristics (Pohunek et al. 2006; Tal et al. 2002; Zimmerman et al. 2004).
Cromolyn/Nedocromil				
Cromolyn	MDI 0.8 mg/puff	Safety and efficacy not established	2 puffs qid	▪ 4–6 week trial may be needed to determine maximum benefit. ▪ Dose by MDI may be inadequate to affect hyperresponsiveness. ▪ One dose before exercise or allergen exposure provides effective prophylaxis for 1–2 hours. Not as effective as inhaled beta$_2$-agonists for EIB. ▪ Once control is achieved, the frequency of dosing may be reduced.
	Nebulizer 20 mg/ampule	1 ampule qid Safety and efficacy not established <2 years	1 ampule qid	
Nedocromil	MDI 1.75 mg/puff	Safety and efficacy not established <6 years	2 puffs qid	
Leukotriene Receptor Antagonists (LTRAs)				
Montelukast	4 mg or 5 mg chewable tablet 4 mg granule packets	4 mg qhs (1–5 years of age)	5 mg qhs (6–14 years of age)	▪ Montelukast exhibits a flat dose-response curve. ▪ No more efficacious than placebo in infants 6–24 months (van Adelsberg et al. 2005).
Zafirlukast	10 mg tablet	Safety and efficacy not established	10 mg bid (7–11 years of age)	▪ For zafirlukast, administration with meals decreases bioavailability; take at least 1 hour before or 2 hours after meals. ▪ Monitor for signs and symptoms of hepatic dysfunction.
Methylxanthines				
Theophylline	Liquids, sustained-release tablets, and capsules	Starting dose 10 mg/kg/day; usual maximum: ▪ <1 year of age: 0.2 (age in weeks) + 5 = mg/kg/day ▪ ≥1 year of age: 16 mg/kg/day	Starting dose 10 mg/kg/day; usual maximum: 16 mg/kg/day	▪ Adjust dosage to achieve serum concentration of 5–15 mcg/mL at steady-state (at least 48 hours on same dosage). ▪ Due to wide interpatient variability in theophylline metabolic clearance, routine serum theophylline level monitoring is essential.

Key: DPI, dry powder inhaler; EIB, exercise-induced bronchospasm; HFA, hydrofluoroalkane (inhaler propellant); MDI, metered dose inhaler

Figure 13-9: Usual Dosages for Long-Term Control Medications in Children (Continued)

Note: Discussion of factors that can affect theophylline levels, see page 13-21.

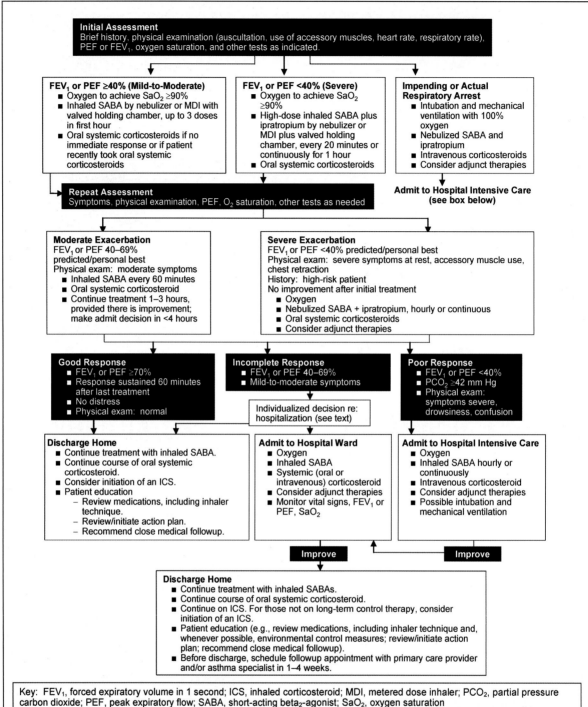

Initial Assessment
Brief history, physical examination (auscultation, use of accessory muscles, heart rate, respiratory rate), PEF or FEV_1, oxygen saturation, and other tests as indicated.

FEV_1 or PEF ≥40% (Mild-to-Moderate)
- Oxygen to achieve SaO_2 ≥90%
- Inhaled SABA by nebulizer or MDI with valved holding chamber, up to 3 doses in first hour
- Oral systemic corticosteroids if no immediate response or if patient recently took oral systemic corticosteroids

FEV_1 or PEF <40% (Severe)
- Oxygen to achieve SaO_2 ≥90%
- High-dose inhaled SABA plus ipratropium by nebulizer or MDI plus valved holding chamber, every 20 minutes or continuously for 1 hour
- Oral systemic corticosteroids

Impending or Actual Respiratory Arrest
- Intubation and mechanical ventilation with 100% oxygen
- Nebulized SABA and ipratropium
- Intravenous corticosteroids
- Consider adjunct therapies

Admit to Hospital Intensive Care (see box below)

Repeat Assessment
Symptoms, physical examination, PEF, O_2 saturation, other tests as needed

Moderate Exacerbation
FEV_1 or PEF 40–69% predicted/personal best
Physical exam: moderate symptoms
- Inhaled SABA every 60 minutes
- Oral systemic corticosteroid
- Continue treatment 1–3 hours, provided there is improvement; make admit decision in <4 hours

Severe Exacerbation
FEV_1 or PEF <40% predicted/personal best
Physical exam: severe symptoms at rest, accessory muscle use, chest retraction
History: high-risk patient
No improvement after initial treatment
- Oxygen
- Nebulized SABA + ipratropium, hourly or continuous
- Oral systemic corticosteroids
- Consider adjunct therapies

Good Response
- FEV_1 or PEF ≥70%
- Response sustained 60 minutes after last treatment
- No distress
- Physical exam: normal

Incomplete Response
- FEV_1 or PEF 40–69%
- Mild-to-moderate symptoms

Individualized decision re: hospitalization (see text)

Poor Response
- FEV_1 or PEF <40%
- PCO_2 ≥42 mm Hg
- Physical exam: symptoms severe, drowsiness, confusion

Discharge Home
- Continue treatment with inhaled SABA.
- Continue course of oral systemic corticosteroid.
- Consider initiation of an ICS.
- Patient education
  - Review medications, including inhaler technique.
  - Review/initiate action plan.
  - Recommend close medical followup.

Admit to Hospital Ward
- Oxygen
- Inhaled SABA
- Systemic (oral or intravenous) corticosteroid
- Consider adjunct therapies
- Monitor vital signs, FEV_1 or PEF, SaO_2

Admit to Hospital Intensive Care
- Oxygen
- Inhaled SABA hourly or continuously
- Intravenous corticosteroid
- Consider adjunct therapies
- Possible intubation and mechanical ventilation

Improve

Improve

Discharge Home
- Continue treatment with inhaled SABAs.
- Continue course of oral systemic corticosteroid.
- Continue on ICS. For those not on long-term control therapy, consider initiation of an ICS.
- Patient education (e.g., review medications, including inhaler technique and, whenever possible, environmental control measures; review/initiate action plan; recommend close medical followup).
- Before discharge, schedule followup appointment with primary care provider and/or asthma specialist in 1–4 weeks.

Key: FEV_1, forced expiratory volume in 1 second; ICS, inhaled corticosteroid; MDI, metered dose inhaler; PCO_2, partial pressure carbon dioxide; PEF, peak expiratory flow; SABA, short-acting beta₂-agonist; SaO_2, oxygen saturation

Figure 13-10: Management of Asthma Exacerbations — Emergency Department and Hospital-Based Care

MedStudy®

Pediatrics Review Core Curriculum

Seventh Edition 2016–2017

7

GASTROENTEROLOGY & NUTRITION

GASTROENTEROLOGY & NUTRITION

Section Editor:

Mark R. Corkins, MD, CNSP, SPR, FAAP
Chief, Division of Pediatric Gastroenterology
Le Bonheur Children's Hospital
Professor of Pediatrics
University of Tennessee Health Science Center
Memphis, TN

Editor:

Mark Yoffe, MD
York Hospital
York, PA

Reviewers:

William E. Bennett, Jr., MD
Assistant Professor of Pediatrics
Indiana University School of Medicine
Riley Hospital for Children at Indiana University Health
Indianapolis, IN

Marian D. Pfefferkorn, MD
Professor of Clinical Pediatrics
Training Director—Pediatric Gastroenterology/Hepatology/
  Nutrition Fellowship Training Program
Indiana University School of Medicine
Indianapolis, IN

Table of Contents
Gastroenterology & Nutrition

NUTRITIONAL DISORDERS

MARASMUS

Marasmus is severe calorie malnutrition in a child. These children have generalized loss of muscle and no subcutaneous fat. They appear to be very emaciated and cachectic. Linear growth is also affected if the malnutrition persists long enough. These patients have very loose wrinkled skin because of the loss of the subcutaneous fat. Facially, they have been described as having the look of a "wizened old man," due to the loss of temporal and buccal fat pads. Note that buccal fat pads are the last to go, indicating long-lasting, severe malnutrition. Because of the prolonged nature of inadequate energy stores, the body tries to adapt, and the child frequently has hypothermia, bradycardia, and hypotension.

KWASHIORKOR

Kwashiorkor is due to insufficient intake of protein. Frequently, it is also associated with an inadequate intake of calories. Kwashiorkor is an African term that means "the disease of the deposed baby when the next one is born." Typically, kwashiorkor appears in young children during the weaning or post-weaning process. Kwashiorkor is epidemic in developing countries, because the main calorie sources are carbohydrates that are low in protein—particularly white rice, cassava, and yams. Those affected are sometimes called "sugar babies." This type of malnutrition can make a child appear fat, but this swelling is primarily edema, caused by hypoalbuminemia and resultant low oncotic pressure.

These children present mainly with soft, pitting, painless edema, usually involving the feet and legs. In severe cases, it can extend to the face and upper extremities. Most affected children have skin rashes that can include hyperkeratosis and pigmentation changes due to desquamation of the epidermis. Their hair is dry and brittle and becomes yellowish-gray. In children who have fluctuating nutrition (some months good, other months poor), you may see a "flag sign" develop, which refers to areas of normal hair alternating with those of depigmented hair.

These children do not gain weight, but the failure to thrive (FTT) is masked by the edema. Their livers are usually large with fatty infiltration. T-cell function and cell-mediated immunity are not normal, and these children are at increased risk for infection.

While the classic distinction between marasmus and kwashiorkor has been taught for decades, the actual mechanism of malnutrition is more complex. A combination of impaired immunity, chronic bacterial gastrointestinal infection, and malnutrition are likely to blame. The line between marasmus and kwashiorkor is often blurred.

ETIOLOGY-BASED MALNUTRITION

Since the old definitions of malnutrition no longer apply to the developed world, in 2013 a multidisciplinary, multisociety task force published a definition that malnutrition can be defined by etiology—either by illness or non-illness (caused by environmental or behavioral factors). The parameters to define malnutrition are based on anthropometric z-scores, which are the number of standard deviations from the means of the growth curves. Acute was defined as < 3 months in duration, and chronic as longer. A BMI z-score of less than –1.0 to –2.0 is mild, –2.0 to –3.0 is moderate, and greater than –3.0 is severe. Once the diagnosis of malnutrition is made, the underlying cause for it must be found. For instance, a child with congenital heart disease and a BMI z-score of –2.3 is moderate chronic malnutrition due to congenital heart disease.

FAT-SOLUBLE VITAMIN DEFICIENCIES

Vitamins A, D, E, and K are fat-soluble vitamins and require carrier proteins for transport. They all require intact mechanisms for fat digestion and absorption for uptake. Vitamins A and D are transported by specific plasma proteins, and vitamins E and K are transported mostly by low-density lipoproteins (LDL). All of these vitamins are responsible for regulating protein synthesis. Know the complications caused by these vitamin deficiencies.

Vitamin A requirements generally are in the 10–30 µg/kg range of body weight, but infants have a higher requirement. Typically, vitamin A deficiency results in night blindness, Bitot spots (keratinization of the cornea), xerophthalmia (dry eyes), corneal opacities, growth failure, increased susceptibility to infection, and even death. If you see a child with vitamin A deficiency on the exam, and that child has clouding of the cornea, this is a medical emergency that requires large parenteral doses of vitamin A. Excess vitamin A can result in scaly skin, pseudotumor cerebri, and hepatomegaly.

Vitamin D is necessary for bone growth and maturation. If it's not available, rickets can occur in children (Image 14-1 on page 14-2) and osteoporosis/osteomalacia in adults. Vitamin D levels are very low in breast milk, so exclusively breastfed infants need to be supplemented with 400 IU of vitamin D daily. For older children with adequate exposure to sunlight, vitamin D supplementation is usually not necessary. Children at risk are those with limited sun exposure, especially those in northern and western countries where sunlight exposure is limited due to the bandwidth of radiation that can pass through clouds. Other risk factors include prematurity and darker skin pigmentation. Rickets can present with poor growth, hypocalcemia, hypophosphatemia, and tetany. Skeletal deformities and bone pain can also occur. Table 14-1 on page 14-2 lists possible clinical manifestations of rickets.

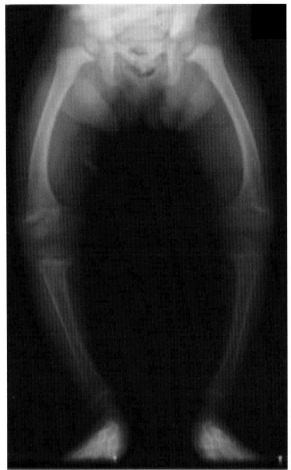

Image 14-1: Skeletal deformation from rickets

Michael L. Richardson, MD

Table 14-1: Manifestations of Rickets
Bone pain or tenderness: • Arms, legs, spine, and pelvis
Skeletal deformities: • Bowlegs • Forward projection of the breastbone ("pigeon chest") • Enlargement of the costochondral joints in the rib cage ("rachitic rosary") • Asymmetrical or odd-shaped skull and craniotabes ("ping-pong ball" consistency) • Spine deformities (including scoliosis and kyphosis) • Pelvic deformities
Increased tendency toward bone fractures
Dental deformities: • Delayed eruption of teeth • Defects in the structure of teeth, holes in the enamel • Increased incidence of cavities
Muscle cramps and weakness
Impaired growth
Short stature

Be aware, however, that the most frequent presenting complaint in infants and children with rickets is "nothing"—physicians most frequently diagnose it through an incidental finding on physical examination.

Laboratory may show:

• Decreased 25-(OH) vitamin D levels. (This is the level that is commonly done to initially test for overall vitamin D status.)
• Decreased calcium (but can be normal until late).
• Decreased phosphorus (but can be normal until late).
• Increased alkaline phosphatase.
• 1,25-(OH)$_2$ vitamin D levels can be decreased, increased, or normal.
• Increased parathyroid (PTH) hormone levels.

Look for a high PTH, low 25-(OH)-D, and a high alkaline phosphatase level. The high PTH is indicative of the hormonal response that tries to maintain normal calcium.

Diagnosis of rickets is usually confirmed by radiographic examination of the long bones, which show rarefied shafts and uneven, blurred ends. Once vitamin D treatment is started, the long bone ends "brighten" on x-ray.

Vitamin E (a.k.a. tocopherol) functions as a membrane-bound antioxidant by inhibiting free radical-catalyzed lipid peroxidation and terminating radical chain reactions. Thus, it serves to protect the body from biologic processes that damage cellular and intercellular structures. Vitamin E deficiency can result in neurologic dysfunction, especially neuroaxonal degeneration and loss of reflexes. In the preterm infant, vitamin E deficiency can present with hemolytic anemia. Vitamin E deficiency is especially common in children with fat malabsorption and is seen particularly in children with cystic fibrosis.

Vitamin K (a.k.a. phylloquinone) is necessary for maintaining prothrombin, Factor 7, Factor 9, and Factor 10. Most vitamin K is obtained in foods, such as dark leafy vegetables, cauliflower, and soybeans. Another nondietary source is bacterial synthesis in the gut. Vitamin K deficiency is uncommon once the intestinal flora is established, except in children with malabsorption, as seen in cystic fibrosis, ulcerative colitis, or history of intestinal resection. Antibiotic use in the newborn or infant can also "sterilize" the intestinal flora, resulting in vitamin K deficiency.

Generally, vitamin K deficiency is most common in these children or in newborns and infants who have not yet developed significant bacterial gastrointestinal flora. Thus, it is routine to give vitamin K prophylaxis at birth (0.5–1 mg IM or 1–2 mg orally).

WATER-SOLUBLE VITAMIN DEFICIENCIES

Vitamin C Deficiency (Scurvy)

Vitamin C (ascorbic acid) deficiency, a.k.a. scurvy, is rare in the developed world. The majority of cases appear in children between 6 months and 2 years of age. Initial symptoms of vitamin C deficiency are nonspecific

Quick Quiz

- What is marasmus? How does marasmus differ from kwashiorkor?
- What are the manifestations of rickets?
- Which vitamins and minerals must be supplemented in patients who are on a strict vegan diet?

and include irritability, digestive disturbances, and anorexia. Classic physical descriptions include follicular hyperkeratosis and "corkscrew-coiled" hairs. Gingival bleeding is also common. Normochromic, normocytic anemia is found in ~ 75% of patients with scurvy.

Vitamin C deficiency results in impaired formation of collagen and chondroitin sulfate. The lack of collagen results in fragile capillaries and gingival hemorrhage; the lack of chondroitin sulfate results in failed osteoid formation by osteoblasts, a process that causes the cessation of endochondral bone formation. In other words, bones become brittle and fracture easily. Most of the abnormalities are found at the metaphyseal zone of tubular bones and at the sternal-rib junctions.

One of the important x-ray findings in scurvy are the white lines of Frankel: a dense band at the growing metaphyseal end, involving the provisional zone of calcification (Image 14-2).

Treat with oral ascorbic acid.

Folate Deficiency

Folate is a water-soluble vitamin and is not stored, so you must have regular intake. Deficiency is associated primarily with hematological problems, including leukocyte and cellular immune dysfunction. Folate deficiency is the #2 nutritional cause of anemia! (Iron is #1.)

Folate deficiency in the pre-pregnant and pregnant woman increases the risk of neural tube defects.

Consider folate deficiency with the finding of anemia and large RBCs (high MCV; similar to B_{12} deficiency). Especially likely in:

- Infant or child who drinks goat's milk (be on the lookout for "non-traditional" feeding practices)

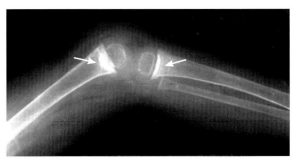

Image 14-2: Scurvy with white lines of Frankel

- Patients with ileal resection—typically from NEC, Crohn disease, or intussusception (these patients also are likely to have vitamin B_{12} deficiency)

Other Vitamin / Mineral Deficiencies

Know:

- **Thiamin (B_1)** deficiency is associated with beriberi: paraesthesias, foot and wrist drop. It is also associated with Wernicke encephalopathy: ophthalmoplegia, ataxia, and confusion.
- **Riboflavin (B_2)** deficiency is associated with cheilosis and sore tongue.
- **Niacin (B_3)** deficiency is associated with pellagra: dermatitis, dementia, and diarrhea.
- **Pyridoxine (B_6):** In infants, seizures that respond to B_6 are associated with a metabolic defect.
- **Cobalamin (B_{12})** deficiency: Most common cause in children is ileal disease (Crohn disease or lack of ileum due to short bowel syndrome). B_{12} deficiency causes megaloblastic anemia.
- **Zinc:** Zinc-containing enzymes are involved in nucleic acid and protein metabolism, so zinc deficiency affects rapidly growing cells. These patients "do not grow" and have diarrhea, a rash (acrodermatitis enteropathica), and hypogeusia (reduced taste).

VEGETARIAN DIETS

Vegetarianism is an acceptable diet for children and other groups as long as appropriate supplements are included (for strict vegans: vitamin B_{12}, iron, calcium, and zinc). Groups especially at risk are infants, children, and pregnant and lactating women. Risks are minimal with a "semi-vegetarian" diet, such as one that includes eggs and milk and/or non-red meat in the nutritional regimen.

Strict vegans must supplement their diet with **vitamin B_{12}**, which is of animal origin only. The supplement can be in the form of vitamins packaged as such, or else vitamin-fortified cereal, yeast, or non-dairy milk. Breastfed infants of mothers who are marginally deficient in B_{12} also are at marked risk for B_{12} deficiency.

Iron is another problem area for the strict vegan child. Iron from plant sources (non-heme iron) is much less absorbable than iron derived from animal sources (heme iron). Coadministering iron-containing foods with vitamin C can enhance the absorption of iron.

Calcium is another element that is of concern for the strict vegan. Calcium-fortified nondairy milk and calcium-fortified juices can provide the daily requirements. Many vegan diets also lack vitamin D; sunlight exposure can help the body synthesize this vitamin.

Zinc deficiency is relatively common in strict vegans; thus, zinc frequently must be supplemented as well.

CALORIE AND FLUID REQUIREMENTS

Many methods are available to treat and diagnose fluid and electrolyte abnormalities. Most are based on body weight and include the basal calorie method, the surface area method, and the Holliday-Segar formula. The first two methods require tables, while the latter formula can be used to answer exam questions on dehydration because this formula relates water loss to the caloric expenditure.

The Holliday-Segar formula for daily kcal required under basal conditions is:

100 kcal/kg for the first 10 kg plus

50 kcal/kg for the next 10 kg plus

20 kcal/kg for the rest of the weight

Example: For a 23-kg patient, the total kcal required per day is:

$$(100 \times 10) + (50 \times 10) + (20 \times 3)$$

or

$$1,000 + 500 + 60 = 1,560 \text{ kcal per day}$$

See Table 14-2 for more on the Holliday-Segar formula.

How do you clinically assess dehydration in infants and young children (Table 14-3)?

Table 14-2: Holliday-Segar Formula for Maintenance of Calories and Fluids		
Weight	kcal/d or mL/d	kcal/h or mL/h
0–10 kg	100/kg/day	4/kg/hour
11–20 kg	1,000 + 50/kg/day*	40 + 2/kg/hr*
> 20 kg	1,500 + 20/kg/day**	60 + 1/kg/hr**
*for each kg > 10 **for each kg > 20		

Table 14-3: Dehydration			
Clinical Data	Severity of Dehydration	Estimated Weight Loss	mL/ kg
Dry mucous membranes Oliguria	Mild	5%	50
Marked oliguria Poor skin turgor Sunken fontanelle Tachycardia Irritability	Moderate	10%	100
Hypotension Poor perfusion Lethargy	Severe	15%	150

Note that rehydration guidelines have changed and IV therapy is no longer standard treatment for most dehydration scenarios; instead, oral rehydration solution is frequently recommended.

For mild dehydration, you should typically prescribe 50–60 mL/kg of an oral rehydration solution (ORS). At the level of moderate dehydration, prescribe 80–100 mL/kg of ORS. For severe dehydration, choose a fluid infusion of normal saline or lactated Ringer's at 40 mL/kg/hr until the pulse and consciousness are normal. The patient then completes rehydration with 50–100 mL/kg of ORS.

VOMITING

OVERVIEW

Vomiting is a coordinated motor response of the GI tract, abdominal muscles, and thoracic muscles, resulting in the forceful expulsion of stomach contents. Nausea often precedes retching, which, in turn, precedes emesis.

The vomiting center is located in the nucleus solitarius and a series of nuclei in the medulla of the brainstem. Stimuli to these areas can come from cortical afferents (migraine, increased intracranial pressure), vestibular afferents (dizziness), and vagal afferents; e.g., posterior pharynx (gagging), the GI tract (distention). Also, the chemoreceptor trigger zone, which is located in the floor of the 4th ventricle, receives stimuli from drugs, toxins, and metabolic products (e.g., acidemia, ketonemia, hyperammonemia).

Some associations can be helpful in suggesting the possible etiology:

• Bilious: GI obstruction beyond the duodenum (e.g., malrotation)
• Red blood or coffee grounds: upper GI bleed
• Fever: gastroenteritis or systemic infection
• Undigested food: achalasia, delayed gastric emptying, rumination
• Projectile emesis: pyloric stenosis, antral web
• Tense fontanelle in infants or headache/neurological symptoms in an older child: increased intracranial pressure due to meningitis or tumor
• Adolescent: pregnancy, drugs, migraine, bulimia

CHRONIC VOMITING

In cases of chronic vomiting, proceed with a careful history and physical and then a stepwise evaluation that may include abdominal ultrasound, upper gastrointestinal contrast x-rays, or endoscopy. In one study, children with vomiting for over a month were evaluated, and a "histologic" diagnosis was made in about 60% of the cases. The main causes were esophagitis and gastritis (including *Helicobacter*-induced). Less commonly found (< 5%) were duodenitis and giardiasis. Endoscopy is the best test for diagnosis of chronic vomiting. Do not forget to think about gastrointestinal disorders like

Quick Quiz

- What are the basal kcal/day requirements for a 17-kg child? A 31-kg child?
- What does bilious vomiting suggest in a neonate?
- What does vomiting of undigested food indicate?
- What is cyclic vomiting?
- The finding of currant jelly stool suggests what possible diagnosis?

Crohn disease, which may be present in multiple areas of the GI tract.

However, many patients have a functional cause for vomiting, including cyclic vomiting syndrome or rumination. These disorders are more common in adolescence, and in children with significant social stressors and/or psychiatric diagnoses such as anxiety or depression.

CYCLIC VOMITING

Cyclic vomiting occurs with paroxysms of vomiting followed by intervals of complete health. It is most commonly seen in girls between the ages of 6 and 7. These children develop intense vomiting episodes that last from hours to days, with vomiting as often as 6 times/hour. The "well spells" last from several weeks to many months between episodes. There is a strong association with a family history of migraine headaches.

Think about the diagnosis when the history is characteristic and the physical examination is normal. If there are signs of other organic disease (especially weight loss), do a workup with all of the following:

- Metabolic screening during an attack
- Upper GI
- Upper endoscopy with biopsies
- Brain imaging

Treatment for cyclic vomiting can be difficult and includes avoidance of triggers plus lifestyle changes. Ondansetron is often used to abort the acute episode. For prophylaxis, use propranolol, amitriptyline, or phenobarbital. Cyproheptadine is the 1st choice for children 5 years old and younger.

RUMINATION SYNDROME

Many patients have episodes of vomiting that occur immediately after eating. This is often semi-purposeful and small in volume, often within seconds or minutes of initiating a meal. If you see an adolescent patient who leaves the table multiple times during dinner to "throw up" mouthfuls of food in the bathroom,

consider rumination. Many patients have comorbid anxiety or depression. Treatment is supportive, relying on psychotherapy and cognitive behavioral therapy.

ABDOMINAL PAIN

HISTORY / PHYSICAL / LAB

Acute abdominal pain is a common complaint in children who present to parents, school nurses, and emergency departments. Less than 5% who present to emergency departments require admission for observation or surgery. It can be very difficult to differentiate the emergencies from the non-emergencies. Usually, careful history and serial physical examination are most important in delineating the etiology. Supplement your investigation with laboratory and diagnostic studies as appropriate to confirm normalcy.

Some clues in the history can be helpful for acute abdominal pain:

- Coincident with psychosocial stress: functional abdominal pain
- Presenting with the acute onset of pain as the 1st symptom: intussusception, midgut volvulus, ovarian or testicular torsion
- Trauma: perforated viscus, hemorrhage, musculoskeletal injury, pancreatitis
- Bilious vomiting: intussusception, volvulus, incarcerated hernia, adhesions
- Peritonitis: appendicitis, cholecystitis, PID
- Adolescent female: PID, pregnancy, ectopic pregnancy, ovulatory pain (mittelschmerz)
- "Currant jelly stool": intussusception
- Melena: upper GI bleed
- Nonbilious vomiting and diarrhea: gastroenteritis

A nonspecific history can occur with many of the above issues (e.g., appendicitis, cholecystitis) presenting at an earlier stage. Also with a nonspecific history, consider gastroenteritis, toxins (e.g., food poisoning), UTI, and even pneumonia (although cough is usually in the history).

Initial laboratory studies for a child with acute abdominal pain include a CBC, U/A, and (for the adolescent female) pregnancy test. These are relatively nonspecific (well, except for the pregnancy test!). If the pain is post-prandial, check for biliary-pancreatic disease (bilirubin, GGT, amylase, lipase; fasting abdominal ultrasound). If the history and physical examination are "classic" for appendicitis, perform surgery. Abdominal x-rays can show obstruction, calcification, ischemia, or free air. You can rule out pneumonia or pneumothorax with chest x-ray.

Perform ultrasound and/or CT scan in patients who do not improve over several hours and do not have defining peritoneal signs. Avoid indiscriminate and routine use of imaging.

FUNCTIONAL ABDOMINAL PAIN

Functional abdominal pain is the most common cause of abdominal pain in children and one of the most common presenting complaints seen by pediatricians. School absenteeism is a major problem in nearly 1/3 of children with functional abdominal pain. Recognizing the difference between an organic disorder requiring intervention and a functional disorder requiring reassurance can be challenging, but it is an essential skill for any practitioner.

Note: There are usually some exam questions that require you to recognize that a child has a benign disorder, so do not be afraid to put "reassurance" for answers when it seems appropriate.

Let's start by defining the common functional causes of pediatric abdominal pain, since these are by far the most common causes of both acute and chronic abdominal pain in children.

The Rome criteria, a catalog of functional gastrointestinal disorders, specify 3 disorders seen in children:

1) **Functional abdominal pain syndrome**: most often seen in school-aged children. Pain is typically periumbilical. Growth is normal and appetite is typically not affected. Symptoms tend to get better on the weekends and during vacations, and it is worse in the morning before school or in the evening before bed. Ask about social stressors such as recent divorce or trouble at school. Treat with reassurance. Workup is usually unnecessary, and medications are not effective. This disorder was previously referred to as "chronic recurrent abdominal pain syndrome." (What a great acronym!)

2) **Functional dyspepsia**: the medical term for "indigestion." Pain is typically in the mid-epigastric area and is strongly correlated with meals. Most patients are school-aged or adolescents. Some children describe a burning sensation. There should not be associated symptoms such as vomiting. (If there is vomiting, consider an organic disorder such as peptic ulcer, gastritis, or esophagitis.) As many as 50% of patients respond to acid suppression, although there is no acid-related damage. Again, growth is normal.

3) **Irritable bowel syndrome (IBS)**: Pain is typically in the lower abdomen or can be multifocal, and it is more common in adolescents. There is a female predominance. The hallmarks of IBS are pain that improves with defecation and frequent changes in stool caliber or frequency. If a patient has constipation one day, normal stools another day, and loose stools another, then it's IBS! Growth and appetite should be normal. Anxiety, depression, and social stressors can greatly influence symptoms. (Everyone will probably have a touch of IBS when studying for Boards!) Treatments and treatment responses vary widely. Treatments include antispasmodic medications, such as hyoscyamine and dicyclomine, SSRIs, a high-fiber diet, probiotics or elimination of certain foods (spicy foods, short-chain carbohydrates called FODMAPs), acupuncture, and caffeine avoidance, to name a few. Nonpharmacologic interventions, such as exercise and psychotherapy, have been shown to be some of the most effective treatments!

You do not need to order a wide spectrum of tests to confirm your clinical suspicions. What are the clues for an organic cause of acute abdominal pain that indicate the need for a targeted workup? Target the workup as follows if a patient has abdominal pain and:

• **Vomiting**: Suspect upper GI problems like gastritis, duodenitis, or esophagitis, as well as anatomic disorders such as malrotation. If brief (a few days), viral gastroenteritis is a very common cause. An upper GI series can confirm normal anatomy. An upper endoscopy is the only way to reliably diagnose any upper GI "-itis." If pain occurs with eating, suspect pancreatitis (order an amylase and lipase) or biliary disease, such as gallstones (order an ultrasound).

• **Weight loss**: Think chronic inflammatory conditions, such as celiac disease (order a tissue transglutaminase IgA antibody) and Crohn disease (look for anemia, hypoalbuminemia, and guaiac-positive stools).

• **Hematochezia**: Think of chronic inflammation, such as inflammatory bowel disease (look for anemia and check a stool guaiac). If brief, have a high suspicion for bacterial colitis (order a stool enteric culture and *C. difficile* toxin assay).

• **Diarrhea**: The most common cause is still IBS, but suspect inflammatory bowel disease. Celiac disease (order an anti-tTG) and giardiasis (order a stool *Giardia* antigen) are also common causes of pain with diarrhea.

• **Nighttime awakening from pain**: Classic test question! Suspect *Helicobacter pylori* infection.

• **Fever, rash, oral ulcers, or joint pain**: Suspect inflammatory bowel disease.

• **Melena** (dark, tarry, pungent stools): Suspect an upper GI bleed, such as bleeding peptic ulcer or gastritis. Most patients need upper endoscopy!

Do not confuse IBS with IBD! Irritable bowel syndrome (IBS) is a chronic, benign, functional disorder that causes no long-term damage and can be managed supportively. Inflammatory bowel disease (IBD) is much more severe and is characterized by chronic inflammatory changes that can cause anemia, weight loss, and malnutrition!

ACUTE DIARRHEA

HISTORY / WORKUP

Acute diarrhea is defined as lasting < 14 days. Almost all diarrhea in children is due to an infectious agent, most commonly rotavirus. For most, aim therapy at rehydration and providing nutritional needs.

Quick Quiz

- What is the most common cause of abdominal pain in children?
- What clues are useful in diagnosing functional abdominal pain?
- What clues suggest an organic cause for abdominal pain?
- What is the most common cause of diarrhea in children?
- When should IV therapy be initiated in a child with diarrhea?
- Do children with resolving diarrhea require special diets?

In most instances of diarrhea, you do not need to search for an etiologic agent since most are self-limited. Certain things, though, prompt you to do further evaluation:

- Infants < 2 months of age (but remember many infants have watery / loose stools, and it's normal!)
- Gross blood in the stool
- WBCs on microscopic exam of the stool
- Toxic-appearing child
- Immunocompromised child
- Diarrhea developing while an inpatient or following a course of antibiotics

If one or more of these are present, order further stool studies to look for invasive bacterial infection. The infant younger than 2 months requires special care because of the risk of quickly developing dehydration, as well as the many noninfectious etiologies that appear in this age group. Depending on your suspicions, stool studies can include a rotavirus ELISA; stool cultures for *Salmonella, Shigella, Campylobacter, Yersinia, E. coli* (including O157:H7), or *Aeromonas*, etc.; *C. difficile* toxin; and *Giardia* or *Cryptosporidium* ELISA. In some cases, use a complete ova and parasite microscopic exam.

Note: *C. difficile* toxin assays in children < 1 year of age are not reliable because enterocytes in infants have not yet developed the receptor for the toxin.

Some associations that can give you a clue to the infectious etiologic agent:

- Recent travel: toxigenic *E. coli* (Montezuma's revenge) or *Giardia*
- Exposure to pet reptiles: *Salmonella*
- Fever and high WBC: *Shigella*
- Hemolytic uremic syndrome: *E. coli* 0157:57
- Swimming in lakes or drinking well water: *Giardia*
- Consumption of pork intestine ("chitterlings"): *Yersinia*

ORAL REHYDRATION THERAPY

Treat acute diarrhea with oral rehydration therapy. Commercial formulations are available and include Enfalyte®, Pedialyte®, and Rehydralyte®; generic products are also available. These are formulated to be iso- or hypotonic with appropriate amounts of electrolytes. Note: Do not recommend using "clear" liquids with these products. Most "clear" liquids (juices, soft drinks, most sports drinks, such as Gatorade®) are hypertonic and have excess glucose. These often result in ongoing diarrhea-like stools even after the illness has resolved.

Certain contraindications to oral rehydration therapy that you need to know:

- Shock
- Stool output > 10 mL/kg/hour
- Ileus
- Monosaccharide intolerance

In patients with these manifestations, you will likely need to initiate intravenous therapy.

Note: Vomiting is not a contraindication to using oral rehydration therapy and does not reduce its success rate. The recommended course with these patients is a clinical trial of oral rehydration.

FEEDING DURING ACUTE DIARRHEA

After you have achieved rehydration, resume the child's age-appropriate diet. The traditional "bland" diet results in a longer recovery time and has never been validated in a clinical trial. Breastfed infants should resume breastfeeding. Infants on solid foods can resume their normal diets. Avoid high-sugar foods, such as juices, which can result in osmotic diarrhea. Also recommend feeding small amounts at frequent intervals.

Children who are on cow's milk or commercial milk formulas can resume their diets, although a small number develop acidosis or recurrent diarrhea. If this occurs, withhold milk/formula for 1–2 days, temporarily using a lactose-free formula instead. There is a higher incidence of transient lactose intolerance in very young infants.

USE OF ANTIDIARRHEAL AGENTS

Antidiarrheal agents are widely available over the counter and by prescription. The most commonly used agents are known as "**absorbents**." These include magnesium aluminum silicate, which is found in over-the-counter brands Donnagel® and Kaopectate®, as well as generic products. They mainly alter stool consistency and do not affect absolute fecal water loss, but they do give the illusion that the diarrhea is better. Bulk-forming agents (methylcellulose, psyllium seed, soy fiber) are also "absorbents" and work like the silicate products. Although the stools appear more normal, they do not shorten the length of the infection.

Antimotility drugs are a 2nd type of agent. Generally, these are opiates, such as codeine, diphenoxylate, or loperamide. They can be quite dangerous in children; thus, do not use routinely. Opiates can induce ileus and worsen underlying bacterial infections.

The 3rd type of available antidiarrheal is **probiotics**. These are microorganisms, which can be taken to modulate diarrhea that is due to bacterial or viral etiologies. *Saccharomyces boulardii* is a nonpathogenic yeast, which is helpful in reducing the recurrence rate of *Clostridium difficile* diarrhea. Studies have shown that *Lactobacillus GG* (previously known as *L. rhamnosus*, sold as Culturelle®) lessens the severity of rotavirus infection.

The 4th main group of agents is the **antisecretory agents**. These include somatostatin and octreotide. They act by stimulating sodium and chloride absorption and inhibiting chloride secretion. These cannot be administered orally and are utilized only in special clinical situations.

Finally, a special type of agent is **bismuth subsalicylate** (Pepto-Bismol®). Bismuth has both antimicrobial and antisecretory properties; it also contains magnesium aluminum silicate, which is an absorbent. Warn parents that this agent results in dark black stools.

CONSTIPATION

DEFINITION

Constipation has no standardized definition and varies from person to person. Note that constipation is a symptom and not a disease or sign. Only a very small minority of children who present with constipation have an organic or anatomic cause. The majority of constipation is due to a functional or behavioral problem. Early on, it is more common in boys, but by adolescence, it is more common in girls.

Some breastfed infants pass a stool only once every 5–10 days; in the absence of other signs or symptoms, they do not need treatment. Some older children pass a stool only every 3–4 days; they do not have any other symptoms, and this pattern continues into adulthood.

"THEY STRAIN WHEN THEY POOP" SYNDROME

A common presentation of infants during the first 10 weeks of life is a parent who comes in and says, "My child strains all the time and cries before every bowel movement." The clinical term is infant dyschezia. This is perfectly normal because some infants have difficulty coordinating an increase in intraabdominal pressure and relaxation of the pelvic floor at the same time. These cries, grunts, and facial expressions are normal and are part of getting this coordinated. For this reason, do not use or recommend enemas or suppositories for these infants! Provide parental reassurance instead.

FUNCTIONAL CONSTIPATION

Etiology and Diagnosis

Functional constipation is the most common nonorganic cause of constipation. It is also responsible for most cases of encopresis in children. The fecal retention is due to voluntary "withholding" of stool secondary to the fear of defecation. The disorder occurs at 2 peaks: toilet-training time and the start of school. It also can develop before toilet training has even been attempted. Causes of the disorder during the toilet-training period are: training at an inappropriately young age, obsessive attitudes toward rectal incontinence, and extreme pressure put on the child to "avoid accidents," although in most cases, there is no clear social or behavioral cause. Some children also have had past experiences with painful defecation, anal fissures, or perianal infections, all of which can cause discomfort to the point that they learn to equate defecation with pain. Also consider child sexual abuse as an etiology if the retentive constipation is a new, sudden onset.

The whole cycle begins with the child voluntarily "holding in" a bowel movement. This accumulates in the rectum, and the child must increasingly contract the pelvic floor muscles and buttocks to prevent stool from passing. As the stool continues to amass, the child's mood and appetite are adversely affected, and the child may experience abdominal pain. Soiling frequently occurs when the child has flatus because the child cannot keep all of the rectal contents intact. The withholding cycle is reinforced when the parent becomes angry at the child for soiling, and the child is actually already trying to prevent any stool passage. Eventually, many develop a negative self-image.

It is important to differentiate functional constipation from other etiologies. Physical examination shows anal fissures and/or perianal fecal staining.

Other causes of constipation, such as Hirschsprung disease, do not typically present with fecal soiling, and the rectal vault is empty instead of full of stool. The finding of a deep sacral pit or a vascular or pigmented hairy patch on the sacrum suggests spinal dysraphism. Consider lumbosacral ultrasound or MRI.

Treatment of Functional Constipation

Treatment of functional constipation requires a mixed behavioral and medical approach, including positive reinforcement schedules and the use of stool softeners. Usually, some sort of "clean-out" of the fecal bolus is required, sometimes with enemas. Occasionally, prokinetic agents are needed and, in very rare instances, disimpaction under anesthesia. Give stool softeners to make stool passage painless, and advise parents to make sure the child has unhurried time on the toilet 2–3 times a day after meals. Instruct parents to have the child sit on the toilet with feet pressed firmly against

GASTROENTEROLOGY & NUTRITION

Quick Quiz

- What is the most common cause of constipation in children?
- Is it rare for a breastfed infant to pass a stool less often than once every 5 days?
- What is the most common nonorganic cause of constipation?
- How do 90% of tracheoesophageal abnormalities present?
- What does VACTERL stand for?
- At the bedside, how do you diagnose esophageal atresia with distal tracheoesophageal fistula?

the floor (or a footstool, if necessary) to help with defecation. Once the fecal mass is cleared, maintenance therapy is necessary to allow the cycle of withholding to be broken. Most commonly used agents include polyethylene glycol, mineral oil, and lactulose. Titrate doses up or down to reach the desired results. After at least 6 months of pain-free and accident-free success, discontinue the agents. Failure rates approach 20% regardless of the treatment used. Relapses are also common in children who were treated for this previously. Avoid excessive oral phosphates and hypertonic enemas.

ESOPHAGUS DISORDERS

TRACHEOESOPHAGEAL FISTULAS AND ESOPHAGEAL ATRESIAS

Overview

Tracheoesophageal fistula and esophageal atresia occur in about 1/4,000 live births. Nearly 90% of tracheoesophageal abnormalities present as a blind, upper esophageal atresia with a fistula between a lower esophageal segment and the lower portion of the trachea, near the carina. The next most common abnormalities include esophageal atresia alone with 2 blind pouches (the esophagus is closed distally, and the stomach is closed proximally, without a connection between the two) and an "H-type" tracheoesophageal fistula, which has a connection between a normal esophagus and a normal trachea. Esophageal stenosis alone can also occur. A clue for esophageal abnormalities can occur prenatally in the mothers of these infants; ~ 50% have polyhydramnios.

Know that nearly 1/3 of these infants also have other congenital anomalies. The most common association is known by an acronym: **VACTERL** (**v**ertebral, **a**nal atresia, **c**ardiac [PDA, ASD, VSD], **t**rach**e**oesophageal fistula, **r**enal [urethral atresia with hydronephrosis], and **l**imb anomalies [humeral hypoplasia, radial aplasia, hexadactyly, proximally placed thumb]).

Esophageal Atresia with Distal Tracheoesophageal Fistula

Esophageal atresia with distal tracheoesophageal fistula is the most common form of anatomical esophageal abnormality. Look for this in the delivery room or early in the nursery. The infant presents with excessive oral secretions and appears to be choking frequently, especially with attempted feeding. Diagnose by trying to place an NG tube into the stomach, whereupon the blind pouch of the esophagus then prevents passage. A simple x-ray of the chest shows the abnormality fairly well, often with the gastric tube coiled in the upper chest. Also, look for a dilated proximal esophagus with air distention of the entire gastrointestinal tract.

See Image 14-3 and Image 14-4. The catheter tip stops in the blind pouch of the esophagus.

Initially in these infants, discontinue all oral feedings, place an orogastric catheter into the blind pouch and tape it into position; then connect it so that there is continuous drainage of the saliva from the pouch to prevent aspiration. Also, it is important to keep the head elevated at about 30 degrees, which prevents stomach contents from being refluxed back into the trachea. After a cardiac evaluation rules out potential cardiac abnormalities, perform surgery as soon as possible.

Optimal treatment is to perform an anastomosis of the distal esophagus and ligation of the fistula. In a very ill or very small infant, you can delay this by doing a gastrostomy and waiting until the child is well enough to perform the definitive surgery. The main complication of surgery is the leakage of material through the anastomosis area. An anastomotic leak can present as tachypnea and

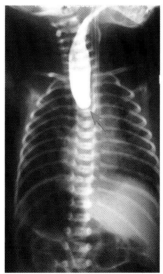

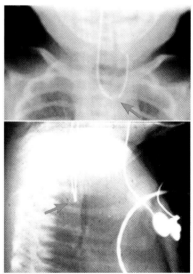

Image 14-3: Esophageal atresia   *Image 14-4: Esophageal atresia*

a sepsis-like picture on the 3rd to 4th day after surgery. Another complication is stricture formation. GE reflux is increased in these patients after the surgical changes required to pull together the esophagus are completed.

Esophageal Atresia without Tracheoesophageal Fistula

Neonates with isolated esophageal atresia have excessive oral secretions with choking and also a flat, gasless abdomen on x-ray, which is not seen in those with a tracheoesophageal fistula. These infants typically have a very wide gap between the two ends of the esophagus, so primary anastomosis is less likely to be an option. Usually, esophageal lengthening, done by bougienage or magnets (!), works only if the gap is less than 3–4 cm. If the gap is > 4 cm, esophageal replacement is necessary. This is generally delayed until after 1 year of age. In this procedure, you bridge the gap with a gastric tube, a colon segment, or a small intestinal segment.

Esophageal Atresia (The H-type Fistula)

Infants with the H-type fistula may present in early infancy with choking during feeding. Others present later with cough, pneumonia, or reactive airway disease. This variant is not associated with maternal polyhydramnios. Diagnosis is tricky; barium swallows frequently miss the H-type fistula. You may need to perform an esophagoscopy and/or bronchoscopy to confirm the diagnosis. Surgery to tie off the fistula is curative. Occasionally, this type of fistula has presented in adults without prior knowledge of their congenital abnormality.

Esophageal Stenosis and Web Diaphragms

Esophageal stenosis and web diaphragms are both rare. They present as dysphagia when solids are introduced to a child. Diagnose with barium swallow or endoscopy. Usually, either can be treated by dilation. A special case is stenosis due to ectopic cartilage known as tracheobronchial remnants. Remove this surgically because it has a high risk of perforation.

In all children with any form of esophageal atresia, long-term outcomes are generally good. However, many present later with anastomotic strictures, dysphagia, or esophagitis because they lose the lower esophageal sphincter tone, or due to abnormal esophageal motility.

ACHALASIA

Achalasia is a disorder of the esophagus characterized by incomplete relaxation of the lower esophageal sphincter (LES) and a lack of normal esophageal peristalsis. Thus, it is a motor problem, not an anatomic problem. Patients present with difficulty swallowing (dysphagia), often with regurgitation/vomiting of undigested food. Weight loss and chest discomfort are often present as well. Recurrent aspiration pneumonia may accompany the presentation of achalasia. Esophageal motility testing is needed to confirm the diagnosis. Achalasia appears to be due to loss of ganglion cells in the esophagus and to dorsal motor nuclei reduction of the vagus nerve. Many patients have antibodies to the Auerbach plexus. Only about 5% of all achalasia cases occur in children; the mean age for presentation in children is 9 years.

If achalasia presents in infancy or early childhood, it may be due to a congenital disorder. One such genetic syndrome is known as achalasia-addisonianism-alacrima syndrome (a.k.a. Allgrove or triple-A syndrome).

There are several therapeutic options for the treatment of achalasia. Options include either a graded pneumatic dilation or, for those physically fit and willing to undergo surgery, a laparoscopic surgical myotomy with a partial fundoplication. Botulinum toxin therapy is recommended in patients who are not good candidates for more definitive therapy. Prescribe pharmacologic therapy, such as with calcium channel blockers, for patients who cannot undergo definitive treatment or who have failed botulinum toxin therapy.

GE REFLUX (GER) AND GE REFLUX DISEASE (GERD)

Overview

GE reflux (GER) is defined as return of gastric contents into the esophagus. This is actually a normal process, and it becomes spitting up or vomiting if the refluxed material passes out the mouth. The age of the patient has an important impact on the need for diagnostic testing and treatment.

Pathologic reflux is rare in normal children; however, it is commonly seen in children with disabilities, especially those with neurological dysfunction, in obese patients, or in patients with reactive airway disease. In infants and children without adequate airway protective measures, reflux is more likely to cause airway complications such as aspiration pneumonia or reactive airway disease exacerbations.

Reflux in Infants

This is normal? Well, yes. 1/2 of infants 0–3 months of age vomit at least once daily, and 2/3 of those 4–6 months old do too! This decreases rapidly after 8 months of age. Most infants with daily vomiting outgrow this problem by 2 years of age and do not require special treatment. This benign presentation of infant reflux is also called physiologic regurgitation.

In a small percentage of infants, GER may become a more pathologic process, at which point it is called GE reflux disease (GERD). This can manifest as FTT due to the inability to consume and maintain enough calories in the digestive tract. There may also be other symptoms caregivers misinterpret as being caused by reflux, such

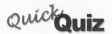

as airway symptoms with hoarseness, laryngitis, cough, pneumonia, and apnea. Intermittent irritability is often blamed on GER, although this is present in many normal infants and is a nonspecific sign.

An upper GI series is often one of the 1st tests done in a vomiting infant. Upper GI can show anatomic abnormalities in the vomiting child, such as malrotation, pyloric stenosis, esophageal stricture, and antral webs. It can also show evidence of esophageal motility problems like achalasia. What upper GI does not do is diagnose pathologic reflux, because—remember—normal children have reflux too, and the upper GI sees a window of only a few minutes. So, the upper GI is good for showing anatomic or motility problems only.

Occasionally, upper endoscopy can be helpful in an infant with GERD who is not growing well, but in most infants without more concerning consequences of GER, no workup needs to be performed.

Since most infantile GER is normal, direct initial therapy toward parental reassurance. For those parents who are upset or having difficulty dealing with the vomiting child, suggest thickening the formula with rice cereal, using 1–2 tablespoons per ounce of formula. The problem with this is that because the thickened formula frequently does not get through the nipple correctly, the parent has to cut the nipple. This may increase the cough or feeding problems the infant is already having. Do not encourage prone sleeping because of the definite increased risk of SIDS in babies who sleep in the prone position. Also, do not give medications to infants with uncomplicated GER. The recent guidelines on GER also recommend a 2-week trial of a low-allergy formula due to the common occurrence of reflux in children with formula protein allergy.

Rule out other causes in infants with GER who have poor weight gain, but know that inadequate caloric intake is the most common cause for FTT in infants the majority of the time. If no other causes are found, therapy is indicated. You can suggest food thickening and/or increasing the caloric content of food. If this is unsuccessful, do a trial of medical therapy. On rare occasions, the vomiting may be so severe that the infant requires NG feedings or postpyloric feedings. Do not recommend surgery (such as a fundoplication) for children when GER is the etiology for their poor weight gain. If there is delayed stomach emptying, promotility therapy may be helpful.

Reflux in Older Children

Older children often have symptoms similar to adults: heartburn, acid brash (a nasty taste in their mouth—some parents report very bad breath), frequent sore throat, or intermittent vomiting. Abdominal pain, especially epigastric pain, is often blamed on reflux, but it rarely proves to be the actual etiology.

Diagnosis of a pathologic reflux disease in children is difficult, and there is no absolute test that defines it.

A **pH probe**, usually inserted by gastroenterologists, records the duration and number of acid reflux episodes that occur in an infant or child. This is performed by inserting an intranasal catheter or a wireless device that is attached to the lower esophagus during endoscopy. The test is helpful for determining the risk of esophagitis. A normal pH probe study does not exclude GER. A positive test also does not always mean that recurrent wheezing or pneumonia is due to the GER detected; it just increases the likelihood that GER is a contributing factor.

Upper endoscopy with biopsy of the esophagus is the only way to definitively diagnose esophagitis. Also use this procedure to diagnose other diseases, such as eosinophilic (allergic) or infectious causes of esophagitis.

Nuclear scintigraphy is another test that can show where formula or food goes after normal feeding. In this case, an isotope-labeled formula or food is given in the normal fashion, and then the patient is monitored for episodes of GER for about an hour after feeding. Remember again, it is normal to have GER, so it is diagnostic only if food material is seen going into the lungs (aspiration). This indicates that airway protective measures are defective, and the child is at serious risk for aspiration. You also can use scintigraphy as part of an emptying study to measure the motility of the stomach, which can be responsible for delayed vomiting.

Treatment of GERD is initially aimed at dietary measures and positioning. The dietary measures include providing small meals, while also avoiding carbonated drinks, high-fat foods, acidic foods, caffeine, and nicotine (usually secondhand in children). Avoid bedtime snacks and treat obesity.

Treat esophagitis with an antisecretory agent, such as a proton pump inhibitor (e.g., omeprazole). Recent guidelines suggest that PPIs are superior to H_2-receptor blockers in healing esophagitis and improving symptoms. If esophagitis is severe and prolonged for many years without therapy, the esophagus can develop strictures, or Barrett esophagus can occur. Barrett esophagus presents with intestinal metaplasia in the distal esophagus. It is a pre-malignant condition requiring surveillance endoscopies and biopsy every 3–5 years. Barrett esophagus is rare in children and normally seen in the context of an underlying neurological disorder or esophageal anomaly.

GASTROENTEROLOGY & NUTRITION

While the use of proton pump inhibitors and H_2-receptor blockers has become common in children with asthma, recurrent respiratory symptoms, or recurrent sore throat/hoarseness, there is little evidence to support this practice.

Long-term acid blockade was previously thought to have few negative consequences, but recent evidence suggests otherwise. Infants taking acid-suppressing drugs have increased rates of pneumonia and viral gastroenteritis; and older children and adults may have increased risk for other gastrointestinal infections, such as *C. difficile*.

Do not use antacids, especially the aluminum-containing compounds, because they can cause toxicity. Bethanechol and metoclopramide are both prokinetic drugs, but neither has been shown to be effective in the treatment of GERD.

Surgical therapy is the final option, especially for those children with severe respiratory or neurologic disease. The most commonly used procedure is the Nissen fundoplication. In this operation, the fundus of the stomach is pulled up and wrapped around the lower esophagus. The parts of the stomach that are wrapped around the lower esophagus are then attached together to form a "valve." The operative mortality from Nissen fundoplication is about 1%, and there are many long-term consequences of the altered anatomy, including "gas-bloat" syndrome and dysphagia from a tight fundoplication. You can now perform this procedure laparoscopically with reduced perioperative morbidity.

Recent studies in adults have shown that prolonged medical therapy is more cost-effective and has lower morbidity.

EOSINOPHILIC ESOPHAGITIS

Eosinophilic esophagitis (often called EOE or EE) is a chronic inflammatory condition of the esophagus, which has become much more common over the past 2 decades.

EOE is now recognized as the most common cause of dysphagia or food impaction in children (60–80% of cases) and is an increasingly common cause for feeding difficulties in infants and toddlers. Suspect this disorder in any child with a history of a food bolus becoming stuck or who describes frequent odynophagia or dysphagia.

The only way to establish a diagnosis is via upper endoscopy. The surface may appear inflamed or ulcerated, but in many cases it may look normal. The key is the biopsy! If you see a large number of eosinophils (usually > 15 per high power field), then the patient has EOE.

Treatment is often difficult, although most experts now recommend high-dose acid suppression with a proton pump inhibitor, food elimination, or swallowed steroids (usually fluticasone or budesonide inhalers, which are swallowed rather than inhaled). Endoscopy is repeated after several months of treatment to determine if inflammation has decreased.

As much as 60% of children with EOE improve symptomatically with the elimination of dietary cow's milk. Some patients require a more complex "six-food elimination diet," which restricts cow's milk, soy, shellfish, wheat, eggs, and legumes (e.g., peanuts). Unfortunately, a specific food can be identified as the cause in only about 1/3 of these patients in this way. Allergy testing (either by serum IgE or by skin-prick test) rarely correlates either positively or negatively with empiric food challenges. The last resort for some patients is nutritional maintenance on an elemental formula.

Many patients with EOE also have some other form of atopy (e.g., asthma, eczema, allergic rhinitis, other food allergies), so this is a strong clue to the answer if a question mentions esophageal symptoms and atopic symptoms in the same patient.

INFECTIONS OF THE ESOPHAGUS

Infections of the esophagus are rare in children, except for those who are immunocompromised. Generally, children at risk are those with HIV, DM, cancer, and long-term, high-dose steroid usage.

Candida, CMV, and HSV are the most common organisms to cause infection in the esophagus. Dysphagia is the most common symptom with which children present. Odynophagia (pain with swallowing) and retrosternal burning are also seen. Diagnose by endoscopy with biopsy and brushings for culture. Treat *Candida* with fluconazole, CMV with ganciclovir and/or foscarnet, and HSV with acyclovir.

INGESTION OF TOXIC HOUSEHOLD PRODUCTS

Ingestion of various products around the house can induce severe esophagitis. The most common products ingested include bleach, laundry detergents, bathroom cleansers, drain cleaners, oven cleaners, and swimming pool products.

Acidic agents taste bad, cause immediate pain, and are rapidly spit or vomited out; because of this, significant ingestions are unusual. They generally cause more injury to the stomach than to the esophagus but can nevertheless cause esophageal damage, although this is rare. Alkaline agents are tasteless and swallowed without consequence initially. The alkalis produce a liquefactive necrosis with intense inflammation of the surrounding tissue. Granular alkalis, like drain cleaners, cause more injury to the mouth, pharynx, and proximal esophagus, while liquid drain openers cause severe injury to the entire esophagus but rarely to the stomach.

Children and infants present with drooling, dysphagia, or abdominal discomfort. Some present with airway symptoms only, including stridor, retractions, and nasal

Quick Quiz

- Which children are at risk for having infection of the esophagus?
- How long after ingestion of a caustic substance should upper endoscopy be performed?
- What are the most common pills that cause pill-induced esophagitis?
- What is the best way to determine if an ingested coin is in the esophagus?

flaring. The symptoms can be immediate or delayed for hours, and the lack of symptoms or the lack of significant oral findings do not necessarily correlate with the amount of esophageal or stomach damage. Severe damage can occur without outward signs or symptoms. Observe the child who has no symptoms and no physical findings—and a questionable history of ingestion—for several hours and give clear liquids to see if the child can tolerate them. Have those with a definite history of ingestion undergo additional tests (see below) no matter what their current symptoms or signs are, and they should remain NPO until after endoscopy.

Upper endoscopy is recommended 12–24 hours after the ingestion, but no later than 48 hours afterward due to increased risk of wall perforation (see Emergency Pediatric Care, Book 1). Doing the endoscopy before 12 hours may not show the full extent of injury. Burn injuries are divided into 3 classes. 1st degree burns are only superficial and consist of mucosal edema or redness. These lesions heal without scars and are well tolerated. 2nd degree burns extend into the submucosa and muscle layers. These lesions cause scarring and can result in strictures of the esophagus. 3rd degree burns extend through the esophagus and/or stomach and are associated with complete thickness burns and perforations. If you suspect perforation, arrange for immediate surgical treatment.

Initial management of ingestion of a caustic product is **observation**. Do not induce emesis, because it leads to further esophageal exposure to the agent. Use of neutralizing agents, milk, and large amounts of water are no longer recommended because of the risk of inducing vomiting. NG tubes are also not recommended because they can perforate damaged areas. If the child has developed upper airway disease, you will likely need to use steroids and/or intubate.

Neither antibiotics nor steroids have been proven to produce benefit in human studies. Nonetheless, some practitioners advocate for using broad-spectrum antibiotics and IV steroids, and most gastroenterologists consider using this combination in 3rd degree esophageal burns. Dilation has been used after stricture formation, and some recommend it after injury, but no studies have proven that it is efficacious as a preemptive method.

PILL-INDUCED ESOPHAGITIS

Pill-induced esophagitis is fairly common in children old enough to take pills, especially adolescents who swallow their pills "dry." The most common location for the pill to become stuck is in the mid-esophagus. Tetracycline, doxycycline, aspirin, NSAIDs, and slow-release potassium are the most common pills implicated. The pills adhere to the side of the esophagus, dissolve, and cause local irritation at the site. Symptoms usually begin soon after ingestion, and patients have retrosternal pain and dysphagia. Look for the adolescent who comes in with chest pain and a history of doxycycline for acne. If the diagnosis is not clear-cut, an endoscopy is helpful.

Symptoms generally resolve in 1–3 weeks. Agents to stop acid production may be helpful for severe cases, but, generally, no specific therapy is necessary other than advising the patient to swallow pills with water.

INGESTION OF FOREIGN BODIES

Ingestion of foreign bodies is common. In younger children, the most common objects by far are coins. In older children, it often refers to the accidental swallowing of chicken bones or fish bones. There are some psychiatric disorders that appear in childhood/adolescence that may lead to swallowing a variety of weird objects. For the most part, foreign bodies pass without incident. Only about 10–20% require endoscopic removal, and less than 1% require surgical intervention. Perforation anywhere in the GI tract after foreign body ingestion occurs in less than 1%. Once in the stomach, nearly 95% of foreign bodies pass without problem.

Symptoms, if they occur, are likely due to the foreign body getting stuck just below the cricopharyngeal muscle. Children may present with drooling, choking, or poor feeding. Older children can usually describe retrosternal pain and/or dysphagia. Respiratory symptoms alone can also occur and are typically due to the foreign body pushing against the posterior tracheal wall.

You can diagnose most with standard chest x-ray, because nearly 90% are radiopaque. Coins have a tendency to lie in the coronal plane ("face forward") in the esophagus and the sagittal plane ("on edge") in the trachea (Image 14-5 on page 14-14). A lateral chest or neck x-ray may be helpful to delineate the exact location of a foreign body. Sometimes you need contrast material or fluoroscopy to show non-opaque items, such as plastic toys or pieces of toys; however, with a good history of ingestion and physical symptoms, you can usually bypass this option.

The child or infant who presents with inability to swallow secretions or who is in respiratory distress requires immediate evaluation and intervention. Fiberoptic endoscopy is the method of choice to grab and remove objects under direct visualization. "Blind" removal with Foley catheters has become popular for removing coins, but you must be careful since some coins have popped over

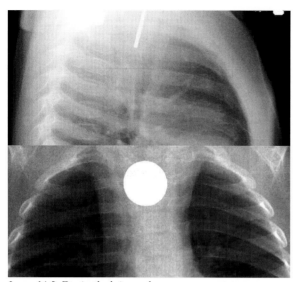
Image 14-5: Foreign body in esophagus

into the trachea in the process of removal, resulting in respiratory distress. Additionally, without direct observation with endoscopy, some foreign bodies turn out to be something more sinister, such as a battery. Observe for 12–24 hours children who are without respiratory distress and can swallow their own secretions. About 1/3 of these pass spontaneously. If the item has not passed into the stomach by 12–24 hours, then retrieve it. Items that are smooth and small and cannot be easily grabbed can be pushed into the stomach, so they can pass normally. Remove items longer than 10 cm, because they cannot easily pass the curve of the duodenum.

Sharp objects are also usually removed because of the increased risk of morbidity, except for straight pins, which can pass safely. Food impaction is a special case in older children and adolescents; it may require intervention if the patient is in respiratory distress or cannot swallow secretions. Without these accompanying problems, it typically passes on its own. Do not use meat tenderizer! It can cause hypernatremia and esophageal perforation.

Foreign bodies in adolescents and older children often indicate an underlying etiology—most commonly eosinophilic esophagitis.

ESOPHAGEAL PERFORATION

Esophageal perforation is rare in children. However, there are a few things you must remember. Spontaneous perforation can occur in patients with Ehlers-Danlos and Marfan syndromes. Pain occurs in the chest and upper back, as does subcutaneous emphysema. Fever and hypotension are common. Do not perform endoscopy in these patients! The safest thing to do is to get plain film x-rays, followed by instillation of a small amount of water-soluble contrast material. If the water-soluble contrast material does not show the perforation, you may have to proceed with a barium examination to better outline the abnormality.

Treat surgically, and then begin IV antibiotics and parenteral feeds. You can do enteral feeds by passing the tube past the healing perforation.

STOMACH DISORDERS

PYLORIC STENOSIS

Pyloric stenosis is fairly common, occurring in 1/750 to 1/200 live births. Boys are affected 6x more often than girls, but do not dismiss a female infant with compatible symptoms. It is more closely associated with smaller family size and higher socioeconomic status rather than with birth order. Caucasian children are 2–3x more likely to be affected than African American children. Asian Americans are less commonly affected. Early (younger than 2 weeks) exposure to erythromycin is also a frequently tested risk factor for pyloric stenosis.

Pyloric stenosis usually presents between 3 weeks and 2 months of age with progressively worsening, nonbilious vomiting. If vomiting is prolonged, hypochloremic metabolic alkalosis can develop, along with dehydration. Hypokalemia can also occur due to exchange of hydrogen ion and potassium in the kidney [Know!].

Studies show that the pyloric muscle is normal at birth but hypertrophies soon after and causes obstruction of the pyloric outlet. The etiology is unknown, although decreased levels of nitrous oxide are present.

Diagnose with physical examination by observing visible peristalsis and palpating for a mobile pyloric mass known as an "olive." Finding the "olive" means you have made the diagnosis because it is pathognomonic for pyloric stenosis. You will typically find it in 60–80% of those affected, although often much more easily once the patient is under anesthesia for their operation! If you cannot diagnose by physical examination, the next step is either an abdominal ultrasound—which will show a thickened and lengthened pyloric muscle, or an upper GI—which will show elongation and thickening of the pylorus, as well as obstruction of the pyloric outlet by thickened mucosa. Many advocate beginning with ultrasound due to its safety and high sensitivity. A memory trick is "pi" (3.14): On ultrasound, if the pyloric channel is thicker than 3 mm and longer than 14 mm, pyloric stenosis is highly likely.

Aim initial treatment at correcting dehydration and electrolyte abnormalities, particularly hypokalemia and alkalosis, before surgery. The surgical procedure of choice is pyloromyotomy, which is curative and has a very low mortality rate (< 0.5%). Full oral feeds can be commenced quickly after surgery. Recurrence rates are less than 1%.

CONGENITAL GASTRIC OUTLET OBSTRUCTION

Congenital gastric outlet obstruction is very rare and occurs in < 1/100,000 births. Pyloric webs are the most common and are areas of extra gastric mucosa and

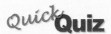

submucosa that prolapse into the duodenum. Patients present with epigastric pain, intermittent nonbilious emesis, or FTT. Perform an endoscopy to define the extent of the lesion.

Some neonates have complete pyloric atresia. They present with polyhydramnios, nonbilious emesis, and an enlarged, gas-filled stomach—with the rest of the abdomen gasless on plain abdominal x-ray. Pyloric atresia is associated with an autosomal recessive disorder in which infants have junctional epidermolysis bullosa. In this condition, simple minor skin friction results in severe vesiculobullous wounds. Diagnose the atresia with an upper GI series.

Treatment for gastric outlet obstruction consists of a surgical gastroduodenostomy or pyloroplasty with local excision, depending on the extent of the lesion.

CONGENITAL MICROGASTRIA

Congenital microgastria is rare and results in a small tubular stomach associated with a large "megaesophagus" and incomplete gastric rotation. It is also associated with asplenia and *situs inversus*, as well as limb and cardiac abnormalities. Children with this disorder present with vomiting and FTT. Diagnose with upper GI. Patients may still gradually develop a functional stomach, so it is best to wait on surgery until later in life. Consider surgery if jejunal continuous drip feeds do not produce gastric growth.

EROSIVE AND HEMORRHAGIC GASTROPATHY

Gastritis vs. Gastropathy

The words "gastritis" (characterized by the presence of inflammatory cells) and "gastropathy" (characterized by the absence of inflammatory cells) are frequently used interchangeably. The words "erosive" and "hemorrhagic" are descriptive of what is seen at the time of endoscopy. There are several causes, although these conditions are relatively uncommon in children.

Stress Gastropathy

Stress gastropathy is due to severe physiologic stress, such as occurs with shock, metabolic acidosis, sepsis, burns, and head injury. (Think sick ICU patient with an upper GI bleed!) Initially, the mucosal ischemia occurs in the fundus and proximal body, and later it spreads to the antrum, resulting in a diffuse erosive and hemorrhagic appearance. Prompt control of the underlying disorder improves the gastropathy/gastritis more than any acid-neutralizing therapy. Because control of the underlying disorder is often impossible, acid suppression is standard clinical practice.

Traumatic Gastropathy (Prolapse Gastropathy)

Traumatic gastropathy is usually due to forceful retching or vomiting (termed "emetogenic gastritis/gastropathy") that causes subepithelial hemorrhages in the fundus and proximal body as the proximal stomach is pulled up into the distal esophagus. The hemorrhages tend to resolve quickly, but large amounts of bleeding can occur in a short time period. Mallory-Weiss tears occur in the distal esophagus at the gastroesophageal junction and can extend into the gastric cardia from profound/extended retching, but note that Mallory-Weiss tears are rare in children. NG tubes and foreign bodies can also cause hemorrhages and erosions.

Drug-Induced Gastropathy

Aspirin and nonsteroidal antiinflammatory drugs are common causes of minor erosions and hemorrhages in the body and antrum of the stomach. Typically, these have little clinical significance. On occasion, NSAIDs can cause more extensive erosions and hemorrhages, resulting in perforation and excessive bleeding. The injuries result from local, as well as systemic, effects. Alcohol is a well-known cause of gastropathy. Corticosteroids are frequently implicated in upper GI bleeding; but this observation often coincides with stress gastropathy, and studies have not shown a clear drug-induced effect.

Exercise-Induced Gastritis

Exercise, particularly distance running, can produce blood loss with anemia from gastritis or gastropathy. GI symptoms may or may not accompany the anemia. The GI disorder can be erosive or nonerosive.

NONEROSIVE GASTROPATHY

Occurrence

Nonerosive gastropathy is the most common gastritis in children and adults. It usually occurs in the antrum and is a histologic diagnosis, since endoscopy may not show anything visually. Etiologies are varied.

GASTROENTEROLOGY & NUTRITION

Nonspecific Gastritis

Nonspecific gastritis is fairly common in children, with no identifiable etiology. On biopsy, the inflammation is chronic and superficial, as well as being focal instead of diffuse. The antrum is commonly involved.

Helicobacter pylori Gastritis

H. pylori is the most common identifiable cause of chronic gastritis in children. An acute infection of *H. pylori* can result in nausea, vomiting, decreased appetite, and epigastric abdominal pain, with a short period of increased acid secretion followed by a marked decrease in acid production. The acute symptoms last only about 1 week. Then, over the next 3–6 months, gastritis resolves and acid secretion returns to normal. Most patients then have a chronic infection with the organism, but in a large majority of individuals this causes no symptoms. The incidence of *H. pylori* is decreasing in the United States, but it remains endemic in many parts of the world, including Africa, the Middle East, India, and Southeast Asia. Note that *H. pylori* is also the primary cause of peptic ulcer disease (PUD), which we discuss later in this section.

Chronic gastritis due to *H. pylori* can cause atrophic gastritis and intestinal metaplasia in adults.

H. pylori is the primary identified cause of gastric adenocarcinoma. However, there appears to be no association between early childhood acquisition of *H. pylori* and the development of gastric cancer in adults. *H. pylori* is also the cause of a rare, slow-growing gastric lymphoma called "mucosa-associated lymphoid tissue" (MALT). MALTomas respond well to antibiotic therapy that eradicates *H. pylori*.

When the pathology is determined with endoscopic visualization and biopsy, a urea breath test (^{13}C or ^{14}C) or a rapid urea test (RUT) on the tissue is done to confirm the cause is *H. pylori*.

Positive gastric biopsies show the gram-negative spiral rods on the surface of the glandular epithelium under the mucous layer. Remember that with nonerosive gastritis, the endoscopic appearance can be normal; therefore, you must biopsy with endoscopy. *H. pylori* gastritis often results in the gastric mucosa appearing nodular.

Treatment and follow-up is essentially the same as for peptic ulcer disease caused by *H. pylori* (see next page).

Crohn Disease

We mention Crohn disease only briefly here; see more under Crohn Disease on page 14-27. Crohn's can cause typical aphthous ulcers in the stomach and duodenum, as well as focal, deep gastritis in the antrum of the stomach. On biopsy, look for giant cells and granulomas.

Allergic Gastritis

Allergic gastritis presents with an eosinophilic infiltrate only in the gastric mucosa; it does not go any deeper. (This is in contrast to eosinophilic gastritis discussed next.) Endoscopy is frequently normal or may show nonspecific swollen folds. It is usually fairly benign. Often, you can identify the allergen, and the patient will be cured if exposure is prevented.

Eosinophilic Gastritis

Eosinophilic gastritis can involve all layers of the gastric wall but frequently may lie in only the mucosa, muscle layers, or subserosa. It is less common than allergic gastritis and is usually much more severe. Biopsy may not be helpful; remember that only the deeper layers may be involved, and the standard mucosal biopsy does not pick up eosinophilic gastritis.

Ménétrier Disease

Ménétrier disease is a protein-losing gastropathy that results in hypoproteinemia. On endoscopy, the stomach fundus and body are folded and swollen. Typically, it presents as peripheral edema with nausea and vomiting, often after an apparent viral illness. Biopsy will show long, tortuous pits and a swollen lamina propria. You will also notice increased numbers of eosinophils and round cells in the lamina propria. It almost always is due to CMV infection. It resolves over several weeks to months in children, but in adults it is a chronic, unremitting disease.

PEPTIC ULCER DISEASE

Overview

Peptic ulcer disease (PUD) is very rare in children, and the majority is caused by *H. pylori* (especially duodenal ulcers) and then NSAIDs (especially gastric ulcers). The cause is unknown in only 20% of affected children.

Diagnosis

Important: *H. pylori* infection in children is common and ~ 80% of those infected are asymptomatic. Only about 20% of these infections cause chronic gastritis (see previously on this page) or PUD. This is why it is important to first diagnose the pathology and only then look for *H. pylori*. Do not test for *H. pylori* initially as an aid for diagnosis of abdominal pain! The presence of *H. pylori* alone is not helpful as a diagnostic indicator.

If you suspect PUD, perform an upper endoscopy. Remember, endoscopy is the best test for children with:

• upper GI bleeding,
• recurrent vomiting, or
• persistent unexplained abdominal pain.

Quick Quiz

- What is the most common identifiable cause of chronic gastritis in children?
- What usually causes Ménétrier disease?
- What organism is responsible for most peptic ulcer disease in children?
- When and how do you diagnose *H. pylori* infection?
- Are antibody tests useful in diagnosing active peptic ulcer disease?
- What is the treatment for *H. pylori* infection?
- What is Zollinger-Ellison syndrome?

An upper GI series is unacceptable in children for diagnosis of PUD.

Just as with chronic gastritis, when the pathology is determined with endoscopic visualization and biopsy, a urea breath test (^{13}C or ^{14}C) or a rapid urea test (RUT) on the tissue is done to confirm the cause is *H. pylori*.

Remember that serum antibody tests confirm only past exposure, not necessarily active, ongoing infection, so do not use them for diagnosis of active *H. pylori* infection.

The stool antigen test can be helpful to determine if a known infection is eradicated, but recent guidelines suggest not to use it for initial diagnosis.

Treatment of *H. pylori* PUD

Treatment of peptic ulcer disease requires both antibiotics and acid suppression. Pharmaceutical agents to reduce acid secretion are helpful to treat symptoms, as well as to heal erosions and ulcers more quickly. Ranitidine is commonly used, as are proton pump inhibitors (PPIs). Antacids are not recommended for most cases.

However, the key in *H. pylori*-induced PUD is to eradicate the infection. Additionally, in the presence of a positive *H. pylori* test, give anti-*H. pylori* therapy only when peptic ulcer disease is proven, or in MALT lymphoma. In children, do not treat *H. pylori* colonization indiscriminately.

Treat *H. pylori* infection with 2 weeks of a PPI plus clarithromycin, plus either amoxicillin or metronidazole. Give all 3 drugs in divided doses, twice a day. Recent evidence suggests that "sequential therapy," which uses antibiotics in a series rather than in parallel, increases the chance of cure with a single course.

Surgery is rarely indicated but may be required if there has been perforation of the stomach or duodenum; active bleeding cannot be controlled; gastric outlet or duodenal obstruction has occurred; or medical therapy has failed, as in hypersecretory syndromes (see below).

Follow-up of *H. pylori* PUD

Ulcers with complications (bleeding, perforation, or penetration) commonly relapse, so confirm healing and eradication of *H. pylori* with follow-up endoscopy.

For uncomplicated ulcers, confirm *H. pylori* eradication with symptom resolution and a follow-up urea breath test or stool antigen test.

Hold off on the follow-up urea breath test or stool antigen test until at least 4–6 weeks after acid suppression therapy has ended. Do not recommend dietary modification.

So, *H. pylori* is the primary identified cause of chronic gastritis, PUD, gastric adenocarcinoma, and MALT. And again, invasive tests (i.e., endoscopic visualization and biopsy) are done only for initial diagnosis, and noninvasive tests are done for follow-up.

PUD Due to Acid Hypersecretory Diseases

Note

There are only a few acid hypersecretory diseases. Note that for the ones discussed next, about 10% present with diarrhea and no ulcers. Mucosal resistance (likely due to genetic factors) prevents ulcer formation in these individuals.

Zollinger-Ellison Syndrome

Zollinger-Ellison syndrome is rare in children. It produces markedly excessive stomach acid due to a gastrin-secreting tumor (gastrinoma), usually located in the pancreas or duodenal wall. Multiple ulcers are common and frequently involve unusual sites for ulcers, such as the esophagus, stomach, or jejunum. The majority of gastrinomas are malignant but slow-growing tumors. A very similar rare syndrome is antral G-cell hyperplasia.

Gastrinomas are strongly associated with MEN1. About 25% of people with gastrinoma have MEN1 (so evaluate them for hyperparathyroidism and adrenal tumors as well!), and 50% of those with MEN1 have gastrinoma.

Perform surgical resection of the tumors if possible, but metastases to the lymph nodes and liver indicate poor prognoses.

Systemic Mastocytosis

Systemic mastocytosis is also associated with acid hypersecretion. It is a disease wherein mast cells accumulate in the skin, marrow, liver, spleen, and GI tract. Hyperparathyroidism is also noted with this disorder.

INTESTINAL DISORDERS

MALROTATIONS OF THE INTESTINE

Malrotation of the intestine can present anytime in infancy or childhood and may be due to nonrotation, incomplete rotation, paraduodenal hernia, or reverse rotation. Malrotation occurs in about 1/6,000 births. Omphalocele and gastroschisis always have malrotation as well. (See page 14-32.)

Nonrotation is the most common malrotation abnormality and presents with the cecum on the left and the small intestine to the right of the superior mesenteric artery. This results in a short mesentery and relatively little fixation of the bowel. The duodenum is small and fuses with the colon, using a common mesentery around the superior mesenteric artery.

Infants with malrotation classically present in the 1st month of life (90% present within the 1st year), with the acute development of bilious emesis. These infants present with abdominal distention and irritability, and, if the bowel strangulates, septic shock is likely. As the bowel necrosis worsens, the infant may develop hematemesis, melena, or both.

In an infant who has bilious vomiting with findings suggestive of malrotation and volvulus, perform an upper GI series for diagnosis. The upper GI series may demonstrate the classic "bird's beak" of the 2nd or 3rd portion of the duodenum, where the gut is twisted (Image 14-6). If the duodenum is partially obstructed, you may see a "corkscrew" pattern. For the older child with intermittent symptoms, the upper GI series can identify an abnormal location of the duodenojejunal junction (the ligament of Treitz). Normally, the ligament of Treitz is to the left of the spine at the level of the gastric antrum and is fixed to the posterior body wall. In malrotation, the ligament of Treitz is on the right side of the spine and is inferior to the duodenal bulb. Thus, in malrotation, contrast from the upper GI fills the jejunal loops on the right side of the abdomen.

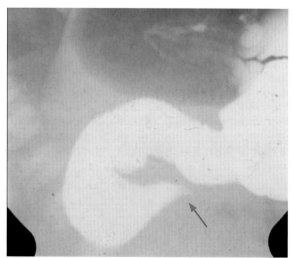

Image 14-6: Volvulus with "bird's beak" sign

After emergent management of the initial shock and cardiovascular compromise, emergent surgery (the Ladd procedure) must be performed. The Ladd procedure consists of opening the abdominal wall and taking out the intestines to inspect the mesenteric root. If the surgeon finds volvulus, they untwist it and inspect the bowel for viability. During surgery, they resect nonviable or necrotic areas, and perform enterostomies. If "questionable" areas of bowel are found, these are generally left in place; then after 12–36 hours, a "2nd look" surgery is performed to assess viability.

If a child is diagnosed with a malrotation but is asymptomatic, most recommend an elective Ladd procedure as quickly as possible.

INTUSSUSCEPTION

Intussusception occurs when one part of the intestine "telescopes" into the lumen of the adjoining bowel. With this telescoping, mesentery is dragged into the process, which can cause venous obstruction, swelling, and/or edema of the bowel wall. Eventually, the edema can cause arterial obstruction, ischemia, and perforation. Intussusception usually occurs between 2 months and 5 years of age, with a peak incidence between 4 and 10 months. Almost all are idiopathic; that is, no pathologic lead point is discovered. Most originate near the ileocecal junction, and many believe these are due to a virus-induced swelling of Peyer patches. The initial rotavirus vaccine was removed from the market due to concerns of an increased rate of intussusception (never proven).

Patients with intussusception present with repeated episodes of severe abdominal pain, with asymptomatic intervals. Vomiting (if obstruction occurs) and hematochezia (if bowel ischemia occurs) are symptoms as well.

An infant with intussusception awakens with crying and has flexion of the knees and hips. Frequently, the pain subsides, and the child appears comfortable. A normal bowel movement is common with the pain; but subsequent bowel movements may look like "currant jelly," and these may occur hours or days after the abdominal pain. Eventually, the pain episodes increase in severity and frequency. Lethargy is a late, ominous sign and likely results from worsening metabolic acidosis. Examination between episodes shows a soft abdomen, and, during an episode, you may be able to palpate a sausage-shaped mass in the right upper quadrant or mid-upper abdomen.

Ultrasound is the best initial imaging study. Look for a "target sign" of telescoped bowel. Plain abdominal x-rays may show a soft tissue mass displacing loops of bowel.

An air-contrast enema is the diagnostic and therapeutic procedure of choice. Nearly 90% may be reduced with the procedure. Peritonitis is an absolute contraindication—and bowel obstruction is a relative contraindication—for an air-contrast enema. Recurrence

Quick Quiz

- At what age do infants with malrotation classically present?
- What does an upper GI series show in an infant with malrotation?
- At what age does intussusception usually occur?
- With what symptoms does a child with intussusception present?
- What is the diagnostic procedure of choice in patients with suspected intussusception?
- What is the "rule of 2s" in Meckel diverticulum?
- What test is preferred to diagnose Meckel diverticulum?

rates are 3–10%, and most recommend admission for 24-hour observation. If the air-contrast enema is unsuccessful, quickly perform a laparotomy. Consult a pediatric surgeon early in the process, because it is helpful to have a surgeon immediately present if air-contrast enema reduction fails.

MECKEL DIVERTICULUM

A Meckel diverticulum occurs when the vitelline (omphalomesenteric) duct fails to become obliterated. It is a "true" diverticulum containing all 3 tissue layers. Ectopic tissue is often present (about 20% of the time), and is typically gastric in origin.

For Meckel diverticula, you must know the "rule of **2**s":

- Present in **2**% of the population (usually asymptomatic)
- Located within **2** feet of the ileocecal valve
- Measures **2** inches in length
- Measures **2** centimeters in diameter
- **2**:1 male-female ratio
- Usually symptomatic before **2** years of age (if and when symptoms are actually present)

In most instances, a Meckel diverticulum is clinically asymptomatic. When found, it is typically an incidental finding discovered during surgery done for a different purpose. The lifetime risk of complication from a Meckel diverticulum, if it is present, is 4%. Symptoms occur more commonly in patients who are less than 2 years of age. The main symptoms are due to gastrointestinal bleeding from ectopic gastric mucosa. In fact, a Meckel diverticulum is the most common cause of serious lower GI bleeding in children.

A Meckel diverticulum is associated with other congenital anomalies, including esophageal atresia (6x risk), imperforate anus (5x risk), neurologic (3x risk), and cardiovascular (2x risk). Patients with a Meckel diverticulum have a 3x risk of developing Crohn disease.

Painless rectal bleeding is the most common presenting symptom. Occasionally, colicky abdominal pain accompanies the bleeding. The color of the blood can be bright red or maroon and has been described on occasion to resemble intussusception with "currant jelly" character. Transfusions are often required because of the large amount of bleeding that occurs. Bleeding tends to stop and start spontaneously.

Diagnosis is difficult. Most prefer a technetium ^{99m}pertechnetate scan (also called the Meckel scan). This scan works because a majority of bleeding Meckel diverticula contain ectopic gastric mucosa. The ^{99m}pertechnetate concentrates in the parietal cells of gastric mucosa and the bladder. A positive scan is indicated when finding isotope uptake outside of the stomach and bladder. Histamine H_2 blockers can enhance the accuracy of the scan. The Meckel scan has an excellent positive predictive value (if a test is positive, a Meckel is likely to be present), but a poor negative predictive value (a negative scan does not rule out the disease very well).

A Meckel diverticulum requires surgical intervention. Fluid and blood are usually required before surgery if the antecedent lower GI bleed is hemodynamically significant. If a Meckel diverticulum is found incidentally during an abdominal surgery in a young child, most pediatric surgeons resect it. For older children or adults, resection is controversial because the risk of bleeding, if the Meckel diverticulum is left alone, is much lower in these older groups.

CONGENITAL INTESTINAL ATRESIAS

Occurrence

Atresias of the gut happen in about 1/5,000 births, with most occurring in the duodenum or other areas of the small intestines.

Duodenal Atresia

Duodenal atresia accounts for over 50% of the intestinal atresias. Duodenal atresia is associated with multiple anomalies, including cardiac, GU, anorectal, and esophageal. About 50% are in premature neonates. 40% of patients with duodenal atresia have trisomy 21 (Down syndrome). Polyhydramnios and a dilated stomach may be visualized on prenatal ultrasound. A majority have their obstruction distal to the ampulla of Vater; so they also have bilious vomiting on the 1st day of life. Abdominal plain x-rays will show the classic "double bubble," (Image 14-7 on page 14-20). This is diagnostic if the rest of the bowel is airless. If there is distal gas, confirm with an upper GI. Surgery is necessary, and most of the complications occur due to the associated cardiac abnormalities.

Jejunoileal Atresia

Jejunoileal atresia is different from duodenal atresia in that jejunoileal atresia is not associated with

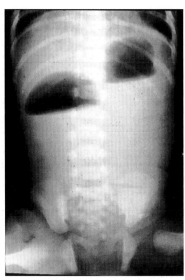
Image 14-7: Duodenal atresia

other congenital anomalies. Prenatal diagnosis is possible with maternal ultrasound. Postnatally, patients present with abdominal distention and bilious emesis. They may or may not have meconium stools. Abdominal x-rays show multiple, dilated loops of bowel with air-fluid levels. Diagnosis is best made with an upper GI or lower GI, and it must be differentiated from meconium ileus, which is seen with cystic fibrosis. Surgery is necessary, with the goal of salvaging as much small bowel as possible.

Colonic Atresia

Colonic atresia is the rarest of the intestinal atresias. If the colon is the only segment involved, patients present with distal bowel obstruction, abdominal distention, bilious emesis, and failure to pass meconium. Confirm diagnosis with a contrast enema, which shows a distal microcolon and the point of obstruction. Surgical reanastomosis is the treatment of choice.

INTESTINAL DUPLICATIONS

Intestinal duplications are rare and may occur anywhere from the mouth to the anus, but the most common location is in the ileum.

3 characteristics are required by definition:

1) Contiguous and strongly adherent to some part of the GI tract
2) 2-layered muscular coat
3) Lined with mucosa or epithelium similar to that of the stomach, small intestine, or colon

Intestinal duplications are located on the mesenteric instead of the antimesenteric side of the bowel and share a common blood supply with the adjacent bowel. This differs from a Meckel diverticulum, which occurs on the antimesenteric side of the bowel. About 1/4 have ectopic mucosa, which is often gastric but

occasionally pancreatic in character. Remember that having ectopic gastric mucosa predisposes to bleeding and peptic ulceration.

Complications from intestinal duplications can include obstruction, intussusception, bleeding, pain, and perforation. It is common for them to present with abdominal pain and frequent vomiting. You can confirm diagnosis with exploratory laparotomy for the symptoms/complications. See Image 14-8, an ultrasound image showing intestinal duplication.

Gastric duplications, another type of intestinal duplication, occur most commonly in girls < 1 year of age. They are much rarer than the ileal location and make up only about 5% of intestinal duplications. Gastric duplications are usually cystic and are located on the greater curvature of the stomach. They do not communicate with the stomach lumen. Major complications include bleeding and ulcerations because they contain gastric mucosa and secrete acid. Treat by resecting the duplication.

Colonic and rectal duplications, additional types of intestinal duplications, are very rare and are associated with GU malformations. Rectal duplications may be confused with rectal prolapse, hemorrhoids, or fistulas.

MECONIUM ILEUS

See The Fetus & Newborn, Book 3, for the discussion of meconium ileus and meconium plug syndrome.

CARBOHYDRATE MALABSORPTION

Lactase Deficiency (Lactose Intolerance)

Lactase deficiency is a common disorder in U.S. patients who are older than 2 years, with prevalence varying substantially by race. Lactase is normally found on the brush border near the tips of the intestinal villi, and it cleaves lactose into glucose and galactose. Primary adult-type

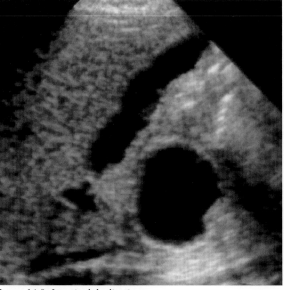
Image 14-8: Intestinal duplication

Quick Quiz

- What do abdominal plain x-rays show in neonates with duodenal atresia?
- Which is associated with other congenital anomalies—jejunoileal or duodenal atresia?
- What is the common carbohydrate metabolism deficiency in the United States that starts after the age of 2 years?
- What is the most common reliable test to diagnose lactase deficiency?

hypolactasia (known as adult-onset lactase deficiency) is the most common genetic cause of carbohydrate malabsorption in the world. It is due to a post-weaning decline in intestinal lactase-specific activity. (Infants are universally able to ingest lactose-containing breast milk and other milk products.) In individuals with this genetic programming, the lactose gene (located on chromosome 2q21) "down-regulates" and produces a much lower lactase level. This can occur as early as the 2nd year of life and may persist into adulthood. Most of the world's population is genetically prone to become "lactase deficient" by early adulthood, except for Caucasian populations of northern and central European descent. As much as 90% of those of Asian descent and 75% of those of African descent are affected. Symptoms of diarrhea and recurrent abdominal pain can occur in those with low levels of lactase who consume a large amount of lactose-containing foods.

Secondary lactase deficiency, sometimes seen in infancy, is usually transient and due to a secondary cause (e.g., infectious diarrhea). In addition, premature infants can have a transient developmental lactase deficiency that resolves as they reach term. And finally, there is also a very rare "congenital" lactase deficiency that presents at birth. It is autosomal recessive and symptoms (most notably severe diarrhea) resolve with complete removal of lactose from the diet.

The diagnosis of lactase deficiency is usually made solely on clinical grounds. However, be familiar with the following tests:

1) Endoscopic biopsy with measurement of mucosal enzyme activity is the gold standard study for disaccharide activity but is rarely done today because of the invasiveness and expense.

2) The breath hydrogen test is the most common reliable diagnostic test. When carbohydrate is malabsorbed, bacteria in the colon produce hydrogen gas, which is then absorbed across the colon mucosa into the bloodstream, transported to the lungs, and expired. In the breath hydrogen test, breath is sampled sequentially after the patient is given a test carbohydrate substance. A rise of more than 10–20 ppm in expired hydrogen indicates that the carbohydrate is not being digested, and then absorbed, properly. If the rise is too early, this typically indicates small bowel bacterial overgrowth. A child on antibiotics may produce a false-negative test, because the bacteria needed for hydrogen production are missed due to the presence of the antibiotics.

3) Measurement of stool-reducing sugars (using Clinitest®) and fecal pH can be useful screening methods. However, these tests usually require a liquid, fresh stool obtained after the patient has consumed the offending carbohydrate. They are rarely used in clinical practice.

Advise older children and adults with lactase deficiency to avoid large quantities of lactose-containing foods (e.g., most commonly milk, ice cream, and soft cheeses) and to limit their intake of lactose to foods like hard cheeses that contain relatively small amounts of lactose. As an alternative, microbial-derived lactase enzyme (e.g., Lactaid®) can be used with meals.

In the past, many recommended lactose avoidance for infants during acute infectious diarrhea (which often causes a secondary lactase deficiency). However, current AAP guidelines advise continuation of a regular diet throughout the diarrheal illness because early refeeding of milk does not prolong diarrhea.

Fructose and Sorbitol Malabsorption

Fructose and sorbitol are used extensively in commercial food products. Fructose is used as a sweetener, especially as high-fructose corn syrup in soft drinks. Sorbitol is a poorly absorbed sugar best known for its use in "diet" foods.

Both fructose and sorbitol may cause malabsorption symptoms if consumed in quantities that exceed the ability of the intestine to break down and absorb these sugars. The transport carrier protein is GLUT5, located on the apical membrane of the enterocyte, and it can be overwhelmed by excessive quantities of these sugars. Fructose malabsorption is associated with diarrhea, abdominal pain, and distention. Fruit juices with high fructose-to-glucose ratios and those with sorbitol (apple, pear) may cause nonspecific diarrhea and recurrent abdominal pain.

Sucrase-Isomaltase Deficiency

Sucrase-isomaltase deficiency is an autosomal recessive disorder that first appears when sucrose-containing formula or fruits are introduced to the older infant. In the U.S., the incidence of this condition is approximately 5/1,000; but in some Canadian populations, it has been reported to occur as commonly as 1/10. These children have low levels of sucrase and maltase and cannot digest starches easily. They can present with mild-to-severe diarrhea and abdominal pain. Sacrosidase, an enzyme derived from *Saccharomyces cerevisiae*, is a potent sucrase and can be taken with meals to overcome sucrase deficiency.

Secondary Carbohydrate Malabsorption

Secondary carbohydrate malabsorption is very common in diseases that cause intestinal mucosal damage or atrophy. Rotavirus is the most common infectious agent. *Giardia* infection and HIV also cause carbohydrate malabsorption. Conditions of bacterial overgrowth can lead to impaired monosaccharide transport. Secondary carbohydrate malabsorption can also affect infants with short gut syndrome who don't have enough surface area to complete carbohydrate digestion. Finally, children with cystic fibrosis or other causes of pancreatic insufficiency cannot absorb starches adequately, due to reduced or absent amylase.

CONGENITAL TRANSPORT DEFECTS

Note

Congenital transport defects are rare. For exam questions, you generally just have to know the "syndrome" and the "defect." But a few require further discussion. (See Table 14-4 and Table 14-5.)

Abetalipoproteinemia and Other Disorders of Fat Transport

Abetalipoproteinemia is an autosomal recessive disorder. In patients with this disorder, there is congenital absence of apolipoprotein B (apo B), which results in an inability to synthesize chylomicrons and very-low-density lipoprotein (VLDL). Patients present with very malodorous steatorrhea and FTT. Fat-soluble vitamins (A, D, E, K) cannot be absorbed, eventually leading to development of problems such as night blindness, sensory ataxia, and nystagmus. Retinitis pigmentosa is present. You will see acanthocytosis on peripheral blood smear because the red blood cells have abnormal membrane lipids. Serum cholesterol is extremely low, and triglyceride levels are just barely detectable. Confirm by observing an absence of plasma β-lipoprotein. Treat by limiting dietary intake of long-chain fatty acids and giving medium-chained triglycerides. Supplement with vitamins E, A, and K. Prognosis is poor.

An autosomal dominant disease known as **hypobetalipoproteinemia** presents in a manner that is similar to abetalipoproteinemia. An autosomal dominant family history (e.g., 1 or more 1st degree relatives with the disease) is a distinguishing feature.

Chylomicron retention disease (Anderson disease) is an autosomal recessive disorder that occurs due to defective exocytosis of chylomicrons. It presents mainly with diarrhea, steatorrhea, and low serum cholesterol without the severe acanthocytosis, retinitis pigmentosa, and neurologic abnormalities (which are more typical of the abeta- and hypobetalipoproteinemias).

Amino Acid Transport Defects

Amino acid transport defects are rare and can involve the small intestine enterocyte, as well as the proximal renal tubule. Clinically, these can be asymptomatic to severe.

Hartnup disease is due to a defect in transport of free neutral amino acids. It results in a deficiency of nicotinamide synthesized from tryptophan and leads to pellagra-type findings. **Blue diaper syndrome** is due to isolated malabsorption of tryptophan. **Lowe syndrome** is due to malabsorption of lysine and arginine and presents with intellectual disability, cataracts, hypotonia, and vitamin D-resistant rickets. You can detect all of these with analysis of urine amino acids. (See Metabolic Disorders, Book 3.)

Congenital Electrolyte Diarrhea

Congenital electrolyte diarrhea can be either a chloride defect or a sodium defect.

For **congenital chloride diarrhea**, the defect involves the Cl⁻/HCO₃⁻ exchange transport system in the ileum and colon. This results in watery diarrhea with a high chloride and low bicarbonate and pH. You can recognize these infants *in utero* with the presence of polyhydramnios due to the excessive diarrhea. Dehydration is common, as is metabolic alkalosis and hypochloremia at birth and in the newborn period. The diarrhea resolves over time, by 3–4 years of age.

Congenital sodium diarrhea presents very similarly but has stool sodium concentrations that are higher than

Table 14-4: Congenital Transport Defects

Name	Defect	Symptom
Abetalipoproteinemia	Apo B	Steatorrhea, FTT
Chylomicron retention	Chylomicron exocytosis	Steatorrhea, FTT
Congenital chloride diarrhea	Cl⁻/HCO₃⁻ exchanger	Low pH diarrhea, alkalosis
Congenital sodium diarrhea	Na⁺/H⁺ exchanger	High pH diarrhea, acidosis

Table 14-5: Congenital Transport Defects

Name	Transport Defect and Result
Hartnup disease	Free neutral amino acids; pellagra-like
Blue diaper syndrome	Tryptophan; bluish urine-stained diapers
Lowe syndrome	Lysine and arginine; intellectual disability, cataracts, hypotonia, rickets
Acrodermatitis enteropathica	Zinc; rash, diarrhea, FTT, alopecia, blepharitis, conjunctivitis

Quick **Quiz**

- What does the absence of apo B result in?
- What is Hartnup disease?
- How do children with abnormal zinc absorption present?
- What dietary protein induces celiac disease?

the chloride, and the stool is alkaline instead of acidic. This is a result of a defect in the Na^+/H^+ exchange transport. This results in a metabolic acidosis instead of a metabolic alkalosis.

Zinc Deficiency

Acrodermatitis enteropathica is an extremely rare autosomal recessive disease with an abnormal chromosome 8q24.3. In patients with this condition, zinc is not adequately absorbed. As a consequence, these patients develop bullous and pustular dermatitis. Additionally, alopecia, blepharitis, conjunctivitis, diarrhea, and FTT are common. Breast milk contains the missing zinc-binding factor, so symptoms won't appear in a breastfed infant until 2–3 weeks after weaning has occurred. Deficiency develops 1–2 months after birth in a non-breastfed infant.

You can confirm diagnosis by the above classic clinical findings and by demonstrating a zinc concentration below 50 µg/dL. Treat with oral elemental zinc 35–100 mg daily for life. Expect prompt improvement (1–2 days) with initiation of therapy.

SHORT GUT SYNDROME

Short gut syndrome is a malabsorption disorder caused by shortened intestinal length, due to congenital anomalies of the gut or to resection of the small intestine. Common causes include necrotizing enterocolitis, volvulus, malrotation, multiple atresias, and gastroschisis. There also exists a congenital short bowel syndrome, but it is not common. Malabsorption occurs because of a lack of mucosal absorptive surface. Other contributing factors may be bile acid deficiency and bacterial overgrowth syndromes.

Just how much bowel is required for normal good health isn't clear. We do know that most infants with at least 38 cm of small intestine survive, and those with less than 15 cm die or require small intestinal transplantation. Normally, infants have 200–300 cm of small intestine. This lengthens to 600–800 cm in adulthood. Recently, there have been reports of survival with shorter bowel lengths, so it appears that a more important factor may be the functional capacity of the remaining bowel.

Some surgical procedures have been shown to improve bowel length in these patients, such as the older Bianchi procedure (bowel is cut lengthwise into 2 segments, which are then sewed end-to-end) or the newer STEP (serial transverse enteroplasty in which a series of alternating cuts are made, turning the bowel into an accordion, which stretches out).

If the defect is in the duodenum, expect decreased iron, folate, and calcium absorption, which results in anemia and osteopenia. If the defect is in the jejunum, there are generally no specific ill effects except the loss of absorptive surface area. If the defect is in the ileum, though, the result is severe, with large fluid and electrolyte losses. Remember that the ileum is responsible for absorption of 2 specific items: 1) bile salts and 2) vitamin B_{12}. Inability to absorb bile salts results in fat malabsorption (and therefore hypovitaminosis A, K, D and E) and vitamin B_{12} deficiency.

If the short gut is due to surgery, adaptive measures in the remaining small intestine usually kick in and eventually result in improved absorption. Again, this depends largely on how much and what part of the small intestine remains, as well as how much functionality of the mucosal area is left. If symptoms do not improve, or TPN is required for lifelong survival, an intestinal transplant is often performed. Unfortunately, intestinal transplant is not curative, and outcomes and survival remain poor even after successful transplant.

GLUTEN-SENSITIVE ENTEROPATHY (CELIAC DISEASE)

Celiac disease, a.k.a. celiac sprue or gluten-sensitive enteropathy, occurs in genetically predisposed children and adults after exposure to specific gluten proteins and resultant intestinal inflammation and damage due to immunological cross-reaction. In susceptible individuals, gluten from wheat products (and similar proteins found in rye and barley) can induce the immune reaction to human transglutaminase and the resulting mucosal damage. Preventing exposure to these products is the only way to make the symptoms go away.

Celiac disease is becoming recognized as an extremely common disorder, and many studies using serology-based screening have determined the incidence to be 0.5–2% (between 1/50 and 1/200) in the developed world, with considerable racial differences. There is also evidence that the incidence has been increasing over the past 20 years.

HLA typing shows only 2 HLA types are associated with celiac disease, DQ2 and DQ8. Penetrance is variable, and people with known genetic markers for celiac disease do not necessarily develop it. You initially see the immune response in the duodenum, but it eventually spreads to the jejunum and ileum. The mucosal lesions are characterized by increased numbers of lymphocytes, plasma cells, and macrophages in the lamina propria, and by increased numbers of intraepithelial lymphocytes.

GASTROENTEROLOGY & NUTRITION

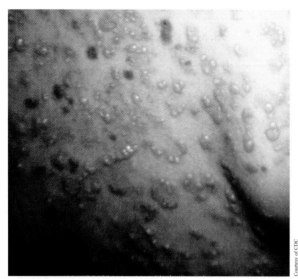

Courtesy of CDC

Image 14-9: Dermatitis herpetiformis

Clinically, patients can present with a variety of symptoms. The "classic" GI form of the disease presents in the child < 2 years of age with symptoms that include malabsorptive diarrhea, poor weight gain, abdominal distention, and proximal muscle wasting. If the malabsorption is significant, look out for resulting vitamin D deficiency and hypocalcemia in the patient who presents with seizures and hypocalcemic tetany. Iron deficiency anemia is common at diagnosis, and unexplained iron deficiency prompts you to look for celiac disease.

Patients with celiac disease may have an associated affective disorder—typically anxiety or depression. Common symptoms include anger, moodiness, and impatience. Sometimes celiac disease is misdiagnosed as ADHD.

In the last 25 years, it has become more apparent that there is a spectrum of presentations of this disease and not all of them are gastrointestinal. The mucosal damage that is occurring can precede the symptoms for many years. Celiac disease today (for reasons that are unclear) often presents with symptoms in the adolescent or adult rather than the young child. When symptoms do occur in this older age group, they can still be gastrointestinal in nature, with diarrhea, abdominal pain, distention, and bloating. More frequently, you may observe extraintestinal symptoms, with delayed puberty and poor growth.

Dermatitis herpetiformis—presenting as extremely itchy, vesicles (i.e., blisters) on the extensor surfaces of the arms, legs, trunk, and on the scalp—can occur with or without gastrointestinal symptoms. The lesion is pathognomonic for celiac disease (Image 14-9).

Autoimmune disorders are common with celiac disease and can include Type 1 DM, autoimmune thyroid disease, Sjögren syndrome, collagen vascular disease, liver disease, and IgA glomerulonephritis. Celiac disease is so common in children with Type 1 DM and selective IgA deficiency that many physicians recommend universal screening in these patients.

Additionally, celiac disease is 50x more common in children with Down syndrome.

Laboratory screening is readily available. The most common tests are antibody tests, along with measurement of a total serum IgA since IgA deficiency may occur in celiac disease. These include:

• IgA antibody to tissue transglutaminase (anti-tTG IgA)
• IgA anti-endomysium antibodies

Most medical centers now screen for celiac disease with an anti-tTG IgA alone. IgA tends to be a better immunoglobulin to test for, since that is the antibody involved in the disease—and is secreted into the gut lumen. The older antigliadin antibodies have poor sensitivity and specificity. If the serologic testing is positive (or if clinical suspicion is high in the face of negative serologic testing), confirm the diagnosis with small intestinal biopsy. Important: Do not place the patient on a gluten-free diet prior to endoscopy.

There are 2 mandatory requirements for diagnosis:

1) Characteristic histology on small intestinal biopsy
2) Complete clinical remission with a gluten-free diet

It is very rare now to undertake the old diagnostic protocol of classic histology that responds to dietary elimination of gluten and relapse of histologic disease with rechallenge. Notice that this requires 3 endoscopies for biopsy!

Treat with dietary exclusion of wheat, oats, barley, and rye. An increasing number of products are becoming available to these patients. You can monitor for low or zero anti-tTG levels to determine if gluten and other products are being effectively excluded from the diet.

CONGENITAL MICROVILLUS INCLUSION DISEASE

Congenital microvillus inclusion disease (a.k.a. Davidson disease, familial protracted diarrhea, or microvillus atrophy) is an autosomal recessive disorder and the most common cause of congenital diarrhea. If the villi of the small intestine are examined under a microscope, they show diffuse thinning of the mucosa without crypt hypertrophy or an inflammatory cell reaction. The characteristic electron microscopy finding is the presence of microvilli within involutions of the apical membrane.

Infants present early in life with severe watery diarrhea and FTT. Fecal water losses can exceed 800 mL/kg/day. The excessive water loss continues even when nothing is given orally. Tests for intestinal absorption are all abnormal, including fecal fat, and infants present with a marked secretory diarrhea with very high stool electrolytes. Death rates are above 80%. No treatment is effective. If children do survive, either they are maintained on parenteral nutrition for life or they must undergo small intestinal transplantation.

Quick Quiz

- How does the classic gastrointestinal form of celiac disease present in children < 2 years of age?

- Children with Type 1 DM and selective IgA deficiency should be screened for what disease?

- What is congenital microvillus inclusion disease?

- What organism causes Whipple disease?

- What part of the gastrointestinal tract does UC affect?

TROPICAL SPRUE

Tropical sprue is mainly seen in long-term visitors (at least 3 months) or inhabitants of endemic regions of the tropics, which include India, parts of Asia, the Philippines, areas of South America, Central America, parts of the Caribbean, and areas of central and southern Africa. Sprue can occur in children but is more common in adults. It is probably infectious, but so far no pathogen has been found.

Malabsorption of sugars, fats, folate, and vitamins A and B_{12} occurs. Early in the disease, fatigue, diarrhea, and anorexia are common. The diarrhea is accompanied by abdominal cramps and flatulence. Nutritional deficiencies eventually occur and present as night blindness, cheilosis, glossitis, stomatitis, and hyperkeratosis. Edema and muscle wasting occur in the final stages of the disease. It can take 6 months to several years for the final stages to occur.

Treat with oral broad-spectrum antibiotics and nutritional supplements, including folate and vitamins A and B_{12}.

WHIPPLE DISEASE

Whipple disease is very rare in children and presents as a multisystem disorder resulting in severe malabsorption. You may frequently note arthritis, polyserositis, and CNS symptoms. Fever is also prominent. The etiology is a gram-positive actinomycete called *Tropheryma whipplei*. The hallmark is finding PAS-positive granules in the lamina propria. You must treat with antibiotics for 6 months or longer for cure.

ULCERATIVE COLITIS

Overview

Ulcerative colitis (UC) and Crohn disease make up the inflammatory bowel diseases. UC occurs less commonly than Crohn disease, and 12 years is its mean age of diagnosis. In UC, the inflammation is restricted to the colon and does not involve the small intestine. (Remember this with a simple mnemonic: UC = **u**nanimously **c**olon.) UC involves only the mucosa—mucosa that is contiguous without skip lesions. It starts in the rectum and spreads into the colon. See Table 14-6 for comparison of UC and Crohn disease.

Presentation of UC

Patients classically present with abdominal pain and bloody diarrhea; however, at onset, many patients have only nonbloody diarrhea. Generally, the more severe the symptoms, the more severe the colonic involvement. Fever and arthralgias/arthritis are the most common extraintestinal findings. The arthritis is migratory, asymmetric, and mainly involves the hip and/or knee. Clubbing is common in prolonged disease. Ankylosing spondylitis, erythema nodosum (Image 14-10 on page 14-26), and pyoderma gangrenosum (Image 14-11 on page 14-26) can all occur. Primary sclerosing cholangitis

Table 14-6: Comparison of Ulcerative Colitis and Crohn Disease		
	Ulcerative Colitis	**Crohn Disease**
Bowel involvement	Colon only	Anywhere from mouth to anus
Pattern of lesions	Continuous, beginning distally, and extending proximally	Skip lesions
Involvement of tissue	Mucosal only (generally)	Transmural disease
Granulomas likely	No	Yes
Weight loss	None or mild	Severe
Hematochezia	Common	Less common
X-ray findings	Superficial disease, loss of haustrations, thumbprinting	Skip areas, string signs
Perianal lesions	None	Common
Aphthous mouth ulcers	Rare	Common
Growth failure	Rare	Common

Image 14-10: Erythema nodosum

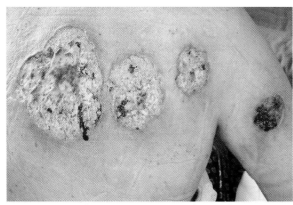

Image 14-11: Pyoderma gangrenosum

occurs in about 3% of patients and sometimes presents before the colonic disease. There is also increased prevalence of deep vein thrombosis and pulmonary emboli.

Diagnosis of UC

You can make a diagnosis with endoscopy and colonoscopy and characteristic endoscopic appearance and biopsies. Ulcerative colitis tends to involve a contiguous area of colon beginning in the rectum, and extending proximally. Involved mucosa is friable (bleeds when you bump into it), erythematous, nodular, and often has mucus or pus oozing from it. Plain films can be done in an acutely ill child, but these are rarely helpful. With severe colitis, you see thickening of the colonic wall ("thumbprinting"). Sometimes, an abbreviated sigmoidoscopy for examination and biopsy is clinically indicated. In the acutely ill child with colitis, perform a flexible sigmoidoscopy rather than a barium enema. The advantage of the sigmoidoscopy is that it allows for mucosal biopsies that are diagnostic.

In children with ulcerative colitis, the histology from colon biopsies tends to show areas of chronic and acute inflammation, often with a mixed population of cells. The crypts in the wall of the colon are often distorted and full of small abscesses, signs of chronic inflammation. Granulomas are not present.

Treatment of UC

Lifelong Treatment

Treatment is lifelong and includes a variety of agents. Overall, medications are either used to induce remission or maintain remission, but some are useful for both.

5-Aminosalicylic Acid (5-ASA)

5-ASA can be used to both induce remission and maintain remission in mild-to-moderate cases. Sulfasalazine was one of the first 5-aminosalicylates used and is composed of 5-ASA linked by an azo bond to sulfapyridine. It is the 5-ASA that is the active antiinflammatory agent. Nausea and headache are common side effects and are related to the sulfapyridine. Newer agents (mesalamine, olsalazine, etc.) without the sulfa component are available but are more expensive. A wide variety of mesalamine-containing formulations exist, none of which has been proven to be more efficacious than any of the others. Removing the sulfa component has reduced the side-effect profile for these agents. Most patients with mild-to-moderate UC respond very well to sulfasalazine. After remission has been attained, many can be maintained on mesalamine. Suppository and enema forms are also available and work well for those children with distal disease.

Corticosteroids

Corticosteroids are very effective in relieving symptoms and inducing remission in moderate-to-severe UC, but they do not have a role in maintenance of remission, and in fact can be quite dangerous if used for long periods of time. Long-term use is associated with significant side effects, including hyperglycemia, osteoporosis, osteonecrosis, myopathy, susceptibility to infection, cataracts, growth retardation, behavioral problems, acne, striae, and cushingoid appearance. You also can use topical hydrocortisone enemas and foam for distal colon disease, but these can still cause adrenal suppression with prolonged use. Newer topical agents, such as budesonide and fluticasone, have much less adrenal-suppressive effects.

Biologic Agents

Infliximab is a chimeric IgG1 monoclonal antibody that is directed against tumor necrosis factor (anti-TNF-α). It is effective at both inducing and maintaining remission. This is now widely used in children with moderate-to-severe disease who are steroid-dependent or steroid-refractory. It is given by intravenous infusion typically at 8-week intervals. Because it is a chimeric protein, the primary side effect is an allergic reaction to the protein. This can be immediate or a delayed serum sickness. The efficacy of the agent also appears to diminish with time in some patients. Other "-mabs" are available, but few are approved for use in children.

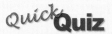

- How do you diagnose ulcerative colitis?
- Which drugs are used for both the remission and maintenance of UC?

Purine Analogs

6-mercaptopurine (6-MP) and azathioprine are very effective in maintaining remission for severe UC and Crohn disease, but do not have a role in inducing remission. They have a very slow onset of action (3–6 months). Both drugs are purine analogs and have cytotoxic and immunosuppressive properties. They inhibit the proliferation and function of leukocytes. Severe complications are rare, but elevated transaminases and/or leukopenia occur in about 15% of patients and resolve with lowering the dose of the drug. Metabolite testing is now available for these agents and can be used to ensure levels are not in a range associated with these complications. Discontinue use if hypersensitivity reactions occur, which present as skin rashes, recurrent fevers, or pancreatitis.

Although there are recommendations to check thiopurine methyltransferase (TPMT) levels prior to initiating therapy, there is no evidence that these levels either predict patient outcomes or are useful for determining the correct dose.

Methotrexate

Methotrexate inhibits dihydrofolate reductase, which impairs DNA synthesis. It also inhibits cytokine production and causes T-cell apoptosis. It works well initially but does a poor job of maintaining remission. Methotrexate is reserved for those who are not surgical candidates for cure and who cannot tolerate or have difficulties with azathioprine or 6-MP.

Cyclosporine A

Cyclosporine A inhibits the production of proinflammatory cytokines by T-helper cells. Most use it with patients who have severe UC that is refractory to standard therapy. Relapse rates, however, are very common in the 1st year, and serious side effects (liver toxicity, neurotoxicity, hypomagnesemia, hypertension, renal toxicity, gingival hyperplasia, and hirsutism) are a concern.

Other Agents

Antibiotics have no beneficial effect in UC unless a specific indication, such as sepsis or abscess, is noted. With the initial presentation or flare of the disease, look for *C. difficile* and treat it if found.

Do not use antidiarrheal agents routinely in pediatric UC due to concern for the development of toxic megacolon.

(Loperamide is an opiate!) Avoid opiates as well for similar reasons.

Bowel rest is not generally indicated unless a patient is at risk for toxic megacolon. Use of fish oils containing omega-3 fatty acids has lessened disease activity in some preliminary reports.

Probiotics

Studies have had conflicting results on the efficacy and safety of probiotics in ulcerative colitis. The overall impact on disease course is variable, and usually modest. Patients with mild disease tend to have greater benefit. Adverse drug events are common, and mild, but it is unclear if this is related to the medication itself or not. VSL#3® (a combination of probiotic bacteria) has shown improvement for patients with both ulcerative colitis and ongoing inflammation after surgical correction (termed pouchitis).

Surgical Therapy

Emergent surgery may be needed as a lifesaving procedure. Emergently, the patient may require an ostomy. Long-term, most now eventually progress to an ileoanal pull-through operation, with creation of a surgical "pouch," which preserves continence. Indications for urgent surgery include uncontrollable massive bleeding, perforation, and toxic megacolon. Most often, though, surgery is done because of failure of standard medical therapy. Consider elective surgery in those with steroid dependence; intolerance of, or complications from, immunosuppressive therapy; long-standing disease; or evidence of colonic dysplasia or cancer.

After pull-through surgery, pouchitis may occur, which consists of increased stool frequency, lower abdominal pain, tenesmus, and hematochezia. Most believe this is caused by colonization of the ileal mucosa-lined pouch with colonic flora. Metronidazole or probiotics (usually VSL#3) are commonly prescribed to manage pouchitis.

Ulcerative Colitis and Colon Cancer

UC predisposes to colon cancer at an increasing rate that is correlated with the duration of active disease. After 10 years of active disease, the yearly risk of colon cancer is about 1%. Have children and adolescents with UC undergo colonoscopy with biopsy every 2 years after having the disease for 7 years. If dysplasia is found, colectomy is indicated.

CROHN DISEASE

Overview

Crohn disease is an inflammatory process that is transmural, involving the GI tract anywhere from mouth to anus. Bowel segments can be inflamed with intervening normal mucosal involvement, referred to as skip lesions. The terminal ileum is the most commonly involved site in patients with Crohn disease, with nearly 70% of pediatric patients also having some colonic involvement (usually the cecum and/or ascending colon). Aphthous ulcers are suggestive of Crohn disease. Extraintestinal manifestations are common and may precede the GI symptoms for years. Crohn disease is seen mainly in adolescent children. It has a higher prevalence among the Ashkenazi Jewish population.

Genetics is a major risk factor. If one parent is affected, the risk of a child having Crohn disease is about 1/8. If both parents are affected, the risk of having an affected child is about 1/3. Monozygotic twin studies show a very strong concordance for Crohn disease—far greater than for UC.

Etiology of Crohn's is still unknown (same for UC). However, variations in the *NOD2* gene, which regulates monocyte response to antigens, is strongly associated with increased risk of Crohn disease.

Weight loss and growth failure are much more common with Crohn disease than with UC. Anal fistulae and abscesses are more commonly seen in Crohn's patients, but most patients do not have perianal or anal disease.

Crohn disease is transmural and can result in fistulous tracts as well as strictures. On microscopic examination, you will see a chronic granulomatous inflammation involving all layers of the intestinal wall. On biopsy, noncaseating granulomas that contain multinucleated giant cells and epithelioid cells are pathognomonic for Crohn disease, although these are seen only 40% of the time.

If the small intestine and the colon are both involved, Crohn disease is the diagnosis. What is difficult is when Crohn disease involves only the colon. In up to 15% of cases, patients may initially be diagnosed as having indeterminate colitis or IBD-unspecified when no granulomas are seen microscopically. Colonoscopy with biopsy is the best means for diagnosis. Infectious etiologies (tuberculosis, histoplasmosis, listeria, CMV, etc.), lymphomas, and sarcoidosis are in the differential.

Treatment

Therapy Basis

Managing Crohn disease is more difficult than managing UC, and, unlike UC, surgical therapy is not definitive. Therapy is based on clinical symptoms and does not necessarily correlate with endoscopic or histologic findings.

5-Aminosalicylates

Recent reviews of the evidence have not shown that 5-ASA compounds are more effective than placebo to induce remission in Crohn disease. However, sulfasalazine and mesalamine have been used for many years to maintain remission in Crohn disease despite the fact that evidence for their efficacy in this setting is weak. There are some mesalamine products targeted to treat the small intestine and colon.

Corticosteroids

Corticosteroid therapy provides marked improvement in patients with active Crohn disease. Most usually give prednisone for 3–4 weeks until remission is achieved and then attempt a gradual weaning, along with maintenance therapy. Steroids for maintenance therapy are not supported by data, and long-term side effects are significant.

Purine Analogs

Use of 6-MP or azathioprine often results in remission and allows patients to avoid long-term corticosteroids. It can take 3–6 months before they become effective, due to their slow onset of action. Many children with Crohn disease are maintained on these agents until early adulthood. Monitor therapeutic metabolite levels to avoid complications, although routine use is still not considered standard.

Methotrexate

Reserve methotrexate for those who fail to respond to, or have significant complications with, 6-MP or azathioprine. Crohn disease can respond very well to methotrexate if other agents present problems.

Antibiotics

Antibiotics are more commonly used with Crohn disease than with UC. Many use metronidazole for fistulae and perianal abscesses. Side effects include nausea, appetite loss, and complaints of a metallic taste. Prolonged use can result in paresthesias, which can persist for years after stopping therapy.

Ciprofloxacin has recently shown benefit comparable to metronidazole. Combination therapy of ciprofloxacin and metronidazole is very effective in treating fistulae and perianal disease.

The therapeutic effect of antibiotics tends to fade with time; therefore, reserve antibiotic therapy for short-term use in the conditions indicated.

Biologic Agents

Infliximab is a chimeric IgG1 monoclonal antibody that is directed against tumor necrosis factor (anti-TNF-α). It is the 1st biologic agent approved by the FDA for clinical use in patients with steroid-refractory intestinal or perianal Crohn disease. It is widely used in those patients refractory to immunomodulators like purine analogs or methotrexate. There are several studies using other biologic agents in Crohn disease, but these are not standard practice at this time. Adalimumab, however, was approved for use in pediatric patients in 2014.

Quick Quiz

- In what part of the gastrointestinal tract does Crohn disease most commonly occur?
- Which is more likely to cause weight loss and growth problems, Crohn's or UC?
- Which is transmural—Crohn's or UC?
- Is surgical therapy curative for Crohn disease?
- What is the most common surgical emergency in children?
- If the pain of appendicitis suddenly resolves, what has likely happened?

Nutrition Therapy

Unlike UC, Crohn disease responds to bowel rest. Recommend an elemental diet for 1 month, excluding other food. Early relapse occurs if the diet is ended. Once remission has occurred, recommend a cycle of elemental diet 1 out of every 4 months. This option requires a highly motivated patient who wishes to avoid alternative therapies.

Supplemental nocturnal nasogastric feedings with elemental or polymeric formulas are used to reverse growth failure. Osteoporosis is also of significant concern in children with Crohn disease, and supplementation with calcium and vitamin D is recommended.

Surgical Therapy

Surgery does not cure Crohn disease, and it eventually recurs. Before more conservative surgical approaches became the norm, Crohn disease was a leading condition leading to short bowel syndrome. Reserve surgery mainly for complications that fail to respond to medical management, such as massive hemorrhage, perforation, and fulminant colitis. In addition, fistulae and strictures may require surgery. Some practitioners resect severely affected areas of the bowel, particularly the terminal ileum, to reduce symptoms. Rectal involvement may require a fecal diversion, such as an ileostomy or colostomy.

Crohn Disease and Colon Cancer

Crohn disease is much less likely than UC to induce colon cancer, but the rate of colon cancer is still 20x higher in patients with Crohn disease compared to the normal population. Current guidelines suggest that you perform a colonoscopy after 8 years of disease, and then regular surveillance every 1 to 3 years afterwards, depending on the degree of colitis. Crohn patients without colitis do not need extra screening compared with normal patients.

APPENDICITIS

Overview

Appendicitis is the most common surgical emergency in children. The peak age of onset is 12 years of age; it is unusual before 2 years. In about 1/3 of cases, the appendix ruptures before surgery; this disease progresses much more rapidly in children.

In children, fatigue and anorexia are frequently the common symptoms at initial presentation. This may accompany indigestion, which is followed by periumbilical discomfort. Soon after, fever between 100° and 102° F, with nausea and vomiting, may occur. Over several hours, the inflammation involves the parietal peritoneum and localizes to the right lower quadrant (RLQ) of the abdomen. But remember, younger children are notoriously poor at localizing pain, and many children with appendicitis do not point to their RLQ. Depending on the location of the appendix, the pain can be in different locations: pelvic appendix—hypogastric pain; retrocecal appendix—psoas and obturator muscle pain (pain with hip flexion or rotation, respectively); and retrocolic appendix—right flank pain.

Pain that suddenly resolves may indicate rupture, which has relieved the appendix's pressure, but remember that most causes of abdominal pain in children may also stop suddenly. Soon, however, high fever, persistent vomiting, thirst, and signs of peritonitis may develop. Signs of systemic infection may occur; or the infection may be "walled off," and a local abscess may form.

Early on, the patient may not have a lot of pain and can be in minimal distress. However, consistent, localized, RLQ tenderness and guarding eventually become prominent. Some authorities recommend you perform a rectal examination to search for pelvic appendicitis. You see psoas irritation with extension of the thigh and obturator irritation with passive internal rotation of the thigh. Rovsing sign occurs when abdominal palpation remote to McBurney point results in RLQ pain.

In children, inflamed appendices perforate within 24–48 hours after onset. CBC is not specifically helpful (WBC is often normal in children), but microscopic pyuria and hematuria may be associated with appendicitis. Abdominal x-ray is rarely helpful.

Admit for observation if the diagnosis is unclear, and preferably have the same physician conduct serial examinations. Ultrasound can sometimes be helpful in the hands of a skilled technician and is the best initial imaging study in most children who are not obese. A CT of the abdomen and pelvis may show enhancement and thickening of the appendix in appendicitis. This test involves significant radiation exposure.

Treatment of Appendicitis

Treat with appendectomy. If the appendix is not ruptured, simply remove it, and patients generally can go home in 12–24 hours. If rupture has occurred, conduct intraoperative anaerobic and aerobic cultures, irrigate the peritoneal cavity, and place drains if abscesses are present. Give broad-spectrum IV antibiotics until the patient is afebrile and clinically improved.

In some patients, perforation occurs days prior to presentation, and you will notice a palpable mass in the right lower quadrant. If the child is well without evidence of peritonitis, manage conservatively with antibiotic therapy and observation. If symptoms respond to the antibiotics, appendectomy can be done in 4–6 weeks. Do the surgery sooner if there is no response to the antibiotics.

Complications are rare today but can include wound infection and intraabdominal abscess.

Neutropenic Enterocolitis (Typhlitis)

Typhlitis is inflammation of the cecum and is mainly seen in patients who are treated for leukemia during periods of neutropenia. It can occur in other immunodeficiencies and after organ transplant. Typhlitis is dangerous in that the inflammation can progress rapidly to gangrene or perforation. Fever and right lower quadrant pain usually suggest acute appendicitis. Abdominal x-ray may show bowel wall thickening or pneumatosis intestinalis. Most use CT to investigate.

Treat with bowel rest, IV fluids, and antibiotic therapy. Some recommend WBC transfusions. Almost all resolve without surgical intervention, unless perforation occurs. Once typhlitis occurs, it has a high risk for recurrence with subsequent episodes of neutropenia.

JUVENILE POLYPS AND JUVENILE POLYPOSIS

Juvenile polyps occur in about 1% of preschool children and account for the majority of all polyps in children. Juvenile polyps are inflammatory polyps, typically pedunculated hamartomas. The classic presentation is a 4- to 6-year-old child who presents with intermittent, painless hematochezia with bowel movements. There is usually not a history of a familial polyp syndrome, and there are typically < 5 polyps. Solitary juvenile polyps of this type are not cancer prone.

On the other hand, juvenile polyposis occurs when there are > 5 polyps, and these have a high, long-term risk of malignancy; affected individuals are 30x more likely to develop colorectal cancer. Juvenile polyposis coli (involving only the colon) refer to polyps that are distributed throughout the colon. If a family member has already been diagnosed with juvenile polyposis, any other member who has even a single juvenile polyp is considered to also have juvenile polyposis.

Most use colonoscopy in children with unexplained rectal bleeding. It allows you to assess for the presence of polyps, as well as the number and distribution, and to get histological data. Unless a large number of polyps

are found, remove all polyps for histology. If you find a single rectosigmoid polyp with typical histology, no further evaluation is necessary. If 5 or more juvenile polyps are found, or if a juvenile polyp with adenomatous changes is found, perform colonoscopy every 6–12 months until no polyps are found; check every 2 years thereafter if no further polyps develop. Monitor children with 2–4 polyps with a repeat colonoscopy. For any child with polyps that show adenomatous changes, you must conduct further investigations.

PEUTZ-JEGHERS SYNDROME

Peutz-Jeghers syndrome (a.k.a. hereditary intestinal polyposis syndrome) is an autosomal dominant disease (mutation of the *STK11* gene on chromosome 19p) with variable penetrance.

It presents with GI hamartomatous polyps and mucocutaneous hyperpigmentation of the lips and gums. The lesions are brown-black macules, 1–5 mm in diameter, and look like freckles. They are nearly universally on the lips and buccal mucosa and are less commonly found on the nose, hands, and feet (Image 14-12). The lesions occur during infancy and childhood and fade during adolescence. Patients have multiple polyps throughout their GI tract. Most commonly affected is the small bowel, followed by the colon and the stomach. Rarely, polyps may be found in the bronchi and genitourinary tract. Histologically, they are distinguished from juvenile polyps by the presence of smooth muscle bands within the polyp.

About 1/3 of patients are diagnosed during childhood, but the mean age of onset of symptoms is around 22 years of age. The most common presentation is intermittent, colicky, abdominal pain with intestinal obstruction from intussusception, GI bleeding, and anemia. Nearly 1/2 of patients develop cancers outside of the colon during their lifetime, with the most common involving the breast, cervix, ovary, testicle, and pancreas. 2–13% develop colon cancer. Adenomatous changes are found in about 5% of Peutz-Jeghers polyps.

Diagnosis depends on finding the hamartomatous polyps, recognizing the skin lesions, and discerning a family history. Remove all large polyps, and perform surveillance endoscopy to continue removing additional polyps as they appear. Also, survey for other tumors, beginning in patients at age 10 or sooner if symptoms

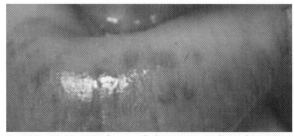

Image 14-12: Peutz-Jeghers synd.; hyperpigmented macules on lips

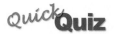

• What is typhlitis?

• How does Peutz-Jeghers syndrome present?

have already developed. Screen all 1st degree relatives regularly after 10 years of age.

SYNDROMES LINKED TO *PTEN* GENE MUTATIONS

PTEN-MATCHS Syndrome

These are rare syndromes known by the term *PTEN*-MATCHS syndrome. *PTEN* refers to the protein tyrosine phosphatase gene and **MATCHS** refers to **m**acrocephaly, **a**utosomal dominant, **t**hyroid disease, **c**ancer, **h**amartoma, and **s**kin abnormalities.

Ruvalcaba-Myhre-Smith Syndrome

Ruvalcaba-Myhre-Smith syndrome is characterized by macrocephaly, pigmented penile lesions, and hamartomatous intestinal polyps. The polyps present with rectal bleeding and sometimes abdominal pain. Additional findings include café-au-lait spots, lipomas, intellectual disability, and a lipid-storage abnormality.

Cowden Syndrome, Bannayan-Zonana Syndrome, and Bannayan-Riley-Ruvalcaba Syndrome

These syndromes are all very rare and are characterized by having multiple hamartomas of the skin, mucous membranes, breast, and thyroid. Hyperkeratotic papillomas of the lips and tongue are characteristic. They are caused by a mutation on the *PTEN* tumor suppressor gene on chromosome locus 10q22-23.

Proteus Syndrome

Proteus syndrome is a rare disorder with hamartomatous polyps and hemihypertrophy, gigantism of the extremities, angiomas, pigmented nevi, and multiple lipomas or hamartomas. Remember this one on an exam if they describe a patient with hemihypertrophy and hamartomas.

FAMILIAL ADENOMATOUS POLYPOSIS SYNDROMES

Incidence

Familial adenomatous polyposis syndromes occur in about 1/10,000 births and are due to mutations on chromosome locus 5q21-22. Most are autosomal dominant and due to mutation in the *APC* gene. Variable penetrance is often observed. A less common variant is

autosomal recessive and is caused by mutations in the *MUTYH* gene. About 1/3 of the cases are due to a new mutation without a family history.

Patients present with hundreds of GI adenomatous polyps, almost always involving the colon. Gardner's (see next) is the most commonly described and is often tested on exams.

Gardner Syndrome

Gardner syndrome is characterized by extra teeth, gastrointestinal polyps, and osteomas. Ampullary and duodenal adenomas are common. Soft tissue tumors include desmoid tumors, sebaceous and epidermoid cysts, lipomas, and subcutaneous fibromas. Osteomas of the skull, maxilla, and mandible are common as well. Other associations include supernumerary teeth and **c**ongenital **h**ypertrophy of the **r**etinal **p**igment **e**pithelium (**CHRPE**).

Diagnosis is established by finding the hundreds of adenomatous polyps in the colon, with genetic testing by sequencing the *APC* gene to confirm.

Management is controversial, but most authorities recommend yearly screening with colonoscopy, beginning between 10 and 12 years of age. Treatment with cyclooxygenase inhibitors has been shown to suppress polyp expression, and patients are now maintained on sulindac. Early colectomy is performed in a majority of patients, usually by the time they are young adults, and it prevents development of colonic adenocarcinoma. Patients are still at risk for malignant transformation of other tumors, especially those in the small bowel. Periodic endoscopic evaluation of the upper GI tract, as well as thyroid testing, is also recommended because of the increased risk of cancers in these areas.

OTHER TUMORS

Neurofibromas

Neurofibromas are commonly associated with café-au-lait spots and skin tumors, but up to 25% of patients with von Recklinghausen disease also have GI tumors. Most commonly, they are in the small intestine. They can cause abdominal pain, bleeding, and anemia.

Adenocarcinoma

Adenocarcinoma is rare in childhood. It typically has histologic features of mucin-producing or signet-ring varieties. Carcinoembryonic antigen (CEA) is not a reliable marker in children. Children usually have a concomitant risk factor, such as a familial polyposis syndrome, inflammatory bowel disease, or ureterosigmoidostomy (performed due to exstrophy of the bladder). The latter develop cancer at a rate of 5%, so perform surveillance endoscopy with biopsy every 2–3 years in these patients.

GASTROENTEROLOGY & NUTRITION

Lymphoma

In children, lymphoma is the most common malignant tumor of the small intestine. These occur in the 2nd decade and are almost always Burkitt lymphoma (non-Hodgkin's). The terminal ileum and cecum are the most common sites. *Helicobacter pylori* is a known risk factor for gastric lymphoma. Unrecognized or untreated celiac disease also predisposes to small intestinal lymphomas. Post-transplant lymphoproliferative disease is associated with Epstein-Barr virus infection.

Carcinoid

Carcinoid is very rare in children. Benign carcinoid tumors of the appendix are more commonly seen than malignant tumors, which predominate in the ileum and have liver metastases. The tumors are made up of neuroendocrine cells that release catecholamines, bradykinins, and serotonin—substances that can result in carcinoid syndrome (flushing and diarrhea). The benign appendiceal form can be cured with appendectomy. The malignant form does not respond well to therapy. You can control some symptoms with octreotide, which is a long-acting analog of somatostatin.

CONGENITAL VENTRAL ABDOMINAL WALL DEFECTS

OCCURRENCE

Abdominal wall defects are varied in appearance and location. They are fairly rare, occurring in only about 1/5,000 live births.

OMPHALOCELE

Omphalocele is a ventral, midline defect in the abdominal wall at the umbilical region, which can contain both hollow and solid visceral abdominal organs. Omphaloceles are larger than 4 cm and are covered by peritoneal membrane internally and amniotic membrane externally. In contrast, umbilical hernias are smaller than 4 cm and contain only intestine.

About 50–75% of neonates with an omphalocele have an associated congenital anomaly, including the thoracoabdominal syndrome (known as the pentalogy of Cantrell), lower midline syndrome, and Beckwith-Wiedemann syndrome. About 25% have major chromosomal abnormalities, including the trisomies.

Omphalocele presents as a central defect of the umbilical ring and has the abdominal contents inside a sac. The umbilical cord inserts into the sac. In about 1/2, the sac contains the stomach, loops of small/large intestines, and liver. "Giant" omphaloceles present with large/small intestines, liver, spleen, gonadal tissue, and bladder in the sac. About 10–20% of omphaloceles rupture *in utero* and may present more like gastroschisis (see next) with

thickened bowel covered in exudate. Midgut volvulus is common in omphalocele.

Manage by keeping the infant warm and hydrated. Cover exposed omphalocele with plastic wrap and warm, saline-soaked gauze. Immediately begin IV antibiotics. Fix the bowel so that circulation is well maintained. Nonoperative management is acceptable if the infant is too ill for surgery. Apply antiseptic agents, such as silver nitrate or povidone-iodine, to the omphalocele. These eventually become an eschar and epithelize, thus protecting the exposed organs. Once this has become granulated, you can place a skin graft, resulting in a ventral hernia, which can be repaired in the future. If primary surgical repair cannot be done, you can attempt a staged repair. Survival of infants with omphalocele is 75–95%; survival is usually affected by the associated congenital anomalies.

GASTROSCHISIS

Gastroschisis presents as a 2–5 cm lateral abdominal wall defect, just to the right of the umbilicus, with exposed (no membrane!) loops of small and large intestines that are short and thick due to an inflammatory reaction of the serosa. The solid visceral organs often are contained in the abdominal cavity, and the umbilical cord is normal. Gastroschisis is more common than omphalocele and is commonly associated with midgut volvulus.

Initial management of gastroschisis is similar to that of omphalocele, with resuscitation, hydration, and temperature control. Perform a similar plastic bag/gauze procedure. For gastroschisis, surgery is mandatory and cannot be delayed. Primary surgical closure is frequently successful in gastroschisis. Early postoperative complications include necrotizing enterocolitis and intestinal obstruction. The survival rate for gastroschisis is 95%.

Many children require bowel resection and end up with short bowel syndrome. Additionally, because the bowel is often fibrous and hypofunctioning from sitting free in the amniotic fluid, many patients have poor motility or absorption of nutrients.

ANORECTAL DISORDERS

OCCURRENCE

Anorectal disorders occur in about 1/4,000 births and can be minor to severe. It is probably easiest to think of these separated out by sex, since the defining characteristics of each disorder depend upon the sex of the patient. Generally, those disorders that cause severe deformity or absence of the sacrum result in serious abnormalities and lack of sphincter tone. Also, absence of 2 or more vertebrae is associated with severe continence problems.

Congenital anorectal disorders are often part of other disorders, including the VATER and VACERL disorders.

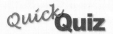

- In children, what is the most common malignant tumor of the small intestine?
- What is an omphalocele?
- If an omphalocele is present, should you suspect another congenital anomaly or is it likely an isolated event?
- What is a gastroschisis?

VATER: **v**ertebrae, **a**nus, **t**rachea and **e**sophagus, **r**adius and **r**enal anomalies. **VACTERL**: **v**ertebral, **a**nal atresia, **c**ardiac (PDA, ASD, VSD), **t**racheo**e**sophageal fistula, **r**enal (urethral atresia with hydronephrosis), and **l**imb anomalies (humeral hypoplasia, radial aplasia, hexadactyly, proximally placed thumb).

MALE ANORECTAL DISORDERS

Perineal Fistula

A perineal fistula presents with a small orifice on the perineum located just anterior to the center of the external orifice. Usually, it is close to the scrotum. Boys have a "bucket handle" malformation or "black ribbon" structure in their perineum that is a subepithelial fistula filled with meconium. Anal dimples are prominent. Less than 10% of those affected have other organ abnormalities. The defect can be repaired without a colostomy.

Rectourethral Fistula

A rectourethral fistula is the most common anorectal defect in males. A rectourethral fistula occurs when the rectum communicates with the lower (bulbar) or upper (prostatic) part of the urethra. Most patients have a well-defined midline perineal groove and an anal dimple. This requires a protective colostomy during the newborn period, with complete surgical repair later in life.

Rectovesical Fistula

A rectovesical fistula occurs when the rectum communicates with the bladder neck. The sacrum is frequently absent. Bowel function is poor, and this requires a colostomy during the newborn period, followed by corrective surgery later in life.

FEMALE ANORECTAL DISORDERS

Perineal Fistula

As in boys, a perineal fistula is the simplest fistula found in girls; however, in girls, the small orifice is located close to the vulva. It does not require colostomy, unlike the other anorectal disorders that affect females.

Vestibular Fistula

Vestibular fistula is the most common anorectal defect in girls. In this instance, the rectum opens in the vestibule of the female genitalia immediately outside the hymenal orifice. The sacrum and sphincter tone are normal, and an anal dimple is present. You must perform a protective colostomy in the newborn period before definitive surgery can be done.

Persistent Cloaca

Persistent cloaca means that the vagina, rectum, and urinary tract meet and fuse as a common channel. There is a single orifice just behind the clitoris. The length can vary from 1 to 10 cm. Those with short channels (< 3 cm) have a well-developed sacrum and good sphincter tone. Those with longer channels (> 3 cm) have a more complex defect and usually have a poorly defined sacrum and sphincter tone. Most girls with a cloaca have an abnormally large vagina filled with mucus (hydrocolpos).

You must perform a colostomy in the newborn period; 90% also have urologic abnormalities requiring emergent attention.

ANORECTAL DISORDERS PRESENTING SIMILARLY IN BOTH SEXES

Imperforate Anus (Anal Atresia) without Fistula

An imperforate anus occurs when the rectum is completely closed off and does not communicate with the anus or skin. On average, the rectum is found about 2 cm above the perineal skin. The sacrum is well developed, and the sphincteric mechanism is intact. Eventual prognosis is good with an initial colostomy in the newborn period and eventual reparative surgery later. Children with trisomy 21 have a much higher incidence of imperforate anus than other children. Some children have much higher defects anatomically, which result in more long-term dysfunction.

Rectal Atresia

Rectal atresia is one of the rarest anorectal abnormalities. Patients have a normal anal canal and a normal anus. You will frequently find the defect when you attempt to use a rectal thermometer. Obstruction is present about 2 cm above the skin level. A protective colostomy is necessary in the newborn period, followed by reparative surgery at a later date.

Rectal Prolapse

Rectal prolapse occurs when 1 or more layers of the rectum protrude through the anus. Usually, it is only the mucosa that prolapses, and it presents as a red-purple, circular protrusion from the anus. It is common for a small amount of rectal mucosa to prolapse after normal defecation. If all layers prolapse, this is known as procidentia. Luckily, it is rare. It presents as a protrusion with circumferential folds due to the contractions of the circular musculature of the prolapsed rectum.

Mucosal prolapse is most common in those < 2 years of age because of the flat sacrum and weak pelvic floor muscles. (There have been reports of massive intestinal prolapse in children sitting on unprotected swimming pool drains!) Cystic fibrosis (CF) is always key to remember with rectal prolapse, but remember: CF is not the most common cause; it actually comes in 3rd overall. Constipation is 1st, followed by infectious diarrhea in 2nd. Other etiologies include various neuromotor disorders, and nearly 20% have no identifiable cause. Most mucosal prolapses reduce spontaneously, but the anus can gap open for up to an hour after reduction. Some require surgical intervention, but these are rare. In children with a history of recurrent rectal prolapse, the anus and anorectal manometry appear normal. Treat any underlying condition (for example, constipation or diarrhea). Again, surgery is rarely needed.

Anal Fissures

Anal fissures are the most common cause of rectal bleeding in children of all ages. Anal fissures are slit-like tears of the anal canal, usually located on the posterior or anterior anal verge. Frequently, they are due to the passage of large stools in a constipated infant or child. After the fissure heals, a small anal tag may remain. In the older child, when the anal fissure does not heal with stool softeners, warm sitz baths, and generous lubrication to the anal skin, suspect Crohn disease. If there are multiple anal fissures or signs of genital trauma, suspect sexual abuse.

Hemorrhoids

Small, asymptomatic hemorrhoids found incidentally on examination are not uncommon in children. Symptomatic hemorrhoids may occur with chronic straining associated with constipation, as a result of an infection spreading to the hemorrhoidal veins, with portal hypertension, or with underlying Crohn disease.

Conservative management of hemorrhoids includes avoidance of straining with defecation, minimizing toilet time, increasing fluids and fiber to relieve constipation, or prescribing a stool softener. Warm water sitz baths may also alleviate symptoms.

Perianal Itching

Perianal itching (a.k.a. pruritus ani) is very common and is frequently due to perianal dermatitis or infection. *Candida* overgrowth commonly occurs after a course of antibiotics for otitis media, etc. Other etiologies include atopic dermatitis, contact dermatitis, perianal streptococcal infection, and anal fissures. Pinworms and tapeworms may present with perianal itching. Some foods—including tea, coffee, chocolate, soft drinks, citrus, tomatoes, and chili—contain chemicals that irritate the skin or have histamine releasers. Urinary tract infection may present in the younger child as itching.

Perianal streptococcal infection, caused by group A beta-hemolytic *Streptococcus* (*pyogenes*) presents as an "angry," bright red, confluent rash around the anal orifice and can spread throughout the entire perineal area. Rectal bleeding may occur, and you may discover that a recent streptococcal disease occurred in the household. Occasionally, the affected child has a concomitant streptococcal pharyngitis. Treat with oral penicillin. Topicals are ineffective.

HIRSCHSPRUNG DISEASE

OCCURRENCE

Hirschsprung disease (a.k.a. congenital aganglionic megacolon) is given special attention here because it is the most common cause of lower intestinal obstruction in neonates! It occurs in 1/5,000 births and is due to the absence of enteric ganglionic neurons (aganglionosis) that begins at the anus and then extends proximally for a varying distance. In 75% of those affected, aganglionosis is limited to the rectum and sigmoid. But about 8% have total colon involvement, and an even smaller number have small intestinal aganglionosis as well. There are also occasional concerns in constipated adolescents and adults for the possibility of "short-segment" Hirschsprung's.

The rectosigmoid form of the disease has a male predominance of 4:1. This form has a multifactorial or a recessive pattern of inheritance. The risk of an affected sibling having the disease is about 7%. Racial differences are not noted. As the affected intestinal segment length increases (for example, involving the total colon or intestine), the sex differences decrease, and the sibling risk increases to nearly 20%. There is an increased association with Down syndrome, Laurence-Moon-Bardet-Biedl syndrome, Smith-Lemli-Opitz syndrome, and Waardenburg syndrome.

PATHOGENESIS

Hirschsprung disease occurs when the craniocaudal migration of neural crest cells to the distal intestine fails to happen. Various factors affect the migration of the neural crest cells, and experts believe that expression of these molecules is controlled by the *Hox* and *Sox* homeobox genes (sounds like a Dr. Seuss book!). In particular, 2 signaling systems have been noted: ret/glial-derived neurotrophic factor and endothelin receptor B/endothelin 3. Many families with Hirschsprung disease have abnormalities in the genes that encode these signals. Additionally, other factors, as yet unknown, also mediate the failure of the neural crest cells to develop and/or migrate properly.

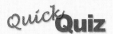

Quick Quiz

- What are the 3 most common causes of rectal prolapse?

- What is the etiology of Hirschsprung disease?

- A term infant is 48 hours old and has not passed meconium. Is it necessary at this point to evaluate for Hirschsprung's?

- How does enterocolitis present in infants with Hirschsprung's?

- What is the gold standard procedure used to diagnose Hirschsprung's?

- A biopsy will show histologic absence of what structures in a patient with Hirschsprung disease?

Because of the loss of normal innervation of the rectum, there is an "overexpression" of extrinsic parasympathetic and sympathic nerves in the lamina propria and muscularis mucosae. This causes the aganglionic segment, internal sphincter, and anal canal to remain constantly contracted, resulting in obstructive symptoms. The area proximal to the aganglionic segment is dilated and hypertrophied. (See Figure 14-1.)

CLINICAL PRESENTATION

The diagnosis of Hirschsprung disease is usually made during the neonatal period, but some are not diagnosed until 3 years of age or later, with reports of patients diagnosed well into adulthood. Two presentation types are noted:

1) Perinatally with intestinal obstruction (delayed passage of meconium, constipation, abdominal distention)

2) At 1 month of age with enterocolitis

90% of normal, full-term infants pass meconium within 24 hours, and 99% within 48 hours. In children with Hirschsprung disease, 94% fail to pass meconium within the first 24 hours. Therefore, evaluate for Hirschsprung disease any term infant who does not pass meconium within 48 hours of birth.

Complete intestinal obstruction can occur in the newborn—or may occur later in the older infant who has a history of only constipation. Intestinal obstruction is accompanied by bilious vomiting, obstipation, and massive abdominal distention.

The most severe complication of undiagnosed Hirschsprung disease is enterocolitis. This usually occurs during the 2nd to 4th weeks and is characterized by fever with explosive, foul-smelling stools. Bloody diarrhea is common, as is abdominal distention. The prognosis for enterocolitis is poor, and the mortality rate can be as high as 33%. The pathogenesis of enterocolitis is unknown, although it is thought to be due to overgrowth of colonic bacteria in an atonic distal colon. Delayed diagnosis is the contributing factor for many cases of enterocolitis.

DIAGNOSIS

Once you suspect Hirschsprung's, proceed quickly with rectal biopsy which is the gold standard procedure for diagnosis. The longer it takes for a diagnosis to be made, the more likely enterocolitis may occur. The most commonly used tool is the suction rectal biopsy, a simple instrument that can be used on infants in the outpatient clinic.

Histologically, the diagnosis is based on the absence of any ganglion cells detected in a biopsy containing adequate submucosa. This appears as an absence of submucosal (Meissner) and myenteric (Auerbach) plexuses and hypertrophied nerve bundles, with high concentrations of acetylcholinesterase between the muscular layers and in the submucosa. If the diagnosis is still questionable, do a full-thickness rectal biopsy to look for aganglionosis in the mesenteric and submucosal plexuses. Barium enema was used in the past, but due to low sensitivity and specificity for Hirschsprung disease, it is now used more often as an adjunct to biopsy to demonstrate a transition zone.

Perform the biopsy no closer than 2 cm to the dentate line to avoid the normal area of hypoganglionosis at the anal verge. Acetylcholinesterase staining shows hypertrophied nerve trunks in the mucosal and myenteric plexuses and their presence in the muscularis mucosa. However, in total colonic aganglionosis, the acetylcholinesterase activity is not uniformly increased, and you may not observe the thickened nerve trunks; therefore, their absence does not rule out disease. Biopsy in this case must contain adequate submucosa to reliably diagnose the absence of enteric neurons.

Additionally, anorectal manometry is extremely accurate in the hands of those experienced with it. Failure of the internal anal sphincter to relax in response to distention of the rectum (rectosphincteric reflex) is diagnostic of Hirschsprung disease.

Other syndromes with a similar presentation are rare and include meconium plug syndrome, other nerve and muscle disorders of the lower colon, hypoganglionosis, and hollow visceral myopathy.

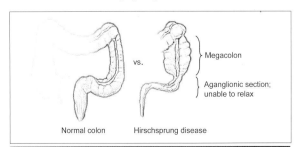

Figure 14-1: Hirschsprung Disease

TREATMENT

Treatment is surgical. If an infant presents with an obstruction, create a stoma proximal to the aganglionic segment. You must treat enterocolitis with IV fluids, broad-spectrum antibiotics, nasogastric decompression, and warm saline rectal washouts to help with colonic decompression. Once the patient is stable, perform a proximal colostomy.

Surgical management of Hirschsprung's usually involves 1 of 3 surgical techniques:

1) Swenson
2) Duhamel
3) Soave procedures

Each involves resection of the aganglionic bowel, then a reanastomosis of the proximal normal bowel to the normal anal canal. The differences depend on how the bowel is reconstructed. Usually, early surgical repair and reconstitution of the bowel is performed, although some specialists wait until the child is 6–12 months of age.

Immediate complications after surgery include stricture or leakage at the anastomotic site, as well as pelvic abscesses. Long-term dysfunction from Hirschsprung disease remains common. Many patients have ongoing difficulty with incontinence, and enterocolitis can still occur despite surgical correction.

PSEUDO-HIRSCHSPRUNG DISEASE

Note

Pseudo-Hirschsprung disease refers to various disorders that can affect the submucosa and myenteric plexuses— and can affect limited or widespread areas of the GI tract. The diseases can be due to defects of the smooth muscle coats or of the GI nerves themselves.

Hypoganglionosis

Hypoganglionosis can be congenital or acquired and occurs when the number of myenteric neurons is decreased. The congenital form likely is due to abnormalities in neural crest cell migration, while the acquired form results from toxic or autoimmune effects on neurons. It occurs as commonly as Hirschsprung disease and presents most commonly as chronic severe constipation.

Diagnosis requires a full-thickness biopsy to see the hypoganglionosis of the myenteric plexus. Treatment is symptomatic.

Intestinal Neuronal Dysplasia

Intestinal neuronal dysplasia is rare compared to Hirschsprung disease. There are 2 types of dysplasia: 1) type **A**, which has sympathetic aplasia, myenteric plexus hyperplasia, and colonic inflammation; and 2) type **B**, in which the submucosal plexus is affected more and there is no sympathetic aplasia. Type B is indistinguishable clinically from Hirschsprung disease; however, it is benign, and the condition eventually resolves spontaneously. Both type A and type B can be localized or disseminated.

Diagnosis for both is made on full-thickness biopsies with findings of hyperganglionosis and giant ganglia.

DISORDERS OF THE EXOCRINE PANCREAS

NOTE

Congenital disorders of the exocrine pancreas are almost always part of a generalized systemic disorder. Thankfully, 98% (!) of the pancreatic functional reserve must be lost before pancreatic insufficiency develops.

CYSTIC FIBROSIS

Cystic fibrosis, the most common cause of pancreatic insufficiency in children, is discussed in considerable detail in Respiratory Disorders, Book 4. Patients who are homozygous for δ-508, the most common mutation in the *CFTR* gene, have a very high risk for pancreatic insufficiency.

SHWACHMAN-DIAMOND SYNDROME

Shwachman-Diamond syndrome, an autosomal recessive disorder, is the 2nd most common cause of exocrine pancreatic insufficiency in children. The lesion of the pancreas is acinar cell hypoplasia, with intact function of the pancreatic ducts. Shwachman-Diamond syndrome is also associated with short stature, intermittent or persistent neutropenia, and skeletal abnormalities. Fetal hemoglobin levels are elevated in most patients. About 1/3 of affected boys develop myeloproliferative malignancies. Because of the neutropenia, recurrent infections are common. Pancreatic dysfunction is less severe than that seen in CF, and about 50% have improvement in pancreatic function over time.

RARE CONGENITAL PANCREATIC SYNDROMES

Johanson-Blizzard Syndrome

Johanson-Blizzard syndrome causes pancreatic acinar cell hypoplasia with preserved ductal function. The syndrome presents with agenesis/hypoplasia of the nostrils, a variable amount of absent secondary dentition, cardiac abnormalities, hair anomalies, deafness, hypothyroidism, GU defects, and developmental delay; presentation is highly variable. It does not have bone marrow or skeletal abnormalities.

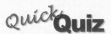

- What is Shwachman-Diamond syndrome?
- What are the commonly identified causes of acute pancreatitis in children?
- What is Cullen sign? Grey Turner sign?
- What radiologic test is usually most helpful in diagnosing acute pancreatitis?

Pearson Pancreatic and Bone Marrow Syndrome

Pearson pancreatic and bone marrow syndrome is a rare autosomal recessive disease in which patients have pancreatic cell atrophy with fibrosis resulting in depressed acinar and ductal function. Associated hematologic abnormalities include macrocytic anemia with varying degrees of neutropenia and/or thrombocytopenia. Hemosiderosis is common.

ACUTE PANCREATITIS

Occurrence / Causes

Acute pancreatitis is more common in children than previously thought. Many cases do not have a recognizable etiology but are probably due to an infectious cause, likely a virus.

Common causes of acute pancreatitis:

- Blunt abdominal trauma (most common)
- Mumps (less commonly seen today) and other viruses
- Multisystem disease
- Congenital anomalies such as an annular pancreas
- Biliary obstruction from gallstones (becoming more common with increasing rates of adolescent obesity)

Less common causes include:

- Drugs, such as didanosine (for HIV), valproate, asparaginase, and azathioprine
- Familial pancreatitis
- Hemolytic uremic syndrome
- Diabetic ketoacidosis
- Kawasaki syndrome
- Bone marrow transplant
- Head trauma

Cystic fibrosis is associated with chronic pancreatitis, although acute pancreatitis can occur. Alcohol has been increasingly recognized as a cause of acute pancreatitis in older adolescents.

Clinical Manifestations

Patients with acute pancreatitis typically present with epigastric abdominal pain and persistent vomiting. The abdominal pain commonly occurs in the midepigastric region and is described as steady and "boring into the back." Children flex their knees and hips and sit upright or lie on their side. The patient appears very uncomfortable and is irritable. Usually, the abdomen is distended and tender to palpation. During the initial 24–48 hours, the pain increases along with the vomiting. Hospitalization is almost always recommended.

A severe form, acute hemorrhagic pancreatitis or necrotizing pancreatitis, is rare in children but is life-threatening. The child is acutely ill with vomiting and abdominal pain. Shock and high fever are common. Classic signs are **Cullen sign** (bluish patchy discoloration around/near the umbilicus) and **Grey Turner sign** (bluish discoloration of the flanks from retroperitoneal hemorrhage—"Turn" to your side to see your flank!). In this severe form, the pancreas becomes necrotic and eventually, without therapy, transforms into an inflammatory hemorrhagic mass. The mortality rate is > 50%.

Diagnosis

Patients with acute pancreatitis usually have laboratory, ultrasound, and/or radiographic evidence. Serum lipase levels tend to be highly sensitive and specific for acute pancreatitis if elevated greater than 4x the upper limit of normal (i.e., in the hundreds). Higher lipase levels are associated with more severe pancreatic inflammation.

Ultrasound of the abdomen is the easiest and best imaging study in children because it can directly visualize the pancreas, showing peripancreatic fluid or an increase in pancreatic size, which supports the diagnosis of acute pancreatitis. Ultrasound also can show gallstones and choledochal cysts and help identify and follow abscesses and pseudocysts of the pancreas (Image 14-13). CT is generally reserved for those cases where ultrasound cannot delineate the anatomy well. See Image 14-14 on page 14-38, showing CT scan with arrow at pseudocyst.

Endoscopic retrograde cholangiopancreatography (ERCP) can be helpful, both diagnostically and therapeutically, in rarer cases, such as a stone in the bile duct, autoimmune hepatitis, sphincter of Oddi (SOD) dysfunction, and other anatomic biliary causes. Additionally, MRI and endoscopic ultrasonography are now available but have not been extensively used in children.

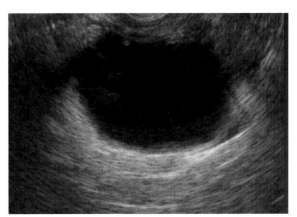

Image 14-13: Ultrasound showing pancreatic pseudocyst

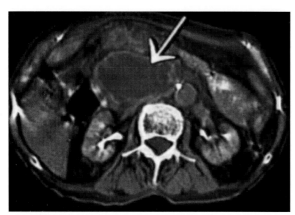

Image 14-14: CT showing pancreatic pseudocyst

Treatment

Treatment consists of pain control, IV hydration, and fasting. Typically, parenteral narcotic pain medications are used, most often morphine, fentanyl, or hydromorphone. Monitor fluids and electrolytes, and replenish as necessary. For those patients who are vomiting, nasogastric suction can be helpful. Low-fat feedings are often recommended, but evidence to support use in all patients is lacking. These can be started as soon as the patient is improving and desires to eat. In severe pancreatitis, transpyloric tube feedings with a semielemental formula are recommended very early in the course of therapy. Antibiotics are not recommended. Most patients respond after 2–4 days of therapy. If pancreatic pseudocysts occur, they usually resolve spontaneously; they rarely require percutaneous drainage or surgical intervention.

CHRONIC PANCREATITIS

Chronic pancreatitis is rare in children. Some cases are due to hereditary pancreatitis, which is an autosomal dominant disorder with incomplete penetrance, but most patients have idiopathic disease. Nearly 80% present before age 20; the mean age of onset is 11 years. Often, there is a strong family history of pancreatitis. A subset of patients with chronic pancreatitis has a defect in the *PRSS1* gene for a trypsinogen protein that makes it hypersensitive to activation. Other defects in pancreatic regulatory proteins, such as the serine protease inhibitor (*SPINK1* gene), have now also been described. Some unique mutations in the *CFTR* gene have also been identified.

Intermittent/repeating episodes of chronic pancreatitis are usually mild to moderate and may resolve over 3–7 days. The frequency and severity of the episodes tends to decrease as the child ages. Acute on chronic episodes can be challenging to manage in these patients because they often have normal pancreatic enzymes. Pancreatic insufficiency occurs in up to 50%, and DM occurs in about 25%. Adenocarcinoma of the pancreas occurs with increased frequency in those affected.

DISEASES OF THE LIVER AND BILIARY TREE

CONGENITAL DISORDERS OF LIVER STRUCTURE

Liver Location Abnormalities

Situs inversus (left-sided) and heterotaxia (central liver) are relatively rare congenital anomalies. Either can occur with other anomalies, such as polysplenia or asplenia syndromes. Many of these patients are without functional difficulties.

Congenital Anomalies of the Portal Vein

Congenital anomalies of the portal vein are frequently associated with cardiac and urinary system abnormalities. Portal vein thrombosis can occur due to umbilical infection; umbilical vein catheterization in the newborn period; pancreatitis; protein C, protein S, and antithrombin III deficiencies; or the presence of anticardiolipin antibodies. You can confirm portal vein abnormalities by Doppler ultrasound, frequently after the patient presents with splenomegaly or esophageal variceal bleeding.

Congenital absence of the portal vein has been described but is very rare.

CONGENITAL ANOMALIES OF THE BILIARY TREE

Extrahepatic Biliary Atresia

Most cases of extrahepatic biliary atresia are acquired, but up to 35% may occur during the embryonic or fetal stage. These infants present with neonatal cholestasis and absence of bile duct remnants. About 20% have other associated anomalies, including cardiac, GI, or GU systems. Pediatric liver transplantation is lifesaving. Extrahepatic biliary atresia is discussed in greater detail later in this section.

Choledochal Cysts

Choledochal cysts are extremely rare. Asian girls are the most commonly affected group, especially Japanese girls. Nearly 40% present before 1 year of age, and an additional 35% present between the ages of 1 and 6 years. The classically described triad of abdominal pain, jaundice, and palpable right upper quadrant mass occurs in only about 25%. Fever, nausea, vomiting, and pancreatitis are classic symptoms. Use ultrasound to show both intrahepatic and extrahepatic biliary tree dilation. Radionuclide scans can show cysts with accumulation of tracer. ERCP or MRCP (magnetic resonance cholangiopancreatography) can be useful for determining the anatomy.

There are 5 different types based on anatomic location as classified by Todani. The most common, however, is type I with diffuse enlargement of the common bile duct.

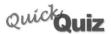

Unfortunately, there is a high incidence of biliary malignancy in patients with choledochal cysts, with rates as high as 17.5%. Most are cholangiocarcinomas. Treatment for the cysts is aimed at early removal of the cysts and gallbladder, with reconstructive surgery based on the anatomic location of the cysts.

Structural Anomalies of the Gallbladder

Congenital absence of the gallbladder occurs in about 1/10,000 births and is of little clinical significance if it occurs in isolation. Frequently, though, absence of the gallbladder is associated with extrahepatic biliary atresia, imperforate anus, GU anomalies, bicuspid aortic valve, and cerebral aneurysms.

Hypoplastic gallbladders are more common and occur in about 1/3 of patients with CF. Additionally, hypoplastic malformations occur in trisomy 18. Gallbladder duplication occurs in about 1/4,000.

"Floating" gallbladder occurs in 5% of the population. These gallbladders lack a peritoneal coat and are suspended and pendulous. This makes them more susceptible to torsion, which results in acute, severe RUQ pain with nausea and vomiting.

Congenital Hepatic Fibrosis

Congenital hepatic fibrosis is the most common abnormality of the ductal plate, which forms at about 8 weeks of gestation and consists of hepatic precursor cells that remodel over fetal life to form the intrahepatic biliary tree. Congenital hepatic fibrosis is usually associated with autosomal recessive polycystic kidney disease.

Neonates and infants present with abnormalities of the renal system, and older children and adults present with hepatic manifestations. The ductal plate abnormality results in dilated bile duct structures and portal tracts without interlobular ducts in the center. In children 5–13 years of age, this leads to portal hypertension and presents typically as hematemesis and/or melena due to esophageal varices. The bleeding can be life-threatening and requires endoscopic intervention. On examination, the child has an enlarged liver, especially the left lobe, and splenomegaly. The liver transaminases are usually normal except for occasional mild elevations. The development of cholangitis is the greatest concern and the prime cause of mortality. Liver biopsy confirms the diagnosis.

Treatment can include portosystemic shunting for portal hypertension and antibiotic therapy for cholangitis. Liver transplantation is beneficial for those with chronic cholangitis or progressive hepatic dysfunction. Some with isolated congenital hepatic fibrosis do well and do not require specific therapy.

Caroli Disease

Caroli disease is another abnormality of the ductal plate and is due to a congenital dilatation of the larger, segmental intrahepatic bile ducts. If Caroli disease occurs in combination with congenital hepatic fibrosis, it is known as Caroli syndrome. Caroli disease and syndrome are autosomal recessive and present in adolescence or adulthood.

Patients present with recurrent cholangitis and abscesses. Liver biopsy can show the hepatic fibrosis, but further diagnosis of Caroli disease requires ultrasound, CT, ERCP, or percutaneous transhepatic cholangiography. These studies show dilatation of the hepatic bile ducts and enlargement of the major intra- and extrahepatic biliary passages.

Treat with antibiotics aimed at the cholangitis. If the disease is confined to 1 lobe, consider a partial hepatectomy. Sepsis is a frequent cause of death. Additional complications include cholangiocarcinoma and amyloidosis.

Alagille Syndrome

Alagille syndrome (arteriohepatic dysplasia, Watson-Miller syndrome, syndromic duct paucity) is an autosomal dominant disorder with variable penetrance that is caused by mutations on chromosome 20p in a single gene, *JAG1*, which encodes protein ligands for *NOTCH1*. It is rare, with an incidence of about 1/100,000. Genetic testing for *JAG1* mutations can identify only 60–75% of patients, however.

Alagille syndrome is associated with peripheral pulmonary artery stenosis, occasionally tetralogy of Fallot, and neonatal cholestasis. Classically, patients present with chronic cholestatic liver disease with a "paucity" of small intrahepatic ducts, "butterfly" vertebrae, abnormal radius/ulna, posterior embryotoxon of the eye (a developmental abnormality marked by a prominent white ring of Schwalbe and iris strands that partially obscure the chamber angle), and characteristic facies. The facies of these children consist of a prominent forehead; moderate hypertelorism; a small, pointed chin; and a saddle or straight nose.

GASTROENTEROLOGY & NUTRITION

Most patients with Alagille have elevated conjugated bilirubin in the neonatal period. In about 1/2 of patients, hepatobiliary scans fail to show biliary excretion of tracer. Liver biopsy shows reduced numbers of small bile ducts with some giant-cell transformation and cholestasis.

Most patients with Alagille syndrome have a benign course. Cholestasis usually resolves or improves over the 1st year of life, and most patients do not develop cirrhosis. Some infants have more severe, sometimes progressive, liver disease. Overall mortality approaches 25% and is typically due to cardiac disease, intercurrent infection, or progressive liver disease.

Do not perform Kasai portoenterostomy in infants with Alagille syndrome! Be aware also that children with Alagille are particularly prone to significant intracranial bleeding with even minor head trauma. This is regardless of their liver function and without a noticeable coagulopathy. Liver transplantation is used only for those with hepatic failure, severe growth failure, or intolerable itching unresponsive to medical therapy.

VIRAL HEPATITIS

Hepatitis A

Hepatitis A is an RNA virus. It is easily transmitted fecal-orally—generally among household and daycare contacts. It can also be sexually transmitted as well. There is no transplacental transmission! There are no carrier or persistent states, although occasionally there is prolonged cholestasis (with increased bilirubin and alkaline phos) for up to 4 months. Incubation period is 15–50 days. (See Figure 14-2.)

Diagnosis of acute infection: high titers of IgM antibodies directed against the hepatitis A virus (anti-HAV IgM) in serum. (IgG indicates only a previous infection.) Symptoms are unusual in young children but very common in adults (70%). Complications are rare—about 1% chance of fulminant hepatitis.

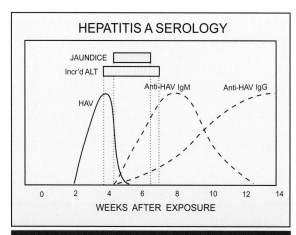

Figure 14-2: Hepatitis A Serology vs. Weeks after Exposure

Give the following groups prophylaxis:

- All household contacts
- Sexual partners
- Needle-sharing partners
- Day care and nursing home attendees and staff in close contact with a case

School, hospital, or workplace day-to-day contact does not warrant prophylaxis.

For prophylaxis, give either hepatitis A vaccine or IG in a dose of 0.02 mL/kg as soon as possible, preferably within 2 weeks of exposure.

Immunoglobulin (IG) is good prophylaxis only against HAV. (Note: Use HBIG [hepatitis B immune globulin] for hepatitis B.)

Hepatitis A vaccine is the preferred prophylaxis for those ≥ 12 months of age, and IG is preferred for those < 12 months of age.

An inactivated hepatitis A vaccine (Havrix® and Vaqta®) is given universally at 1 year of age in 2 doses, 6 months apart. Virtually all those completing the series develop protective levels of antibody to hepatitis A virus (anti-HAV). Based on what is now known of the antibody levels, protection persists for up to 20 years in those who complete the series.

Even though the HAV vaccine is universally recommended in the U.S., many people may not have received it as a child. Be on the lookout for people who are at high risk for hepatitis A infection or complications:

- High-risk sexual behavior or IV drug use
- Children > 2 years old living in communities with high rates of HAV infection
- Chronic liver disease
- Travel to high-risk countries
- Patients with hepatitis B or C (because these patients are at risk of fulminant disease if they get hepatitis A)

Hepatitis B

Hepatitis B is the only hepatitis virus composed of DNA. The incubation period is 1–6 months. It is transmitted by sexual contact (most common way in adolescents and adults!), contaminated body fluids, and contaminated needles. Clinical: First are prodromal constitutional symptoms, which typically resolve at the time jaundice becomes apparent. Occasionally (10–15%), the prodromal symptoms are serum sickness-like, with fever, arthritis, urticaria, and angioedema. This seems to be caused by circulating immune complexes (especially HBsAg+ complexed with anti-HBs) activating the complement system. With the onset of jaundice, the patient usually feels much better but may have liver swelling and tenderness and cholestatic symptoms. The likelihood of developing chronic HBV is inversely proportional to age. Chronic HBV occurs in 90% of infants infected at birth, in 25–50% of children infected between the ages

Quick Quiz

- How is hepatitis A transmitted from person to person?

- What laboratory test will diagnose acute hepatitis A?

- What can be given to household contacts to prevent spread of hepatitis A once a case has been identified?

- How is hepatitis B transmitted?

- Once infected with acute hepatitis B, who is more likely to develop chronic hepatitis B—an infant or an adolescent?

- In adults, chronic hepatitis B is associated with what 2 serious conditions?

- What laboratory test indicates immunity to hepatitis B?

- Which laboratory test correlates with increased infectivity of the patient with hepatitis B?

- What is the window period for hepatitis B infection?

of 1 and 5 years, and in 5% of older children and adults who become infected. There is now universal pre-school vaccination in the U.S. Overall, less than 1% of patients with hepatitis B develop fulminant hepatitis, but about 5–7% develop chronic carrier states. There are 3 types of carrier states:

1) Asymptomatic
2) Chronic persistent hepatitis
3) Chronic hepatitis B

The first 2 carrier states are benign. You must do a liver biopsy to differentiate chronic persistent hepatitis from chronic hepatitis B. Chronic hepatitis B is a serious illness—in adults, it often progresses to cirrhosis and is strongly associated with hepatocellular cancer. There have been poor results with liver transplantation so far, and chronic hepatitis B is not considered an indication for transplant. There are some treatment protocols with antivirals, interferons, and other agents.

Know the 3 main antigenic markers in hepatitis B and their corresponding antibodies (follow along in Figure 14-3):

1) Hepatitis B surface antigen (HBsAg): If an asymptomatic patient has HBsAg in the serum, it means either the patient is a carrier or the patient has early hepatitis B—so initial action is only to follow closely. Once a patient is infected, neither vaccination nor HBIG helps. Finding IgG antibodies to the hepatitis B surface antigen (anti-HBs IgG) in the serum indicates past exposure to either hepatitis B virus or the vaccine and indicates immunity to the virus.

2) Hepatitis B core antigen (HBcAg): HBcAg+ protein is the core particle (inner shell) of the virion. This protein is retained in the hepatocyte until it is covered with an HBsAg+ nucleocapsid outer shell, which then incorporates the DNA. Free HBcAg+ protein does not circulate in the serum. However, antibody to HBcAg appears early in the disease (initially IgM, then IgG) and persists for life, so anti-HBc IgG is the most reliable marker for previous exposure to HBV.

3) Hepatitis B e antigen (HBeAg): HBeAg is a soluble protein made from the same gene as HBcAg; however, unlike HBcAg, which does not circulate in the serum, HBeAg is secreted from the hepatocytes and does circulate in the serum. HBeAg correlates with the quantity of intact virus and, therefore, with infectivity and liver inflammation. The hepatitis B antibody (anti-HBe) appears several weeks after the illness. Detecting HBsAg and HBeAg indicates active virions and high infectivity (more so than HBsAg+ and HBeAg–). The tests for HBeAg and anti-HBe are often not available locally.

Once infected, the 1st marker detectable in the serum is the antigen, HBsAg. This is followed by the appearance of antibody to the core antigen. After HBsAg becomes undetectable, there is a period of several weeks before the anti-HBs antibody becomes detectable. This is called "the window," and you must measure an anti-HBc IgM during this period to confirm acute hepatitis B.

Removal of HBV is T-cell mediated, and the only purpose of anti-HBsAg is to prevent reinfection or initial infection with the use of vaccine.

Hepatitis B immunoglobulin (HBIG; anti-HBs) provides some protection against hepatitis B, although it appears to only decrease the severity of illness rather than protect the patient from disease. It is effective as prophylaxis and when given in early infection.

The 2 hepatitis B vaccines are composed of HBsAg. They are equally effective, and they are safe for pregnant patients. It is best if the hepatitis B vaccine is given

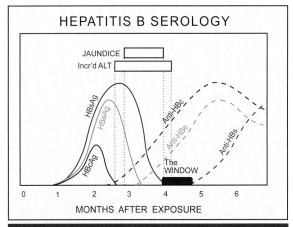

HEPATITIS B SEROLOGY

JAUNCICE
Incr'd ALT

HBsAg
HBeAg
HBcAg
Anti-HBc
Anti-HBe
Anti-HBs
The WINDOW

MONTHS AFTER EXPOSURE

Figure 14-3: Hepatitis B Serology vs. Months after Exposure

HBsAg	Anti-HBc	Anti-HBs	Interpretation
+	−	−	Acute infection
+	+	−	3 possibilities: 1) Acute infection (IgM anti-HBc) 2) Chronic hep B (high ALT, IgG anti-HBc) 3) Inactive carrier (normal enzymes, IgG anti-HBc)
−	−	+	2 possibilities: 1) Remote infection 2) Immunized
−	+	+	Remote infection
−	+	−	3 possibilities: 1) Window disease 2) Remote infection 3) False positive
+	+	+	More than 1 infection; e.g., IV drug user or renal dialysis patient with both acute and chronic hepatitis B (infected with different strains of hepatitis B).

Table 14-7: Hepatitis B Scenarios

	Anti-HAV IgM	Anti-HAV IgG	HBsAg	Anti-HBs IgG	Anti-HBc IgG	Anti-HBc IgM	HBeAg	Anti-HDV
Acute hepatitis A	+	−				−		
Previous HAV	−	+				−		
Acute HBV			+early	−	−	+	+	−
Acute HBV—window			−	−	−	+	−	−
Chronic active HBV			+	−	+	−	usu+	−
Remote HBV (immune)			−	+	+	−	−	−
Vaccinated (immune)	−		−	+	−	−	−	−
Acute hepatitis D (w/ acute HBV)			+early	−	−	+	+	+
Acute hepatitis D (w/ CAH)			+	rarely	+	−	usu+	+

Table 14-8: Types of Viral Hepatitis and Their Serological Tests

before the patient is exposed to HBV. 95% of immunocompetent patients develop antibodies, whereas only about 50% of dialysis patients do. Because these vaccines are surface antigens, to ensure effectiveness after the course of vaccine has been given, check for anti-HBs—there will be no anti-HBc.

Hepatitis lab scenarios and serologic tests are listed in Table 14-7 and Table 14-8.

Give HBIG and hepatitis B vaccination to the newborn of a mother with hepatitis B. There is a 5–10% transplacental transmission of HBV. In high-prevalence areas (e.g., Alaska, northern Canada, and other places with a high number of Asian immigrants), the transplacental transmission is the main route of transmission. In low-prevalence areas, HBV is mainly acquired during adolescence and adulthood.

If a person has possible blood exposure to a person with an acute HBV infection and the HBsAg is still negative, the CDC recommends giving that person HBIG, followed by a complete course of HBV vaccinations.

Note: Several months after an episode of hepatitis B, check for loss of HBsAg and HBV-DNA to ensure that it has not become chronic.

Hepatitis B is strongly associated with polyarteritis nodosa (PAN). The surface antigen is found in 20–30% of these patients. It appears that the hepatitis B infection precipitates an autoimmune reaction resulting in PAN. Chronic infection with hepatitis B is a strong risk factor for hepatocellular carcinoma.

Hepatitis C

Hepatitis C, a parenterally transmitted single-stranded RNA virus, is the most common bloodborne disease in the United States. It is also the most common infectious cause of liver disease in the U.S. The prevalence of HCV infection in children is 0.1–0.2% compared to 1.8% in adults. Most HCV infections in the U.S. are genotype 1, which happens to be less responsive to treatment.

In most instances, the source of the infection in individual patients is unknown. However, the following are associated with an increased risk of hepatitis C:

- IV drug use
- Prison exposure
- High-risk sexual behaviors: STDs, prostitutes, > 5 sexual partners a year
- Blood transfusion before 1990
- Tattoos and body piercings
- Snorting cocaine
- Infants born to HCV-infected mothers

While only 1% of adults with hepatitis B develop chronic disease, 70–80% of acute HCV infections become chronic! Also, hepatitis B has high virus counts, whereas hepatitis C has low virus counts. These low virus counts are consistent with the more insidious nature of hepatitis C:

- Only 25% of acute infections are symptomatic.
- HCV infection has an increased likelihood of becoming chronic.
- The chronic form is relatively benign. (25% are only carriers; 50% have no symptoms but have abnormal LFTs; 25% have chronic active disease with symptoms.)

It is also consistent with the low rates of sexual transmission seen in monogamous couples: only 5% after 10–20 years. This is low but does occur, so recommend safe sex.

Needle-stick transmission rate from a known infected patient is about 5–10%.

Transplacental infection is < 5%.

Extrahepatic disease includes small vessel vasculitis with glomerulonephritis and neuropathy, mixed cryoglobulinemia, and porphyria cutanea tarda ([PCT]; Image 14-15). Mixed cryoglobulinemia presents as a small vessel

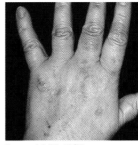
Image 14-15: PCT

(leukocytoclastic) vasculitis with a rash consisting of "palpable purpura" or "crops of purple papules."

70–80% of patients infected with HCV develop chronic hepatitis—and about 25% of these get end-stage cirrhosis after 20–25 years! And 1–4% of patients with cirrhosis develop hepatocellular carcinoma (HCC) each year. Chronic HCV infection has become the #1 cause of adult liver transplants in the U.S. It must be assumed that many of these were infected during childhood.

There is no vaccine for hepatitis C.

Lab tests:

- In a person positive for anti-HCV, confirm positive antibodies with RIBA (recombinant immunoblot assay) test (to exclude a false-positive test). If the RIBA is positive, check for active virus by ordering an HCV-RNA viral load. This is necessary because the anti-HCV does not confer immunity (as does the HBV antibody).
- Within 2–4 months after an episode of hepatitis C, recheck for loss of HCV-RNA (PCR) to ensure that it has not become chronic.

Protocols for treatment are interferons and ribavirin, although the response rate is at best nearing 50%.

Mixed cryoglobulinemia can result from chronic hepatitis B or C (in addition to various other occult viral, bacterial, and fungal infections).

Hepatitis D

Hepatitis D is an RNA virus that requires a concomitant or previously existing hepatitis B virus infection to become pathogenic. It is usually found among IV drug abusers and high-risk hepatitis B surface antigen (HBsAg) carriers. It typically does not make an acute HBV infection much worse, but, if acquired as a superinfection in an HBV carrier, the infection can be very severe, even fulminant. If acquired acutely, HDV does not increase the risk of chronic hepatitis B. Immunity to hepatitis B implies immunity to hepatitis D. Diagnosis: anti-HDV IgM.

See Table 14-8 for a review of the serologic tests done with hepatitis A, B, and D.

Hepatitis E

Hepatitis E is a single-stranded RNA virus, which is spread through the fecal-oral route just like hepatitis A virus. Found in the Far East, Africa, and Central America, it frequently is due to contamination of water supplies after monsoon flooding. Recently, anti-HEV has been found in pigs in midwestern U.S. states and in rats in Maryland, Hawaii, and Louisiana.

Like hepatitis A, hepatitis E has no known chronic form. Unlike hepatitis A, however, it carries a very high risk for fulminant hepatitis in the 3rd trimester of pregnancy—with a 20% maternal fatality rate. Think of acute hepatitis E infection in a returning traveler from endemic areas who presents with acute hepatitis and whose hepatitis A, B, and C serologies are negative.

Hepatitis G

Hepatitis G is bloodborne, like hepatitis B and C. Mode of transmission is not well defined but is similar to HCV. There is evidence of infection in 1.5% of blood donors. It causes < 0.5% of community-acquired hepatitis. There is no evidence that HGV causes chronic liver disease.

Epstein-Barr Virus

Epstein-Barr virus (EBV) is a DNA virus that is transmitted by close person-to-person contact with infected secretions, most commonly saliva. Infectious mononucleosis is an EBV infection characterized by fever, pharyngitis, and lymphadenopathy. Liver involvement is common and presents with hepatosplenomegaly, mild-to-moderate elevation of transaminases, and occasional jaundice. The liver disease tends to be mild and transient but can be severe and long lasting, particularly in those who are immunocompromised. A small number of patients can have fulminate liver failure. The normal course, however, is to document acute infection by serum EBV IgM and allow the disease to resolve on its own. The heterophile antibody test (Monospot®) is often done acutely to diagnose EBV, but antibody testing is preferred, especially with liver involvement. Findings of EBV as an etiology for severe disease include a liver biopsy (rarely needed) showing portal and lobular inflammation with sinusoidal infiltration of mononuclear cells.

Some recommend short courses of prednisone to help alleviate the liver dysfunction if it is severe. Antiviral agents are not helpful in the treatment of EBV infection of the liver.

Cytomegalovirus (CMV)

In adults, CMV infection usually causes a presentation similar to infectious mononucleosis (EBV), typically with mild hepatic involvement. The course is usually benign. Acute infection can be confirmed with CMV IgM (but this is rarely done). Treatment is supportive.

In neonates, CMV infection of the liver can be quite severe and resembles idiopathic neonatal hepatitis—which can eventually lead to cirrhosis. This is why testing for CMV infection is typically necessary only in pregnant patients presenting with mono-like symptoms.

Classic cytoplasmic inclusions in the biliary epithelium and hepatocytes occur in only 5% of those affected, but these are virtually pathognomonic when they are found.

Other Viruses

Parvovirus B19 rarely causes liver involvement, but recent case reports have implicated it as an etiology for fulminant liver failure, especially in infants. Mumps and measles (paramyxoviruses) can occasionally cause liver damage.

Final scenario on viruses and the liver: You are presented with a patient who has evidence of acute hepatitis. What screening serologic tests do you order to determine if hepatitis A, B, or C is involved?

Answer: for hepatitis A, IgM HAV; for hepatitis B, HBsAg (hepatitis B surface antigen) and IgM HBc (IgM antibody to hepatis B core); and for hepatitis C, anti-HCV antibody. These are the usual constituents of a "viral hepatitis panel."

METABOLIC LIVER DISEASES

Overview

Galactosemia, fructose intolerance, glycogen storage diseases, hereditary tyrosinemia, and disorders of fatty acid oxidation are discussed in Metabolic Disorders, Book 3.

There are 3 disorders of bilirubin conjugation that result in varying levels of unconjugated hyperbilirubinemia. It is helpful to think of Gilbert, CN II, and CN I as points on a spectrum with mild, moderate, and severe deficiencies in conjugation of bilirubin. They are all the same disease (not enough glucuronosyltransferase), but with different mutations causing different enzyme levels:

1) Gilbert syndrome (mild deficiency; most common)
2) Crigler-Najjar syndrome type II (mild-to-moderate deficiency in conjugation)
3) Crigler-Najjar syndrome type I (severe deficiency in conjugation)

These are all due to mutations in *UGT1A1*, the gene that codes for uridine diphosphate glucuronosyltransferase (UDP-GT), which conjugates bilirubin. These mutations lead to a less active, relative deficiency of glucuronosyltransferase, and thus, less conjugating ability.

Gilbert Syndrome—Mild

Gilbert syndrome occurs in 2–10% of the population. It is often caused by a less severe mutation in *UGT1A1* or its promoter. This results in a mild, indirect

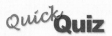

- How is hepatitis E transmitted?
- In whom is hepatitis E most virulent?
- Can EBV cause significant liver disease?
- What is Gilbert syndrome?
- How does Crigler-Najjar syndrome type I differ from Crigler-Najjar syndrome type II?
- What is Dubin-Johnson syndrome?
- What drug is associated with Reye syndrome?
- How does α_1-antitrypsin deficiency present?

hyperbilirubinemia, usually < 5 mg/dL. It is often discovered incidentally when bilirubin is measured for some other reason (typically on a comprehensive metabolic panel). There is no associated hemolysis or hepatocellular damage. Typically, it becomes apparent during episodes of stress or fasting, when the patient becomes mildly jaundiced. No treatment is required, and no morbidity or mortality is associated with it. Infants with prolonged physiologic jaundice or breast milk jaundice often have polymorphisms in *UGT1A1* as well.

Crigler-Najjar Syndrome Type II—Moderate

Crigler-Najjar syndrome type II results in partial activity of bilirubin UDP-GT. Hyperbilirubinemia of < 10 mg/dL is usual. It resolves with phenobarbital and other inducers of cytochrome P450, but phenobarbital is not recommended for long-term therapy due to its neuro-developmental complications from long-term use. Hyperbilirubinemia from this disorder does not require specific therapy and is not associated with increased morbidity or mortality.

Crigler-Najjar Syndrome Type I—Severe

Crigler-Najjar syndrome type I is more severe than type II and is due to a complete absence of bilirubin UDP-GT activity. It presents in the newborn period with severe indirect hyperbilirubinemia and requires phototherapy and/or exchange transfusions. There is no conjugated bilirubin. Kernicterus is a major concern. DNA testing can confirm the diagnosis pre- and postnatally. Mainstay of therapy is phototherapy, although this is difficult to maintain long-term. Liver transplant can be curative.

Dubin-Johnson Syndrome

Dubin-Johnson syndrome causes conjugated (unlike Gilbert and Crigler-Najjar, which are unconjugated) hyperbilirubinemia and is due to a deficiency in the *cMOAT/MRP2* gene, which encodes the canalicular transporter of conjugated bilirubin. It presents with mild conjugated hyperbilirubinemia of 3–8 mg/dL. It is not associated with any evidence of hepatocellular injury. It does not require specific therapy and is not associated with increased morbidity or mortality.

Reye Syndrome

Reye syndrome is an acute liver disease with hyperammonemic encephalopathy. It appeared to be associated with aspirin use in children with an intercurrent viral infection, such as influenza or chickenpox. The incidence of Reye syndrome peaked in the 1960s and 1970s and is very rare today.

Vomiting is a common presenting finding, and, soon after emesis, AST/ALT values rise. Jaundice is not a specific finding of this disorder, but an elevated prothrombin time (PT) is common. Elevated ammonia is usual. The prognosis is determined by the neurologic rather than hepatic findings, the latter of which frequently resolve over several days.

Treat by correcting metabolic abnormalities and minimizing intracranial hypertension. Most specialists now believe that Reye syndrome was a heterogeneous disorder that probably represented the effect of aspirin use on patients with an underlying metabolic disorder, such as a fatty acid oxidation defect.

α_1-Antitrypsin Deficiency

α_1-antitrypsin deficiency, the most common genetic cause of liver disease in children, can cause progressive liver disease and occurs with an incidence of 1/2,000 live births. Suspect this diagnosis in any child with chronic liver disease. To diagnose, measure α_1-antitrypsin concentration and determine the alleles in the *Pi* locus (and hence the phenotype). The 3 alleles occur in different frequencies and are helpful in determining risk of liver disease:

1) M: normal allele
2) S: mildly low α_1-antitrypsin
3) Z: severely low α_1-antitrypsin

Those with ZZ are most severely affected with both lung and liver disease. Heterozygotes (MS or MZ) have an increased chance of lung and liver disease, especially with concurrent environmental exposure (such as smoking or alcohol use).

The liver disease can present as neonatal jaundice, juvenile cirrhosis, chronic hepatitis, or hepatocellular cancer (HCC). Cholestatic jaundice occurs in 10–15% of infants who are homozygous for the deficiency, and nearly 50% of infants who are homozygous have abnormal liver tests. Giant-cell hepatitis is the classic histologic finding in neonates. Periodic acid-Schiff-positive staining of the liver is classic also, showing that hepatocytes containing the abnormal protein α_1-antitrypsin deficiency are associated with emphysema in young adults.

Most infants with neonatal liver disease improve by 4 months of age for reasons that are unclear. A majority remain healthy throughout childhood. A few present later in life with cirrhosis or HCC. If patients progress to liver failure, liver transplant is curative.

Wilson Disease

Wilson disease is an autosomal recessive disorder of copper metabolism that occurs with an incidence of about 1/100,000 to 1/500,000 births. The disease results from the excessive accumulation of copper in the eyes, liver, kidneys, and brain. This results in degenerative changes in the brain and liver and formation of Kayser-Fleischer rings in the cornea (Image 14-16). These are copper deposits in the inner lining of the Descemet membrane and are almost always found in those with neurologic symptoms. The relevant gene is mapped to chromosome 13.

The disease begins with accumulation of copper in the liver. The clinical presentation varies widely. Most children do not present before the age of 5, and those who present in childhood usually do so with hepatic manifestations, including hepatomegaly and/or acute hepatitis. Hepatic insufficiency occurs later. Fulminant hepatitis is rare before adolescence.

Adolescents may present with mostly neurologic and psychiatric dysfunction. These can include falling grades in school, behavioral changes, tremors, and slurred speech. If left untreated, dysarthria and dystonia eventually develop.

The Kayser-Fleischer rings are frequently absent in children who have only hepatic disease.

Suspect this disorder in children and adolescents with unexplained acute or chronic liver disease, neurologic symptoms of unexplained origin, acute hemolysis, psychiatric illness, behavioral change, Fanconi syndrome, or unexplained bone disease.

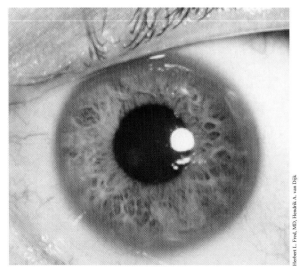

Image 14-16: Wilson disease, Kayser-Fleischer rings

Know all of the following regarding Wilson disease:

- The best screening test is the serum ceruloplasmin level, but, remember, it is not diagnostic. Most patients with Wilson disease have low ceruloplasmin levels.
- Early in the disease, serum copper levels may be high, and 24-hour urinary copper excretion is increased, sometimes to 1,000 µg/day. (Normal urinary copper excretion is < 40 µg/day.)
- If you are still uncertain about the diagnosis, you can give a dose of D-penicillamine, which increases urinary excretion of copper to nearly 2,000 µg/day in those with Wilson disease.
- Liver biopsy is the gold standard for diagnosis and shows markedly elevated hepatic copper content. (But you have to order it!)

Screen family members of those with proven cases. This usually includes checking a serum ceruloplasmin and 24-hour urinary copper excretion. If abnormal, perform a liver biopsy.

Treat with copper-chelating agents such as D-penicillamine, which should lead to a rapid excretion of excess copper. With therapy, hepatic and neurologic functions improve, and Kayser-Fleischer rings disappear. If the patient cannot tolerate penicillamine, try triethylene tetramine dihydrochloride. Limit oral intake of copper to < 1 mg/day. Have patients avoid foods such as liver, shellfish, nuts, and chocolate. If the copper content of the local water supply is elevated, suggest a demineralizer.

Treatment is lifesaving; those without treatment die. For the patients who already have fulminant liver failure or decompensated cirrhosis, liver transplant is necessary. Some recommend liver transplant for those with progressive neurologic disease, but this indication is controversial. In screened siblings who are asymptomatic with the disease, implement penicillamine therapy.

Hemochromatosis

Hemochromatosis is a disease of excessive storage of iron, mainly in the form of hemosiderin in the parenchymal cells of multiple tissues. It can result in abnormalities in the function and structure of the liver, heart, pancreas, skin, joints, gonads, and other endocrine organs.

There are 3 forms of this disease:

1) Hereditary hemochromatosis
2) Transfusion-induced hemosiderosis
3) Neonatal hemochromatosis

Hereditary hemochromatosis is most commonly due to a mutation in the *HFE* gene, but it is variably expressed. This is not a disorder of childhood, but children can have elevated iron studies. Adults develop cirrhosis, bronzing of the skin, and diabetes mellitus (often called "bronze diabetes"). If families are screened, you can

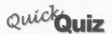

prevent disease in affected individuals by periodic phlebotomy; for children, this is usually not necessary until adolescence.

Transfusion-induced hemosiderosis occurs in those patients who repeatedly receive red cell transfusions. It most commonly occurs in those with congenital or acquired anemias who require frequent transfusions. (Look for a patient with sickle cell anemia and evidence of liver damage!) Monitor iron overload and treat with chelation therapy (deferoxamine).

Finally, neonatal hemochromatosis is an acquired syndrome due to severe fetal liver damage likely caused by maternal alloimmunity. Mortality is > 90%. These children present with cholestatic jaundice with coagulopathy and/or ascites at birth. Treatment is supportive.

Progressive Familial Intrahepatic Cholestasis (PFIC)

Progressive familial intrahepatic cholestasis refers to a group of inherited disorders in which bile is not formed properly. PFIC1 (formerly known as Byler disease) and PFIC2 are characterized by normal serum GGT (γ-glutamyl transpeptidase) but with severe cholestasis. PFIC3 has elevated serum GGT levels (know this difference!).

PFIC1 usually presents between 3 and 6 months of age with conjugated hyperbilirubinemia and severe, unremitting pruritus—but remember: GGT is normal! It is due to a mutation in the *FIC1* gene on chromosome 18. Fat-soluble vitamin deficiencies (A, D, E, and K) are common, secondary to lack of available bile salts to facilitate absorption in the small intestine. These children have persistent diarrhea with fat malabsorption and protein loss. Poor growth is common. Cirrhosis develops in early childhood and requires liver transplant. Even after liver transplant, bouts of pancreatitis and diarrhea are still common.

PFIC2 differs from PFIC1 in that the gene mutation is *SPGP* and occurs on chromosome 2. These children do not have pancreatitis or diarrhea, but they have prominent liver disease with normal GGT. It is most commonly seen in Middle Eastern Europeans.

PFIC3 differs from the other two progressive familial intrahepatic cholestasis diseases in that the cholestasis is associated with an elevated GGT. Jaundice is generally less prominent, but the pruritus is still severe. Patients with PFIC3 present later and have a slowly progressive disease process.

DRUG-INDUCED HEPATOTOXICITY

Acetaminophen is the most common cause of acute liver failure in the United States. Its toxicity is dose-dependent and due to shunting down a minor pathway that produces a toxic metabolite when the glucuronidation pathway is depleted. N-acetylcysteine replenishes glutathione stores and allows the liver to metabolize acetaminophen without generating toxic metabolites. There are nomograms you can utilize to determine the risk of hepatotoxicity based on the time since ingestion and measured metabolite level. In severe toxicity, emergent liver transplant may be required. Most cases occur in toddlers (accidental ingestion) or adolescents (intentional overdose). Look for co-ingestion which is common and can make liver toxicity worse, especially alcohol. (See more on acetaminophen ingestion in Emergency Pediatric Care, Book 1.)

Idiosyncratic hepatotoxic reactions have been reported with many drugs, but a few are noted with great frequency. These include phenytoin, sulfasalazine, and halothane. Various antibiotics, including erythromycin and trimethoprim/sulfamethoxazole, can cause hepatic injury.

Oral contraceptives are associated with hepatic vein thrombosis (Budd-Chiari syndrome) and liver adenomas. Use of androgens by adolescent athletes to enhance performance is also associated with liver toxicity.

Except for acetaminophen overdose, no specific therapy is useful for most liver toxicities. Usually, supportive care and stopping the offending agent are the only means to potentially reverse the course.

AUTOIMMUNE HEPATOBILIARY DISEASE

Autoimmune Hepatitis

Autoimmune hepatitis refers to a variety of distinct diseases that affect the liver and frequently overlap with disorders that affect the bile ducts and other hepatic elements. The etiology of autoimmune hepatitis is unknown, but it appears to have genetic features. It is likely that a viral infection or drug exposure may initiate the disorder in those susceptible. Other autoimmune comorbidities are common (like PBC, PSC, and autoimmune thyroiditis).

There are 3 types of autoimmune hepatitis:

- **Type I** is known as the "classic" form and affects females > males between 10 and 20 years of age and also between 45 and 70 years of age. It is associated with the presence of smooth muscle antibodies and/or antinuclear antibodies (ANA).

• **Type II** occurs in younger children (males = females) and is characterized by the liver-kidney microsomal-1 antibody (anti-LKM-1). These children present with more severe liver disease than those in Type I.

• **Type III** occurs in adults primarily and is characterized by the antisoluble liver antigen (anti-SLA).

Any of these 3 types can present in various ways. Most commonly, patients initially have only malaise, weight loss, and/or anorexia. Serious complications may not present until cirrhosis and portal hypertension have already occurred, and the child/adolescent presents with variceal bleeding. Jaundice can be quite variable. Always look for a family history of other autoimmune diseases, such as thyroiditis, arthritis, and inflammatory bowel disease. Many older patients come to attention due to new onset of jaundice and are then found to have evidence of hepatitis on routine laboratory testing.

Diagnosis depends on finding the serum antibody markers in the face of elevated aminotransferases with an elevated total protein (due to hypergammaglobulinemia). Always evaluate for viral hepatitis, especially hepatitis C, which can lead to elevated ANA or LKM antibodies. Usually, you must perform a biopsy to show portal lymphoplasmacytic infiltrates that can extend to the surrounding hepatic lobule.

Initial treatment is immunosuppression with corticosteroids. Some patients remain in remission on a low dose of steroids. Other agents used to maintain remission include azathioprine, cyclosporine, and tacrolimus. Liver transplant may be useful in refractory cases, but autoimmune hepatitis can recur in the transplanted liver too!

Primary Sclerosing Cholangitis

Primary sclerosing cholangitis is a disease of unknown etiology that is characterized by chronic fibrosing inflammation of the intra- and extrahepatic bile duct. Secondary sclerosing cholangitis has the same findings but is due to choledocholithiasis, postoperative stricture, toxin-induced bile duct injury, AIDS, or Langerhans cell histiocytosis. Primary sclerosing cholangitis is associated with inflammatory bowel disease (especially ulcerative colitis!) and occasionally is ANCA-positive, both of which indicate a possible immunological etiology.

Clinical presentation is variable. Patients can be asymptomatic or have fatigue, jaundice, hepatosplenomegaly, or abdominal discomfort with itching. For some children, cirrhosis and portal hypertension may be the first clues. Always consider primary sclerosing cholangitis in any child with inflammatory bowel disease if there is evidence of hepatobiliary dysfunction.

Laboratory testing shows elevated alkaline phosphatase and GGT (cholestatic pattern) in most patients. Low titers of anti-SM or anti-LKM antibodies may be present. The best test to confirm the diagnosis is endoscopic retrograde cholangiography, which will show alternating normal, strictured, and dilated portions of the biliary tree, known as "beading." Most experts perform MRCP first, prior to the more invasive ERCP, but the results are less precise. On histologic examination, the classic "onion-skin lesion" is pathognomonic but not common.

Treat with endoscopic management of biliary strictures and supportive care for chronic liver disease if it is present. Some recommend using ursodeoxycholic acid to stimulate bile flow, but this does not improve survival and is associated with frequent adverse drug events. Recommend liver transplant if cirrhosis and portal hypertension have occurred.

IDIOPATHIC NEONATAL (GIANT-CELL) HEPATITIS

Idiopathic neonatal hepatitis is a catchall phrase for newborns with liver damage where known infectious and metabolic etiologies have been ruled out. The liver disease presents histologically as multinucleated giant cells and can occur in 40% of infants with cholestasis. Jaundice often occurs in the 1st week after birth but can take 1–3 months to appear. Acholic (clay-colored or gray) stools and dark urine are common. Hepatomegaly is universal; splenomegaly occurs in 50%. Laboratory testing shows an elevated bilirubin of about 8–12 mg/dL, of which over 50% is conjugated. Albumin and GGT are usually normal.

Diagnosis relies on excluding other etiologies and finding giant-cell transformation around the central veins on liver biopsy.

Except for supportive care and fat-soluble vitamin supplementation, no specific therapy is helpful. 70–80% will have a complete recovery by 6–8 months. Those who don't improve will likely develop cirrhosis and portal hypertension.

AAGENAES SYNDROME

Aagenaes syndrome is very rare (except on exams). It is an autosomal recessive disorder of Norwegian families. It presents as severe cholestasis in Norwegian newborns. Lymphedema of the lower extremities is a characteristic finding. Histologically, it resembles giant-cell neonatal hepatitis. Children gradually improve without specific therapy.

BILIARY ATRESIA

Although biliary atresia is uncommon, it is nonetheless the most common reason for pediatric liver transplantation in the United States. The cause of this condition is unknown. The condition leads to the destruction of bile ducts, progressing from extra- to intrahepatic which, in turn, results in fibrosis, biliary cirrhosis, and eventual liver failure.

Clinically, cholestatic jaundice usually appears during the 2nd or 3rd week of life but can present at birth as well. Look for clay-colored (acholic) stools and dark urine as clues to biliary atresia. Hepatomegaly is common. Laboratory evaluation reveals hyperbilirubinemia (both conjugated and unconjugated) and hypertransaminasemia. The gallbladder is frequently not seen on ultrasound.

These infants must be evaluated and treated quickly to increase the odds of a favorable outcome.

Do the following tests:

- Abdominal ultrasound.
- HIDA scan: Hepatobiliary scintigraphy is frequently performed in this setting, but it is not recommended for routine use.
- Operative cholangiography and liver biopsy.
- If these tests are suggestive of biliary atresia, do an intraoperative cholangiogram.

If the intraoperative cholangiogram confirms the diagnosis, the surgeon continues with the Kasai procedure, a bile drainage procedure making a hepatoportoenterostomy (HPE). In this procedure, a loop of the intestine is attached to the porta hepatis. This allows bile to flow from the liver. Typically, it must be done before 3 months of age. A successful Kasai procedure can avoid or delay the need for liver transplantation.

Prognosis varies. In those in whom bile flow is not reestablished and jaundice never resolves, hepatic failure ensues, usually before 1 year of age. In a large majority, however, bile flow is reestablished and jaundice slowly resolves over several months. In these patients, cirrhosis develops over time.

Ultimately, liver transplantation is required in all patients with biliary atresia. Only a small minority achieve apparent permanent drainage post-Kasai without progression of the disease in the liver itself. Once the Kasai is done, these children are at risk for ascending cholangitis and must be followed carefully for signs of fever and worsening jaundice.

CHOLELITHIASIS

Cholelithiasis (gallstones) in healthy children and infants is likely more common than previously thought. Most are asymptomatic and are incidental findings on radiological studies. Follow them. Classic symptoms of biliary colic include RUQ pain, vomiting, and jaundice, without fever. Pain can occur with or without meals and may resolve once the stone has passed.

Certain children are predisposed to developing gallstones, including those children with hemolytic disease (particularly sickle cell), those on chronic TPN, those with short bowel syndrome, and adolescent pregnant females. In the U.S., where there is increasing prevalence of obesity, rates of hospitalizations for pediatric cholelithiasis have also increased. The most common complication in children with cholelithiasis is pancreatitis due to an obstructing stone or stones in the common bile duct.

Plain x-rays may reveal stones with high calcium content, but RUQ ultrasound is the best initial imaging study. A majority of pediatric gallstones are pigment stones and do not respond to oral bile acid therapy. If stones are picked up incidentally, many pediatricians recommend observation only. Cholecystectomy is recommended in patients with biliary colic, cholangitis, cholecystitis, or pancreatitis.

Gallstones are a common finding in adults, and many families will ask you if this is the cause of their child's abdominal pain. Even in children who do have gallstones, it is usually not the cause of pain. Routine removal of a gallbladder because of gallstones without evidence of obstruction is not generally recommended. Many clinicians order a radionuclide hepatobiliary iminodiacetic acid (HIDA) scan to assess the gallbladder in a patient with biliary pain, but without stones. A low gallbladder ejection fraction on a HIDA scan is the diagnostic finding for biliary dyskinesia. This disorder is poorly described in children, and a large number of patients who have a cholecystectomy due to an abnormal HIDA scan still have abdominal pain after the operation.

ACUTE CHOLECYSTITIS

Acute cholecystitis is bacterial inflammation of the gallbladder; it can occur with or without stones (acalculous cholecystitis), although it rarely occurs in children at all. RUQ pain and tenderness on palpation of the gallbladder are common. If the pain worsens with inspiration, this is known as Murphy sign. Other things can cause similar pain, including hepatitis, hepatic abscess, Fitz-Hugh-Curtis syndrome (gonococcal perihepatitis), pancreatitis, appendicitis, pneumonia, pyelonephritis, and renal stones.

Most patients have an elevated WBC count with a left shift and mild increases in bilirubin and transaminases. Markedly elevated bilirubin, alkaline phosphatase, and/ or GGT levels indicate obstruction of the biliary tree with a stone. Ultrasound is best to visualize stones or a thickened gallbladder. Hepatobiliary (HIDA) scan can demonstrate poor or no visualization in the presence of an inflamed gallbladder.

Children have a 30% complication rate, which includes perforation, abscess, and empyema. Most recommend hospital admission with intravenous fluids, antibiotics, and bowel rest. Perform cholecystectomy in patients with acute calculus cholecystitis.

Acalculous cholecystitis can be acute (< 1 month duration) or chronic. It presents acutely, similarly to calculous cholecystitis, except there are obviously no visible stones. It occurs most commonly after a life-threatening illness, burn, or trauma. The chronic form is also known as biliary dyskinesia.

BILIARY DYSKINESIA

Biliary dyskinesia is poorly coordinated gallbladder contraction, usually in the setting of a fibrotic or inflamed gallbladder. It is commonly diagnosed in adult patients, but is less common in children. The HIDA scan can show poor excretion (a "low ejection fraction") from the gallbladder. In adults, this is one of the most common indications for cholecystectomy. A large percentage of patients still have pain after cholecystectomy.

SPHINCTER OF ODDI DYSFUNCTION

Sphincter of Oddi dysfunction (SOD) is a common cause of upper abdominal pain in adults. This condition needs to be considered in pediatric patients with unexplained upper abdominal pain. Think of it as "IBS of the bile ducts"! It is more common after cholecystectomy. If there is evidence of obstruction of the biliary tree (Type I or Type II SOD, less common), then sphincterotomy using ERCP may be helpful. If there is no obstruction (Type III, more common), sphincterotomy is not helpful.

HYDROPS OF THE GALLBLADDER

Hydrops of the gallbladder refers to an acute noncalculous, noninflammatory enlargement of the gallbladder. It is associated with Kawasaki syndrome, streptococcal pharyngitis, prolonged fasting, TPN, and Henoch-Schönlein purpura. Patients complain of RUQ pain with a palpable mass. Fever, vomiting, and jaundice are common. Ultrasound shows a markedly dilated, stone-free gallbladder. Acute hydrops rarely requires cholecystectomy. If performed, a laparotomy will show a large, edematous

gallbladder that contains white, yellow, or green bile. Usually, treating the underlying condition results in the gallbladder returning to normal over several weeks.

TUMORS OF THE LIVER AND BILIARY TREE

Tumors of the hepatobiliary system are rare in children, comprising about 1–4% of all solid tumors. If they occur, they are most common in the right lobe of the liver. In children, benign tumors are much more frequent than malignant ones. The common benign tumors include hemangiomas, adenomas, focal nodular hyperplasia, and mesenchymal hamartomas.

Hepatoblastomas are the most common malignant liver tumors in children. They are single masses found in infancy. The serum α-fetoprotein level is markedly elevated in these children and is useful for diagnosis and monitoring after therapy (for recurrence). With complete resection and postoperative chemotherapy, survival rates approach 50%. Liver transplant has been used successfully in cases where complete resection cannot be done.

FOR FURTHER READING

[Guidelines in blue]

NUTRITIONAL DEFICIENCIES

Craig WJ. Health effects of vegan diets. *Am J Clin Nutr.* 2009 May;89(5):S1627–S1633.

Lanska DJ. Chapter 30: historical aspects of the major neurological vitamin deficiency disorders: the water-soluble B vitamins. *Handb Clin Neurol.* 2010;95:445–476.

Mehta NM, Corkins MR, et al; American Society for Parenteral and Enteral Nutrition Board of Directors. Defining pediatric malnutrition: a paradigm shift toward etiology-related definitions. *JPEN J Parenter Enteral Nutr.* 2013 Jul;37(4):460–481.

National Institutes of Health Office of Dietary Supplements. Zinc. *Fact sheet for health professionals.* 2011.

National Library of Medicine. Kwashiorkor. *A.D.A.M. Medical Encyclopedia* [Internet]. Atlanta (GA): A.D.A.M., Inc.; ©2005; [updated 2012 Feb 1].

Sathe MN, Patel AS. Update in pediatrics: focus on fat-soluble vitamins. *Nutr Clin Pract.* 2010 Aug;25(4):340–346.

FLUIDS AND ELECTROLYTES

King CK, et al. Managing acute gastroenteritis among children: oral rehydration, maintenance, and nutritional therapy. *MMWR Recomm Rep.* 2003 Nov 21;52(RR-16):1–16.

VOMITING

Khan S, Di Lorenzo C. Chronic vomiting in children: new insights into diagnosis. *Curr Gastroenterol Rep.* 2001 Jun;3(3):248–256.

Moses S. Pediatric vomiting. *Family Practice Notebook*. 2013.

Li BU, Lefevre F, et al; North American Society for Pediatric Gastroenterology, Hepatology, and Nutrition consensus statement on the diagnosis and management of cyclic vomiting syndrome. *J Pediatr Gastroenterol Nutr*. 2008 Sep;47(3): 379–93.

ACUTE ABDOMINAL PAIN

Chiou E, Nurko S. Management of functional abdominal pain and irritable bowel syndrome in children and adolescents. *Expert Rev Gastroenterol Hepatol*. 2010 Jun;4(3):293–304.

Leung AK, Sigalet DL. Acute abdominal pain in children. *Am Fam Physician*. 2003 Jun 1;67(11):2321–2326.

Ross A, LeLeiko NS. Acute abdominal pain. *Pediatr Rev*. 2010 Apr;31(4):135–144; quiz 144.

American Academy of Pediatrics Subcommittee on Chronic Abdominal Pain. Chronic abdominal pain in children. *Pediatrics*. 2005 Mar;115(3):812–815.

ACUTE DIARRHEA

American Academy of Pediatrics. Managing acute gastroenteritis among children: oral rehydration, maintenance, and nutritional therapy. Centers for Disease Control and Prevention. *Pediatrics*. 2004;114(2):507.

CONSTIPATION

Constipation Guideline Committee of the North American Society for Pediatric Gastroenterology, Hepatology and Nutrition. Evaluation and treatment of constipation in infants and children: recommendations of the North American Society for Pediatric Gastroenterology, Hepatology and Nutrition. *J Pediatr Gastroenterol Nutr*. 2006 Sep; 43(3):e1–e13.

ESOPHAGUS DISORDERS

Chuah SK, et al. 2011 update on esophageal achalasia. *World J Gastroenterol*. 2012 Apr 14;18(14):1573–1578.

Sarathi V, Shah NS. Triple-A syndrome. *Adv Exp Med Biol*. 2010;685:1–8.

Solomon BD. VACTERL/VATER association. *Orphanet J Rare Dis*. 2011 Aug 16;6:56.

Wu JT, et al. Esophageal perforations: new perspectives and treatment paradigms. *J Trauma*. 2007 Nov;63(5):1173–1184.

Vaezi MF, Pandolfino JE, et al. ACG clinical guideline: diagnosis and management of achalasia. *Am J Gastroenterol*. 2013 Aug;108(8):1238–1249.

Vandenplas Y, et al. Pediatric gastroesophageal reflux clinical practice guidelines: joint recommendations of the North American Society for Pediatric Gastroenterology, Hepatology, and Nutrition (NASPGHAN) and the European Society for Pediatric Gastroenterology, Hepatology, and Nutrition (ESPGHAN). *J Pediatr Gastroenterol Nutr*. 2009 Oct;49(4):498–547.

STOMACH DISORDERS

Jones VS, Cohen RC. An eighteen year follow-up after surgery for congenital microgastria—case report and review of literature. *J Pediatr Surg*. 2007 Nov;42(11):1957–1960.

Lambrecht NW. Ménétrier's disease of the stomach: a clinical challenge. *Curr Gastroenterol Rep*. 2011 Dec;13(6):513–517.

Lee JK, et al. Gastrointestinal manifestations of systemic mastocytosis. *World J Gastroenterol*. 2008 Dec 7 14(45):7005–7008.

Osefo N, et al. Gastric acid hypersecretory states: recent insights and advances. *Curr Gastroenterol Rep*. 2009 Dec;11(6):433–441.

INTESTINAL DISORDERS

Ball S, et al. Breast cancer, Cowden disease and PTEN-MATCHS syndrome. *Eur J Surg Oncol*. 2001 Sep; 27(6):604–606.

Baum M, et al. Nucleotide sequence of the Na+/H+ exchanger-8 in patients with congenital sodium diarrhea. *J Pediatr Gastroenterol Nutr*. 2011 Nov;53(5):474–477.

Blumer SL, et al. Sporadic adenocarcinoma of the colon in children: case series and review of the literature. *J Pediatr Hematol Oncol*. 2012 May;34(4):e137–141.

Durno CA. Colonic polyps in children and adolescents. *Can J Gastroenterol*. 2007 Apr;21(4):233–239.

Eng C. *PTEN* Hamartoma Tumor Syndrome (PHTS) 2001 Nov 29 [Updated 2014 Jan 23]. In: Pagon RA, Bird TD, et al, editors. *GeneReviews®* [Internet]. Seattle (WA): University of Washington, Seattle; 1993–2015.

Ghimire P, et al. Primary gastrointestinal lymphoma. *World J Gastroenterol*. 2011 Feb 14;17(6):697–707.

Fernández-Bañares F, et al. Fructose-sorbitol malabsorption. *Curr Gastroenterol Rep*. 2009 Oct;11(5):368–374.

Half E, et al. Familial adenomatous polyposis. *Orphanet J Rare Dis*. 2009 Oct 12;4:22.

Hammer HF, Hammer J. Diarrhea caused by carbohydrate malabsorption. *Gastroenterol Clin North Am*. 2012 Sep;41(3):611–627.

Heitlinger LA, Lebenthal E. Disorders of carbohydrate digestion and absorption. *Pediatr Clin North Am*. 1988 Apr;35(2):239–255.

Kere J, et al. Genetic disorders of membrane transport III. Congenital chloride diarrhea. *Am J Physiol*. 1999 Jan; 276 (1 Pt 1):G7–G13.

Loi M. Lowe syndrome. *Orphanet J Rare Dis*. 2006 May 18;1:16.

Maverakis E, et al. Acrodermatitis enteropathica and an overview of zinc metabolism. *J Am Acad Dermatol*. 2007 Jan;56(1):116–124.

McCarville MB, et al. Typhlitis in childhood cancer. *Cancer*. 2005 Jul 15;104(2):380–387.

Patel AB, Prabhu AS. Hartnup disease. *Indian J Dermatol*. 2008 Jan;53(1):31–32.

Robertson RG, et al. Carcinoid tumors. *Am Fam Physician*. 2006 Aug 1;74(3):429–434.

Treem WR. Clinical aspects and treatment of congenital sucrase-isomaltase deficiency. *J Pediatr Gastroenterol Nutr*. 2012 Nov;55 Suppl 2:S7–S13.

Urbach DR, Rotstein OD. Typhlitis. *Can J Surg*. 1999 Dec;42(6):415–419.

Waite KA, Eng C. Protean PTEN: form and function. *Am J Hum Genet*. 2002 Apr;70(4):829–844.

GASTROENTEROLOGY & NUTRITION

Williams VC, et al. Neurofibromatosis type 1 revisited. *Pediatrics*. 2009 Jan;123(1):124–133.

Farraye FA, Odze RD, et al; AGA Institute Medical Position Panel on Diagnosis and Management of Colorectal Neoplasia in Inflammatory Bowel Disease. AGA medical position statement on the diagnosis and management of colorectal neoplasia in inflammatory bowel disease. *Gastroenterology*. 2010 Feb;138(2):738-745.

ANORECTAL DISORDERS

Kaidar-Person O, Person B, et al. Hemorrhoidal disease: a comprehensive review. *J Am Coll Surg*. 2007;204:102–117.

Levitt MA, Peña A. Anorectal malformations. *Orphanet J Rare Dis*. 2007 Jul 26;2:33.

Solomon BD. VACTERL/VATER association. *Orphanet J Rare Dis*. 2011 Aug 16;6:56.

HIRSCHSPRUNG DISEASE

Feichter S, et al. The histopathology of gastrointestinal motility disorders in children. *Semin Pediatr Surg*. 2009 Nov;18(4):206–211.

DISORDERS OF THE EXOCRINE PANCREAS

Durie PR. Inherited and congenital disorders of the exocrine pancreas. *Gastroenterologist*. 1996 Sep;4(3):169–187.

DISEASES OF THE LIVER AND BILIARY TREE

Corness JA, et al. The portal vein in children: radiological review of congenital anomalies and acquired abnormalities. *Pediatr Radiol*. 2006 Feb;36(2):87–96, quiz 170–171.

Correa KK, et al. Idiopathic neonatal giant cell hepatitis presenting with acute hepatic failure on postnatal day one. *J Perinatol*. 2002 Apr–May;22(3):249–251.

Faingold R, et al. Hepatobiliary tumors. *Radiol Clin North Am*. 2011 Jul;49(4):679–687, vi.

Faure JP, et al. Abnormalities of the gallbladder, clinical effects. *Surg Radiol Anat*. 2008 Jun;30(4):285–290.

Fradin K, Racine AD, et al. Obesity and symptomatic cholelithiasis in childhood: epidemiologic and case-control evidence for a strong relation. *J Pediatr Gastroenterol Nutr*. 2014 Jan;58(1):102–106.

Halata MS, Berezin SH. Biliary dyskinesia in the pediatric patient. *Curr Gastroenterol Rep*. 2008 Jun;10(3):332–338.

Jonas MM, et al. Treatment of children with chronic hepatitis B virus infection in the United States: patient selection and therapeutic options. *Hepatology*. 2010 Dec;52(6):2192–2205.

McKusick VA, Kniffin CL. Cholestasis-lymphedema syndrome. *OMIM®*. 1986 [Updated 2007].

Misra S, Treanor MR, et al. Sphincter of Oddi dysfunction in children with recurrent abdominal pain: 5-year follow-up after endoscopic sphincterotomy. *J Gastroenterol Hepatol*. 2007 Dec;22(12):2246–2250.

Zimmermann A. Pathobiology of hepatobiliary neoplasms in children. *Journal of Gastroenterology and Hepatology*. 2004 Dec;19(Suppl 7):S372–S376.

American Academy of Pediatrics. Recommendations for screening, monitoring, and referral of pediatric chronic hepatitis B. *Pediatrics*. 2009 Nov;124(5):e1007–e1013.

Benson AB 3rd, Abrams TA, et al. NCCN clinical practice guidelines in oncology: hepatobiliary cancers. *J Natl Compr Canc Netw*. 2009 Apr;7(4):350–391.

Fiore AE, et al. Prevention of hepatitis A through active or passive immunization: recommendations of the Advisory Committee on Immunization Practices (ACIP). *MMWR Recomm Rep*. 2006 May 19;55(RR-7):1–23.

Mack CL, et al. NASPGHAN practice guidelines: diagnosis and management of hepatitis C infection in infants, children, and adolescents. *J Pediatr Gastroenterol Nutr*. 2012 Jun;54(6):838–855.

Mast EE, et al. A comprehensive immunization strategy to eliminate transmission of hepatitis B virus infection in the United States: recommendations of the Advisory Committee on Immunization Practices (ACIP) part 1: immunization of infants, children, and adolescents. *MMWR Recomm Rep*. 2005 Dec 23;54(RR-16):1–31. Erratum in: *MMWR Morb Mortal Wkly Rep*. 2007 Dec 7;56(48):1267 and *MMWR Morb Mortal Wkly Rep*. 2006 Feb 17;55(6):158–159.

U.S. Preventive Services Task Force. Screening for hepatitis B virus infection in pregnancy: reaffirmation recommendation statement. *Am Fam Physician*. 2010 Feb 15;81(4):502–504.

Weinbaum CM, et al. Recommendations for identification and public health management of persons with chronic hepatitis B virus infection. *MMWR Recomm Rep*. 2008 Sep 19;57 (RR-8):1–20.